SEX MATTERS FOR WOMEN

Sex Matters for Women

A Complete Guide to Taking Care of Your Sexual Self

Sallie Foley
Sally A. Kope
Dennis P. Sugrue

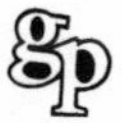

THE GUILFORD PRESS
New York London

A Division of Guilford Publications, Inc.
72 Spring Street, New York, NY 10012
www.guilford.com

The information in this book is offered to assist you in making informed choices about your sexuality. It is not intended as a substitute for competent medical care. If you suspect that you have a medical problem, we urge you to consult a qualified healthcare professional.

Printed in the United States of America

This book is printed on acid-free paper.

Last digit is print number: 9 8 7 6 5 4 3 2 1

Library of Congress Cataloging-in-Publication Data

Foley, Sallie
Sex matters for women: a complete guide to taking care of your sexual self / Sallie Foley, Sally A. Kope, Dennis P. Sugrue.
p. cm.
Includes bibliographic references and index.
ISBN 1-57230-700-5 (cloth) — ISBN 1-57230-641-6 (pbk.)
1. Women—Sexual behavior. 2. Sex. I. Kope, Sally A. II. Sugrue, Dennis P. III. Title.
HQ29.F65 2002
306.7′082—dc21

2001045050

In the clinical cases reported in this book all names and identifying characteristics have been altered.

To my husband, Steve, and our children, Lauren, Jessica,
and Rob, whose support and patience were invaluable.
With all my love.
And to Nancy M. and Bernard J. Podurgiel,
whose work and vision have helped so many.

—SALLIE FOLEY

To Marty. You have grown old along with me, and we
know what the best is. It's celebrating the branches
of our mighty family tree. All my love, Sally.

—SALLY A. KOPE

To Bernadette, who has brought passion, joy,
and meaning to my life. *Ja cie kocham.*

—DENNIS P. SUGRUE

Acknowledgments

For the last five years, the three of us have persisted in our belief that we could create a book that would be a comprehensive guide to women's sexuality. It has been a lively collaboration, rich in both argument and agreement, and more dedicated than we could have imagined. We have profoundly influenced each other's thinking as the book has taken shape, and the book and the three of us are the better for it. Many colleagues have been generous in their assistance at every phase of the book's development. We wish to thank those individuals who so generously contributed their knowledge and skill.

For reading and providing invaluable commentary on many parts of the manuscript, we thank Carita Anderson, PhD; Sheila Crowley, PhD; Jeannette Godfrey, PhD; Dennis Hacker, MDiv; Sandra Jordan, PhD; Michael Kaplan, MSW; JoAnn McFall, MSW, RN; Anne Segall, MSW; Russell Stambaugh, PhD; Bernadette Sugrue, MA; Pat Warner; Beverly Whipple, PhD, RN; Daniela Wittmann, MSW; and Mary Louise Yurik, MSW. For reviewing the manuscript for medical accuracy, our gratitude to Evan Eyler, MD; Riad Farah, MD; Hope Haefner, MD; Elisabeth Quint, MD; Beverly Whipple, PhD, RN; and Max Wicha, MD. We are grateful to Doug Davies, PhD, MSW; Steven Foley, PhD; Martin Kope, MDiv, MS; Michael Kope, JD; Laura Nitzberg, MSW; Claudia Kraus Piper, MSW; Margaret Punch, MD; Caren Stahlberg, MD; Peg Tewksbury, MS; Alice Um, JD; and our colleagues at the University of Michigan, who provided countless hours of sound advice and listened patiently as we developed our ideas. We are also indebted to our students and clients who have shared their experiences and trusted our guidance in better understanding the remarkable complexity of human sexuality. For excellent technical assistance, we thank Jacob Balazer, Scott Lynn, and Elisa Wares. The book would not exist if it were not for our editors at The Guilford Press—Kitty Moore, for her amazing vision and organizational sensibility, and Christine Benton, for her editorial incisiveness and insistence that we not stop till we got it right.

Most of all, we are indebted to our partners—Steve, Marty, and Bernadette—and our families. They made the book possible because they not only loved us but also respected and believed in the importance of this work. You hold it in your hands because of them.

Contents

Introduction

In 1960, the birth control pill launched a revolution that promised to free women from sexual restraints and inhibitions. Women were told that they now had the right to celebrate their sexuality and openly take care of their sexual selves. It was to be the end of an era of sexual repression, secrecy, and ignorance.

Forty years later, women have more opportunities than ever before in history, but their educational, occupational, and political advances have not been accompanied by comparable advances in their sexual comfort and satisfaction. Although women are told they are sexually liberated, cultural messages about women are still confusing. The sexual revolution, it appears, failed to deliver real sexual change for women. Instead, a paradoxical gap emerged between the perception of unlimited sexual choices for women and the reality of limitless sexual dilemmas. The perception of how far women have come is quite different from the reality of how far women have to go.

MOVING FROM SEXUAL PERCEPTION TO SEXUAL REALITY

From the very beginning, the sexual revolution created new dilemmas for women. Although women supposedly had more freedom to explore their sexuality, they also experienced less freedom to make choices without pressure or coercion. In the decades preceding the sexual revolution, women who avoided premarital sex were seen as prudent and moral. But starting in the sixties, the advent of the pill, legalization of abortion, and the growing acceptance of premarital sexuality changed the sexual climate. Women who chose not to be sexually active were perceived as prudish rather than prudent, frigid rather than moral. They were supposed to be enjoying themselves and often felt like failures if they weren't. Instead of choices being widened, one kind of tyranny was replaced with another.

The highly respected National Health and Social Life Survey (Laumann, Gagnon, Michael, & Michaels, 1994), a nationwide survey of adult sexual behavior, revealed many incongruities between perceptions and realities about sex. For instance, we may assume that women were eager for their first intercourse experience, but 30% of all women interviewed reported that they did not want, or were forced to have, their first intercourse. In an overwhelming number of these forcible acts, the woman knew the man. The survey captures other surprises in the reality of women's sexual behavior.

- In the 1960s, Masters and Johnson encouraged masturbation as a form of sexual pleasure and self-awareness. Yet fewer than 20% of the women reported masturbating more than three times a month, and 58% of the women had not masturbated at all during the preceding 12 months.
- Women of the baby boomer era think that theirs is the generation that broke down the barriers of sexual repression, but statistics show that even though more women in their 30s masturbate (48%) than women in their 40s (40%), only about 35% of women aged 18–24 masturbate in a given year.
- Despite increased efforts in education about sexually transmitted diseases (STDs), about one person in six (19%) reported having had a sexually transmitted disease. Women are twice as likely as men to have genital warts and chlamydia and three times as likely to have genital herpes.
- In the aftermath of the sexual revolution, 43% of American women between the ages of 18 and 59 reported having a sexual dysfunction.

Additional examples of the gap between the promise and the reality of the sexual revolution abound. Ironically, despite growing up during the 1960s and 1970s, the women and men who were products of the Age of Aquarius continued to raise their daughters differently from their sons. Developmental psychologists point out that while boys are taught to explore, compete, and dominate, girls are still encouraged to accept, cooperate, and accommodate. These differences in upbringing affect sexual development. Men will talk about sex in terms of desires, triumphs, and conquests, while women—when they do talk about sex—speak about disappointments, fears, and complaints.

Women are raised not only to be more cooperative but also to be warier. Despite our wishes to the contrary, misogyny continues to exist in our culture. Girls are reminded of their defenselessness by parental warnings to avoid strange men, to stay in groups, to be cautious on dates, never to leave a drink unattended, and to be vigilant against the ever-present dangers of pregnancy, STDs, date rape, sexual abuse, and violence. Early messages about sexuality are clear: it is something to be feared rather than embraced. Women learn to make their way in the world aware of their vulnerability. They associate sex not only with pleasure but with the danger of exploitation and harm. Sadly for adult women, sexual vigilance often replaces sexual responsiveness.

Over the last 35 years, our knowledge about the body and how it responds sexually has increased dramatically. At the same time, more women today have a college education than ever before in history. Yet despite the availability of sexual information and the educational advances women have made, sexual ignorance remains rampant. In our clinical practices we frequently encounter highly educated women who are unaware of their sexual anatomy. Despite widespread publicity about the existence of the "G spot," most women have never explored the recesses of their vagina to discover how to increase sexual arousal. Old messages that good girls shouldn't be "too interested" in sex and that they shouldn't touch their vagina unless it's absolutely necessary continue to linger in the background of many women's psyches. Even women who have learned to derive pleasure from clitoral stimulation are often reluctant to insert their fingers into their vaginas. Their mothers' early warnings persist: "Never put anything in there."

The struggle for gender equality has produced important advances, but vestiges of male dominance remain in our culture, including the bedroom. Lovemaking often follows a male script of arousal, penetration, and orgasm. When women make love to women, on the other hand, lovemaking is far less genitally focused and instead reflects a strong emphasis on holding, caressing, and dialogue.

Far too often, women seek sex therapy not because of personal dissatisfaction but because they are pressured by their partners or simply want to please them. Even though the belief that "normal" women always climax during intercourse was disproved more than 30 years ago, women continue to seek professional help because they can't reach orgasm through intercourse alone. When pressed, they often acknowledge that this pattern is not problematic for them but represents a severe blow to their partners' pride.

The rhetoric of the 1960s affirmed that it is okay for women to assert their own sexual needs rather than serve exclusively as sex objects for men. Women have made little progress on this issue. Men tend to experience sexual desire in terms of how attracted they are to their partner, but women often say that they *themselves* need to feel attractive in order to feel sexual desire. A woman who communicates her own sexual needs to her partner is the exception.

Madison Avenue cheers women on by proclaiming "You've come a long way, Baby"—but the media also incessantly remind women that their bodies are imperfect and that the quest for happiness is synonymous with a quest for youthfulness and beauty. Imagine the blow to the economy if one day magically every woman awoke, looked in the mirror, and was completely satisfied with what she saw! Contentment does *not* sell products. Women may complain about this tortuous standard, but individually they continue to try to achieve the body impossible. It is clear that holding out an unobtainable goal for women is good for business but bad for self-esteem, self-acceptance, and sexual health.

The gap between the ideal of sexual liberty and the reality of sexual negativism is perhaps at its widest point when considering the elderly, the sick, and the disabled. Although women often wish to remain sexually active in older age, they are not encouraged to do so. Yet the more they engage in sexual stimulation, the more sexually responsive they can become. This ability to experience and even increase erotic focus as women age is not valued by our culture. Elderly women who speak about their interest in sex are considered, at best, cultural curiosities and, at worst, dirty old women with dementia. A common complaint of women with chronic illnesses or disabilities, whatever their ages, is that they are not seen as sexual persons.

TAKING ACTION ON YOUR OWN BEHALF

Where does the failed promise of the sexual revolution leave women? All too often, disappointed, conflicted, and confused—yet hungry for information and guidance. The immense popularity of the television show "Sex in the City" results, in part, from the delight we take in watching women who don't follow cultural norms and seemingly don't have to pay a price for breaking the rules. We derive vicarious pleasure from watching TV characters live out a sexual lifestyle marked by comfort and self-assurance. Most of us want the same sexual comfort and self-assurance for ourselves, but we don't know how to achieve it.

There is no lack of information about sex, but there is a lack of *relevant* information for women. Women's magazines regularly offer lists on how to find time for sex, how to please partners, how to heighten arousal, but rarely do these magazines ground the advice in the imperfect contexts in which most women find themselves. Before tips and techniques can be useful, women must expunge the common sexual myths they have absorbed, understand the gender roles they juggle, and deal head-on with the unfair "stigma" of having a real rather than an ideal body. They need to figure out how their sexuality can flourish in their lives, given religious heritage, health status, past sexual experiences, and idiosyncrasies of their relationships. They have to find ways to overcome the gap between the promise of sexual fulfillment and the reality of sexual negativism. But how?

Sex Matters for Women: A Complete Guide to Taking Care of Your Sexual Self is a self-help book that gives you the information and guidance to maximize your sexual health, overcome cultural challenges, and solve many of the problems that arise throughout your sexual life. Through accurate information, examples from the lives of other women, and detailed self-help exercises, this book can help you succeed where the sexual revolution failed—you can make sexual fulfillment a reality rather than merely a perception.

The sexual revolution was right on one count: sexuality is an essential part of every woman's identity. But the revolution didn't know how to deliver on that promise. *Sex Matters for Women* puts the promise into words: know your story, understand and make peace with your body, create better sexual relationships, and overcome your sexual difficulties.

In this book, we cover five important ways for you to take care of your sexual self:

- *Knowing your sexual story.* Your history influences your sexuality throughout your life. It has shaped your sexual attitudes and identity and affects how you respond sexually as an adult. By understanding your personal story and the impact it has had on your sexuality, you're better able to free yourself of negative influences and learned inhibitions. In Part I we discuss how childhood, adolescent, and adult experiences can impact your sexuality. The Appendix offers journaling exercises to help you better understand the story of how your sexuality has evolved.
- *Understanding your body.* Research routinely points out how little most women know about their own anatomy and sexual functioning. Understanding your body and how it functions helps you develop a positive sexual identity and gain greater comfort with sexual behavior. In Part II you'll find detailed, user-friendly information about anatomy, hormones, and sexual functioning. In the Appendix you'll be guided through exercises to help you become not only more familiar with your sexual anatomy but also more comfortable touching, exploring, and enjoying your own body.
- *Making peace with your body.* Body image has a dramatic impact on a woman's sexual identity. Cultural messages about the importance of being youthful, shapely, thin, or light-skinned can prevent a woman from feeling sexually desirable and, in turn, sexual desire. Learning to feel empowered by your physical appearance, coming to terms with your uniqueness, and feeling comfortable in your body can contribute to a healthy sexual identity. Accepting your body can be complicated if you've been sexually abused, have vaginal pain, contracted an STD, or live with a serious illness or disability. In Part III and the corresponding section of the Appendix, you can address these challenges with specific self-help strategies, helping you move from the negative to the positive and from victimhood to sexual resilience.
- *Creating a better sexual relationship.* Most women, heterosexual or lesbian, are interested in establishing a meaningful relationship that includes mutually enjoyable sex. To create such a relationship, you will need skills in communicating, the ability to foster positive sexual experiences with your partner, and the savvy to avoid the pitfalls that typically beset long-term partnerships. If you're heterosexual, you'll also benefit from understanding how your partner's sexual response may differ from your own. Part IV describes the steps that lead to a satisfying sexual relationship, and the Appendix provides exercises to help you and your partner talk about your sex life together and experiment with ways to supercharge your lovemaking.

• *Overcoming sexual difficulties*. In the final section of the book, we discuss ways you can overcome sexual problems such as low desire, lack of arousal, and inability to orgasm. Common medical and psychological causes for these problems are described, and self-help techniques for overcoming dysfunctions are provided. Part V offers guidance for determining when sex therapy might be helpful and how to find a qualified therapist.

Sex Matters for Women is written by three sex therapists. We have worked with hundreds of women and their partners as they have sought ways to take better care of their sexual selves. The stories we present in this book are composites of our clients' experiences. We think these examples are representative of the common themes we've encountered in our professional work. Above all, they reflect the remarkable effort that individuals take to make sense of their sexual lives.

Although the treatment of women's sexuality has not been one of the more cheerful aspects of human history, we've chosen to focus not on discrimination, torment, and abuse that women have had to endure but instead on the stories of personal triumph, growth, and celebration of sexuality that serve as a testament to, and reminder of, women's resilience and strength. It's inevitable that we've overlooked or under-appraised some aspects of women's sexuality, but we've tried to be sensitive to the many ways that women are sexual, acknowledging the diversity of women's lives, orientation, and sexual choices. Although much of the book speaks of heterosexual relationships, lesbian relationships are discussed as well.

Writing this book has been a long but incredible experience for all three of us. We are grateful to many people for their support and inspiration along the way, especially the women who, over the years, have entrusted us with their care. Even for a writer there are some things that are very difficult to put into words. One of those things is the profound sense of respect that we hold for the people with whom we've worked. They've trusted us and allowed us to be part of their quest for greater self-understanding. In the end, it is they who have inspired us to write about women and sex. It is they who have taught us how much sex matters to them.

PART I

Knowing Your Sexual Story

Are *you* comfortable with your sexual self? Many women instinctively answer yes until we ask more specific questions, such as: Do you feel at ease when you undress before your partner or stand naked in front of a mirror? Are you truly relaxed during lovemaking, able to focus on your body's sensations without distractions, worries, or guilt? Do you feel completely free to explore your sexuality, try new things, talk openly with your partner, and feel confident when educating your children about sex? Being comfortable with your sexuality means a lot more than just enjoying sex. It means all of the above and more. Discomfort, uncertainty, or confusion about any facet of your sexuality can have negative or limiting repercussions for *all* of your life, in all *parts* of your life.

In our experience, many women wrestle with myths and misconceptions about their sexuality and how it is formed. Today, at this very moment, your sexual attitudes, beliefs, and comfort level are the cumulative result of your past life experiences. How your early caregivers held you as an infant, how you made love with your partner last night, and countless experiences in between have helped shape how you now experience yourself as a sexual person. In addition to these life experiences, you have been exposed to continuous mixed messages in your environment that have further shaped and influenced your sexual growth and development.

If sex matters to you, you may welcome the opportunity to review the sexual story that is such an important part of your life and to learn how other women have navigated the passages of sexual development. Upbringing that ignored sex or put it in a negative light, faulty sex education, confusing cultural messages about sex, constant exposure to media that foster dissatisfaction with real bodies, and double standards for men and women are but a few of the challenges that many women have faced and are still facing today. We have a lot to gain from the stories of women who have emerged from these challenges with a healthy, fulfilling sexuality.

Once you understand why you feel awkward, ashamed, distrustful, or inferior, you're finally in a position to challenge the negative thinking that underlies these feelings. Once you realize how your beliefs have been shaped by misinformation and cultural propaganda, you can take steps to replace these faulty beliefs with accurate information. Once you discover why sex intimidates you and why you hold back in sexual situations, you're in a better position to experiment with new, more fulfilling behaviors. Once you know what is joyful, fulfilling, and inspiring to you as a sexual being, you can look for similar ways to enhance your sexual growth.

To accomplish these tasks, you need to know and understand your sexual story. In the next two chapters we talk about how girls grow and develop sexually and common sexual experiences of adult women, both the challenges and the pleasures. The Appendix offers exercises to help you reflect on your personal life story. We hope that these exercises and reflections will give you a clearer understanding of what factors have shaped your sexuality and that, armed with these insights, you'll be able to make better use of the information and suggestions in the remainder of this book. In Chapters 1 and 2 we look at common questions like these:

- Is my attitude toward sex normal?
- Why do I keep making the same bad decisions about sex?
- At what age is masturbation normal?
- Why does it seem so much easier to *have* sex than to *talk* about it?
- Is there such a thing as too much sex education?
- Who decides what's sexy—me or my partner?
- Can a young girl fall in love with another girl and still be heterosexual?
- How can I live by the values about sex that are important to me when everything around me says the opposite?
- Shouldn't the "first time" be a romantic fantasy come true?
- How can I tell my daughter what's important about her sexuality when I don't understand my own?

CHAPTER ONE

Every Story Has a Beginning

Children are sexual beings from birth, and their adult sexuality is influenced by childhood experiences. In this chapter, we explore the common milestones of childhood and adolescence that impact a woman's sexuality. It's not our goal to write the definitive treatise on development and sexuality—entire books have been devoted to that theme. Instead, we want to provide you with the opportunity to reflect on how an important period in your life—the time between birth and young adulthood—influenced where you are today on your sexual journey so that you can better decide how you want to live your life now and in the future. The knowledge you gain may lead to sexual growth and greater satisfaction.

WHEN DOES THE STORY BEGIN?

Annie raced back home after playing with Mary, Phil, and Junie. She dumped her things in her fort, a place she had constructed of plywood and old junk. She tried not to step on the tiny row of lilac bushes her mother had planted in front of the fort in a futile attempt to disguise her daughter's shack.

Annie sat down, resting her back against the pine tree. Her shirt felt sweaty and sticky; she pulled it off and leaned back on the rough bark, scratching a few choice places as she relaxed. Just last summer her mom had made her start wearing a shirt all the time. Phil and Junie didn't have to wear shirts on hot summer days. But Annie's mother had told her that girls were different—they had to "cover up" or someone would think that they weren't nice girls.

Annie didn't want to be nice; she wanted to be free. She wondered about places she'd seen in the *National Geographic* magazines. There were pictures of girls who didn't have to wear shirts. Annie decided that when she grew up, she would live someplace where she could take off her T-shirt whenever she wanted.

This pine tree fort was Annie's favorite place, and late afternoon was her favorite time of day. Drawing her knees up to her chest, she wrapped her arms around them and rested her head there. She breathed in and smelled the piney smell, then rubbed her face across her forearm. She thought how much she loved her body. She liked how her skin was so taut and smooth across her bones. She examined those tiny hairs that grew on her arms. She rubbed her cheek against them, feeling her skin's smoothness underneath that soft, fuzzy hair. Then she smelled her skin. More than anything, Annie loved these private, special smells of her body. She thought the skin on her forearm smelled the best: a clean, sweet smell only humans had.

She slid her hands along her legs and arms, scratched where a pine needle poked her in the neck, and then stood up and rubbed her hands over her body, making her feel cool and shivery. She looked down at her chest. There, too, her skin was smooth. There were few hairs to see, and her nipples were flat and round and pink and interested her.

Looking down at her body, Annie felt for the bones just under the skin and watched as her breath made her stomach suck in and out. Her ribs disappeared and reappeared. The muscles on her chest seemed to spread all the way out to her arms. She tightened her fist and flexed her arm like a strongman. The muscle bulged. *Boy, I'm strong!* she thought.

Annie was an eight-year-old girl, an explorer, and at that moment, a person at peace with her body and herself.

When does a woman's sexual story begin? The first time she makes love? The moment she discovers orgasm? Puberty?

A woman's sexual story starts in infancy and continues throughout her life. Early childhood experiences that most people would never consider to be sexual are, in fact, fundamental to being a sexual person. Young Annie, reveling in the wonders of her body, is learning to become a sexual person because she's learning how to live in her body, how to be at peace with herself, and how to find pleasure from her senses. Each of these discoveries is part of a lifelong sexual journey.

EARLY CHILDHOOD

Even during the first years of life, a girl's sexuality is being shaped and scripted. Biology assigns her gender, but people around her quickly assign her the role that is supposed to go with that gender—a role that will influence how she views and values herself and how she will relate to others for years to come. During these earliest years she also will learn whether she can trust other people to love her and to respect her body and her emerging sexuality. The foundation for bonding and trust is established even before a child takes her first steps. Finally, as an infant and toddler, a girl will make important discoveries about her body that will influence her self-acceptance and her capacity to experience pleasure well into her adult years.

It's a Girl!

Sociologists have studied the reactions adults have to newborn babies. By the time babies are one minute old, they are treated differently depending on their sex. Think about the observations that people make: "Look at those delicate fingers." "Such big, strong hands!" "Check out the size of those feet!" Actually, most newborns look remarkably alike. But right from the beginning, people viewing a newborn will respond differently depending on the baby's gender. Parents will hold a girl more gently and speak to her more softly than they would to a baby boy.

This pattern continues as a baby girl grows into a toddler and begins exploring her world. If a little girl takes a tumble while running, she'll be consoled more quickly and allowed to cry about it longer than if she were a little boy. She'll be held more often than a boy toddler. Girl toddlers are often encouraged to be gentler and less aggressive than boys, to get along and resolve conflicts quickly. Even though today's young girls are getting muddy playing soccer, they're still far more likely than their brothers to get an American Girl doll.

While the seeds of many wonderful attributes will be implanted by the age of four or five, such as sensitivity, nurturing, and an orientation toward cooperation and constructive problem solving, so also will the seeds of characteristics that conform to the dictates of cultural sexism, myths, and double standards—such as an emphasis on being pretty, staying neat and clean, and being a "good girl." These latter characteristics may make it difficult to separate self-worth from personal appearance. They may also make adult relationships more complex because a woman's traditional gender role and identity may come into conflict with her attempts to gain autonomy, be assertive, and act competently. They may make the natural desire to enjoy sexual passion difficult because "good girls don't do that." Perhaps you can relate to what one woman told us:

> "Sometimes when I get really turned on during sex, I want to moan and thrash about because it feels so great. But I don't—I keep hearing my mom's voice saying, 'That's not very ladylike.' "

Peek-a-Boo: Where Trust Begins

An important part of our sexuality is how comfortably we relate to a partner. The abilities to bond, to trust, and to freely touch and be touched are essential for a successful sexual relationship, and the foundation of these abilities is established in infancy. Even before a baby girl can speak, she's spoken to. Even before she can hug, she's hugged. Children's earliest experiences are shaped by their adult caregivers. When the child is hungry or in distress, she cries. If a parent or caretaker responds and tends to the child's need, a foundation of trust is formed. If parents treat a baby with love, nurture, and respect, the baby receives important information not only about trusting others but also about self-worth. Because her needs are met, she feels important and valued. And by feeling valued by others, she learns to value herself. Without early nurture and loving touch, a girl may grow up wary of trusting others, uncomfortable with physical contact, or feeling unworthy and unlovable. One woman recalled,

> "I wasn't 'grown up,' I was 'thrown up.' My family was so alcoholic and chaotic, I was never attended to. It's amazing that I can look at myself in the mirror without disgust."

Junior Scientists in Action

Our bodies are the epicenter of our sexuality. It is by means of our bodies that we experience sexual pleasure and connect with other people. This relationship between our bodies, pleasure, and connecting with others begins within minutes of birth. Sucking is the child's first experience of satisfaction. Whether breast-fed or bottle-fed, the child derives pleasure from her mouth, and this pleasure is associated with close physical contact with the parent or caregiver. This association between physical contact with another person and pleasure derived from the body becomes the basis for all future sexual relationships.

Later, a girl makes further discoveries about her body's ability to produce pleasure. During early childhood, children are junior scientists. They love to learn and explore. They are naturally curious about themselves and their world. One woman recalled:

> "When I saw a woman nursing her baby, my mom did a great job of explaining breast-feeding to me. But when I came home and tried to get my baby doll to suck my breast, she freaked out."

This curiosity includes their bodies. After all, children spend an enormous amount of time trying to learn how to do things in their bodies, from potty training to tying shoes, from skipping to whistling. It's normal and natural for children, girls and boys alike, to explore their own bodies with all their senses: sight, hearing, touch, taste, and smell. Part of that exploration will include their genitals. They will touch themselves for the pleasure of it. This isn't sexually stimulating in the erotic way that adults might think of it. Rather, it is a normal expression of interest and an experience of pleasure in a part of the body that feels good when touched. Many women remember playing in the bathtub as little girls and touching and looking at their genitals.

Look What I Found!

Little girls are at a disadvantage compared to little boys in developing long-term familiarity with their genitals. Little boys have "outies"—their penis is right there for them to explore, stroke, and tug. If a small girl attempts to probe her vagina in an exploratory way, her parent will most likely interrupt her and make it clear that she shouldn't do this. Little girls are far less clear about the source of their pleasure because they have "innies." They probably have no idea that the pleasure they feel when rubbing their vulva comes from their clitoris, a part of their body largely unseen and, in all likelihood, unnamed. They may have been told that they have a vagina, but that's a part of their body they don't have ready access to, and it will be years before it will become fully biologically functional.

She may not know what to call it, but free of parental shaming or restrictions, a little girl will quickly learn that touching and rubbing her vulva can be very pleasurable. It's natural and normal that she will want to reproduce these pleasant feelings, especially when she's tired, nervous, or bored.

> "Even now, in my 60s, I can still remember the pleasure I got from masturbating as a little girl. I would go to bed and tuck my hand between my legs and rock back and forth, feeling great, until I fell asleep. Before sex was arousing, it was soothing."

When this natural curiosity and self-pleasuring is allowed to occur without shame or embarrassment, the child will have a fairly good start toward developing a healthy sexuality. Unfortunately, some girls receive a message that their body is shameful and that genital pleasuring is bad at the same time they are discovering that it feels good to touch their vulva. All too often these messages are carried into adulthood and influence many women's sexual experiences.

Where do these messages come from? How does a little girl pick up negative attitudes about her body and genital pleasure?

Shame on You!

> "I remember I was watching TV and idly rubbing my vulva because it felt good. My mom came into the room, saw me, and screamed. I thought someone had died. What 'died' was my interest in pleasuring myself."

Consider what happens when a little girl is caught rubbing her vulva or exploring her vagina. All too often parents react with anger or embarrassment. Not surprisingly, the girl associates touching her vulva with upsetting people and doing something wrong. All children rely on adults for love, and if faced with the fear of displeasing her parents, a young girl will readily give up the good feelings that come from touching herself so that she can hold on to parental approval. She will deny her own pleasurable experience because she's too young to determine that her parents are wrong; her connection to her parents at this stage of life is stronger than her connection to pleasuring her body.

Sometimes parents' reactions aren't meant to shame but to protect. Children must learn that orifices—ears, noses, vaginas, and anuses—aren't meant to have things put into them. But some parents go overboard by promoting a "hands-off" approach to the genitals. It's normal for a young child to ask questions about sex, to explore her genitals, and to be curious about other children's genitals. Because masturbation is a healthy part of development, forbidding or punishing self-pleasuring makes no more sense than forbidding a child to read books or punishing a child for eating healthy food.

What's in a Name?

Do you remember the names that you were given for your genitals? Were they even *remotely* close to the accurate names for the vulva, clitoris, or vagina? Girls will pick up negative attitudes about their bodies and their sexuality in a number of other subtle ways. When parents refer to a girl's genitals as her "wee-wee," "tinkle," or "place down there," a girl is left wondering, *Why don't people like talking about that part of my body?* It's a small leap from this kind of thinking to *My body must be shameful or bad because no one will mention it.*

It isn't just that people aren't comfortable teaching children the accurate names of genitals but that most adults wouldn't know what to do if the children started to use them.

> "When I was three, my mom told me all the names of my genitals. I was so proud I wanted to tell everybody. I showed my genitals to my friend Evan, pointing and naming. Then he showed me his and we named them together. I still remember the feel of his penis when I touched it. When Grandma came over later in the day, I enthusiastically asked her if she had a vulva just like mine!"

Don't Forget to Wipe!

Most of us don't remember toilet training, but we do have our "habits" in the bathroom, habits that often got an early start. Little girls are usually toilet-trained differently from little boys. They miss out on the thrill of arching their stream at a floating target but, instead, are expected to sit quietly and to take thorough steps to wipe themselves clean afterwards. The strong emphasis on staying clean after voiding can reinforce a notion that there must be something dirty about their genitals. One woman remarked that every time she got aroused, her underpants would get wet with discharge, and she'd feel embarrassed about "messing her underpants." Another woman reported feeling like she has to thoroughly wash her genitals before sex with her partner, afraid that her natural smell is "dirty."

Private Property

As children grow, so does their need for privacy. While three-year-olds want to show off what they did in the toilet, seven-year-olds want to be alone in the bathroom! There is a natural, increasing desire to be private about one's body. Most of the time, this is what kids also see modeled in their homes. Mom and Dad request privacy for toileting, bathing, dressing, and other personal times. A child initiates her own need for privacy as she grows. Women recall very different experiences.

> "I was a wild, intense little girl, very high-spirited. My parents had to work with me to close bathroom doors. I'd masturbate in the living room 'til my mom helped me to finally understand the difference between 'public' and 'private.' "

> "I was a painfully shy girl. I'd undress in my closet because I didn't want anyone to see me in my underwear. Annual trips to the doctor's office were agony. I could only get through them if my mom stayed right with me the whole time."

> "I live on my own, and because of a physical disability, I have a personal attendant to help me with toileting and bathing. As a girl, my mom did all that. You have a different relationship with your mom when you're arguing about whether you can watch *Pretty Woman* at the same time she's wiping your butt and changing your menstrual pad."

It's important that the child learn about privacy and modesty, but often the lesson can go too far and the girl learns to associate nakedness with shamefulness. Some women report that they can't undress in front of their partners because they feel ashamed of their bodies. Other women say that they don't want to let anyone, not even their partner, see them in their underwear.

Caught in the Act

Did you ever have the experience of stumbling in on your parents while they were having sex? Those moments when a child catches the parents in the act of lovemaking can also reinforce negative ideas about sexuality. It's not the fact that the child sees the parents naked but the parents' reaction to being discovered that can confuse and frighten the child. If the parents react with panic and anger, such as diving under the covers and yelling for the child to leave the room, the child could conclude that her parents are up to no good.

Notice that, in the example above, negative attitudes were reinforced not by abusive parents, sexual trauma, or emotionally impoverished environments but by normal parents relying on common, almost universal, child-rearing practices. Most parents do the best they can, and they, too, are products of a culture that views sexuality with suspicion and wariness. As a result, this suspicion and wariness is passed along to children at a very early age.

PREPUBERTY: THE AGE OF MASTERY AND MYSTERY

A school-age child knows there is a whole world beyond her home and family, a world in which she is not the center, but only one of many players, and people other than her parents—teachers and peers—are important influences. She must figure out how she fits into this bigger world and how to thrive in it.

This is the age of mastery: What can my body do? How fast can I run? Can I ride a bike? Do I know all my "times tables"? Do the other kids like me? At school, there are countless opportunities for testing mastery by comparing and contrasting. Fitting in is the all-important quest; being excluded or feeling different or inferior can be traumatic. If things go badly, a young girl may feel she did something wrong—even if the circumstances are out of her control. Because she failed to master the situation, she feels responsible. This is especially true if a girl is sexually abused. She may feel she is responsible for the abuse, that it was somehow her fault. This may also occur if a girl is teased about her size or how she looks. She may feel that she is a failure.

Long after they've grown up, women remember the painful experiences of childhood when they felt responsible yet utterly powerless. Instead of mastery, they remember misery. This may affect how they feel about their sexuality as adult women.

> "When I was young, my older sister made me dress up and 'model' all my school clothes each year. Then she critiqued how I looked. It was agony. To this day, I hate to shop."

> "At family reunions, our older boy cousins would grab us little girls and feel our bottoms and flat chests. We'd scream and everybody else would laugh. I still hate to be held."

> "Because I was heavier, I got teased a lot at school. I couldn't run very fast in gym and the kids called me 'chubbette' and 'tiny.' I've never stopped being sensitive about weight. I don't like to be naked during sex because I don't want my husband to see my body."

That's Gross, Tell Me More

For the most part, girls during the early school years are not very interested in the mystery of sexual behavior. Sexual feelings and curiosity are largely submerged, with an emphasis instead on accomplishment and social skills. This does not mean that sex is entirely ignored. School-age girls masturbate and can be orgasmic. Mild same-sex play is not unusual or abnormal, and many women remember some "show and tell" games or peeking at each other's changing bodies. You may remember being curious about sex and feeling dissatisfied with the sex education you received in schools. Perhaps you prowled around your parents' bedroom looking for information about sex, or eavesdropped on the conversations of your older siblings.

> Nine-year-old twins Ruth and Hannah giggled as they looked at their parents' book on sex. "It looks like a hairy mouth," Ruth whispered, pointed to a drawing of a woman's vagina, then burst into nervous laughter.
>
> "You think that's weird, look at the man's thing," Hannah said, flipping through the pages, then stopping to stare at the drawing of a couple having intercourse.
>
> "I would never do that to have a baby," Ruth declared.
>
> "Me neither," answered Hannah, "but let me show you the picture of their butts. . . ."

There can be many ways a girl will react to sexual information before she enters puberty. Some women remember feeling disinterested or annoyed by this intrusion on their childhood. Others felt sexuality was fascinating and exotic. Some women recall that they were upset by the information and mourned that, as girls, their bodies would have to change, that menstrual periods would be monthly, and that they'd have to grow up and have "sexual relations." If the subject of sex was treated differently from other family topics, some women, mimicking their parents, learned never to discuss sex or confront sexual issues.

Unfortunately, for some girls lessons about sexuality don't come from innocent curiosity or parental instruction but from terrifying first-hand experience. One of every four girls is sexually victimized in childhood. For many of these girls, their victimization will sensitize them to sex in disturbing ways. Some will desperately avoid any sexual talk and recoil if anyone attempts to touch them. Others will become sexually preoccupied and provocative, reenacting their own exploitation. They may say sexy things excessively or persistently masturbate in public areas of the house. They may be too sexual in their play responses with other kids.

If a woman was sexually abused as a girl, knowing her own sexual story will require grieving and courage. Most adult survivors of childhood sexual abuse find counseling an important part of healing. Chapter 10 may also be helpful.

PUBERTY: A GIRL FROM THE INSIDE OUT

By the time hormonal levels begin to change, a young girl in her preteen years has come a long way from her junior scientist days of exploring her world with abandon, and her fourth-grade days of trying to master everyone's social schedule. She will head into puberty approximately *24 months* ahead of the boys in her class. With the onset of puberty, she begins a phase when she's more aware of herself as being separate from others. On the surface, she has friends and loves school and all the social activities. But under the surface, she is discovering more about herself and is trying to come to terms with the changes taking place in her body.

Invasion of the Body Snatchers

The time period from ten to 12 years of age covers a lot of territory in a girl's development. As she begins to undergo changes in her hormones, her body will change also. Pubic hair may appear. She may have breast buds as early as age eight. The onset of menstruation can be as early as nine or ten or as late as 16 or 17. The average age is about 11 or 12 years old.

The first period is called *menarche*. Typically this will be experienced as a rite of passage, marked by pride mingled with some anxiety. Cultural slang like "being on the rag" can create negative attitudes about her body. It is within this context that a girl faces the challenge of learning to relate to her body and her sexual parts in a healthy manner.

A woman may remember not only when she started her period but also where she was, what she was doing, and her first immediate rush of feelings. She remembers whether her mother and other women prepared her for this first period. She may feel sadness if she was not helped with this entry into puberty. Perhaps she remembers feeling confused, even angry, with her body for betraying her into adulthood.

> "I was at my friend's at a sleepover when my period started. I had no idea what was happening."

> "I remember when my period started, I was at summer camp. I looked down and saw the brown spot on my underwear. Fifty years later, I can still recall that I felt a rush of excitement and thrill. But I was scared because it seemed such a permanent change."

> "When my period started, I wanted to avoid the whole thing. I went around ignoring it for three days, wadding up my bloody underwear and stuffing them under my bed. My mom had to come and talk to me. It made me anxious."

A girl may feel out of control because of all that is happening to her body. Although there can be pride and excitement about physical changes, she may grieve that her body is no longer familiar to her. Breasts may be so tender that it hurts to be bumped or jostled. Menstruation can be accompanied by painful cramps. Oily pores and hair seem to need constant attention, and acne can feel like leprosy. Some girls become plump and round, while others appear all feet, elbows, and limbs. Mothers smile in remembrance and talk about ducklings who will someday become swans. Unfortunately, peer ridicule can be so cruel and unrelenting during this vulnerable stage that, years later, a swan can look in a mirror and still see only a duckling. The embarrassment and self-criticism that develops as a result of body changes during puberty can impact a woman's self-image well into adulthood.

I "Vant" to Be Alone

With puberty comes a heightened interest in sexuality. Girls may experiment with smutty jokes and vulgar language, especially when around boys. Many girls masturbate during these years. Self-discovery, self-pleasuring, and even orgasm are normal parts of this stage of development. Finding time to be alone and explore their bodies is important.

> Tamecca liked to be alone in her room. She'd lock her door and, in total privacy, touch herself. Using a mirror, she'd look at her genitals. She liked to rub her clitoris, especially when she lay on her stomach. She would place her hand cupped against her vulva and rub back and forth. Sometimes while rocking like this she would feel more excited and tension-filled. She'd rock harder until she had a tingly, pulsing sensation in her genitals. She didn't know that what she was doing was called *masturbation*—she simply thought of it as her special, private time.
>
> Sometimes Tamecca thought about a movie star when she was touching herself. She was beginning to fantasize, and imagining herself grown up and involved with him made her feel even more excited when she masturbated.
>
> Tamecca thought her genitals were lovely. She liked all the colors of her skin in her vulva. When she pulled back her labia, she could see her vagina, making it open and close by tensing her muscles.
>
> When changing clothes, Tamecca noticed that her underpants sometimes had dried white mucus on them. Her mom explained that it was normal and called it "discharge." The next time she was alone, she reached her finger a little way inside her vagina and felt the wetness; it was moist, like the inside of her mouth. She pulled out her finger and brought it to her nose, breathing in the musty, comforting smell of her vagina. When she tasted the wetness on her finger, it was a little disappointing, a little chalky and bland. Nevertheless, she felt that she had the most interesting body ever made.

Leaving Childhood

As a girl enters puberty, she may alternate (sometimes rapidly) between extreme sociability and intense solitariness. In the years to come, she will no doubt learn how to handle her own unique emotional coloring. In her current daily life, however, she has had no prior experience with such intense moods, no language yet to describe what she is feeling. Physiology seems to have taken over what was a familiar mastery of her body. She may feel that she fits in neither the world of children nor that of adolescents. It is a time in between the two, and some girls feel nostalgia for childhood even when they still seem a child.

> On a quiet summer day just before seventh grade, Annie headed to her fort. The lilac bushes, now taller than Annie, partially hid the old fort's warped and weathered boards. Annie ducked under the branches crouching, and noted that she could no longer stand in her old hiding place. How small it seemed.
>
> Reaching out, she pulled on the boards nearest her; they came apart with only a little tugging. Knowing it was time, Annie solemnly took the fort apart, her strong arms easily stacking the lumber aside, until only the branches of the pine tree sloped vacantly to the ground. The emptiness made her nervous, and she wanted to get away from what had once been her sanctuary.

Young girls approaching their teen years are becoming biologically mature, capable of reproduction. Their gender role and identity have been firmly established. For better or worse, they are imbued with attitudes and beliefs about sexuality that will influence their sexual comfort and satisfaction for years to come. What they do not have is the life experience and the emotional maturity that will help them integrate their biology, gender role, and sexual beliefs into a balanced, wholesome sense of being a sexual person. Much of this necessary experience and the time to mature further will occur in their next stage of life—adolescence.

ADOLESCENCE

Our society is fascinated by adolescence. This stage of life is the subject of countless books, the focal point of hundreds of movie and TV plots, and the topic of constant commiseration among parents. Perhaps this is because adults look back on this period as a poignant time in life, teens need reminders that their struggles are not unique, and preteens look forward to the excitement of this major turning point. It is during these years that girls (and boys) make startling discoveries about sex, struggle with self-esteem, develop crushes, and are crushed by rejections. It is a time that helps define who we are, how we relate to others, and how we experience ourselves as sexual people.

An adolescent girl is a young woman, and she quickly learns that sex can be incredibly complex and perplexing. Some young women are cautioned against any sexual exploration and warned that, if they get pregnant, they'd better not come home. Some hear this threat so young, they don't even know how pregnancy occurs. Young women are told that looking sexy means they're "asking for it." Sometimes these same young women are sexually abused within their own families. Some are told they will burn in hell if they feel any sexual urges. But they're *not* told what they're supposed to do with the strong, hormone-driven sexual feelings they are already having in their bodies.

A complex matrix of factors defines adolescent sexuality. Internal and external forces interact with a young woman's sexual experiences in ways that can be both confusing and profound. These factors will influence how an adult ends up experiencing herself as a sexual person: whether she is comfortable, confident, and sexually satisfied. Most of us don't perceive this process as it unfolds and don't have any idea how we became the sexual beings we are today. Looking back on the factors at work in adolescent sexuality can help us see whether where we are today is where we want to be and, if not, which factors in our adult sexual lives we might address.

Biology

"I'm too tall and geeky looking."
"My boobs and hips are huge."
"Everyone hates me."
"No one thinks I'm pretty."

During adolescence, a young woman undergoes significant biological changes that affect her appearance, emotions, self-esteem, and self-confidence. Most young women's periods have begun, although it's still normal for menstruation to begin as late as 16 or 17. Breast development continues, height can shoot up, and oily skin makes life miserable. Sudden mood shifts only add to the inner turmoil.

Prior to puberty, children are curious about their bodies, responsive to pleasurable genital sensations, and aware of sexual taboos surrounding them. But during adolescence, sex becomes up-close and personal. A young woman is no longer merely curious about sex; she is often drawn to it, fascinated by it, afraid of it. She suddenly has physical sensations that go beyond mere genital tingling. She finds herself drifting into daydreams and fantasies that excite her. She finds herself so attracted to other people, both male and female, that at times she can't take her mind off them. These new experiences are very different from childhood ones of playing doctor, sneaking a peek at nude pictures, or giggling over new sexual information. This is the real thing—adult sexuality is becoming biologically hard-wired into a young woman's body *and* psyche.

This heightened sexual awareness has a disquieting impact on a young woman, especially in early adolescence when self-awareness steadily increases. Nakedness becomes both fascinating and scary; a young adolescent woman in a bathing suit can be a mass of nervous energy—giggling, silly, and anxious. Because most early teens don't feel in command of their fluctuating sexual awareness and physical sensations, they often confuse sexual feelings with feelings of affection and love. As a result, one minute a young teen can hug Mom and Dad with abandon because she loves them, and the next minute she recoils from any touch because it feels weird. *Nothing* feels the same anymore.

Self-Esteem

> Barbara ducked into the school bathroom and squeezed her way to the mirror. Her thick, bushy red hair never seemed to lie flat. Next to her, Keisha wasn't any happier as she tried to tame a wandering wave of her own soft black hair. They both glanced enviously at Beth, who was smoothing her long straight blond hair over her shoulders.
>
> *I'd give anything to look like that,* Barbara thought to herself.
>
> Beth muttered under her breath, "I look like a freak."
>
> "What are you talking about?" Keisha asked, dumbfounded. "Beth, you always look *perfect.*"
>
> "No, I have these bumps on my head where my ears stick out under my hair. Look, you can see it in the mirror." Beth tried to flatten her ears with her hands. "I feel like Dumbo."
>
> The bell rang and a dozen teens heaved their backpacks on their shoulders and left the bathroom for class, preparing to do another day of internal battle with their own critical voices.

Teenagers compare themselves to the standards of beauty they see in advertising and the media. Even with the benefits of Title IX and a plethora of strong female role models, many adolescent women still place more value on appearance than on competence, intelligence, or accomplishments. They struggle with self-scorn, convinced that their bodies just don't measure up.

A young woman's self-esteem affects her sense of sexuality. As a child, a girl might have been comfortable in her body, touching herself and masturbating without awkwardness or discomfort. Now when masturbating, physical sensations have to break through a barricade of self-criticism. A girl rubs her skin and wishes it were darker or lighter. She slides her fingers over her vulva and is distracted, thinking other girls have prettier thighs than hers. If she looks at her breasts, she feels disgust over their size or shape. After this sort of once-over, it's a wonder she has any pleasurable sensations whatsoever.

Self-esteem can impact sexual development in other important ways. A young woman who lacks confidence and feels self-conscious about her body may pull away from opportunities to socialize and "hang out." As a result of her shyness, she misses out on opportunities to develop social skills, one of the building blocks for later success in relationships. A young woman struggling with self-esteem issues may engage in sexual behavior that is risky and beyond her ability to manage, believing that being sexually accommodating is the only way she can possibly hold the interest of a boyfriend. Another young woman may be so worried about the feelings she is having for other females that she throws herself at guys in a frantic attempt to figure out her orientation. These young women run the risk of carrying into adulthood sexual attitudes marred by feelings of shame and/or resentment.

The relationship between self-esteem and sexuality goes both ways. Not only does a young woman's self-esteem affect her sexual comfort and growth, but sexual experience also can influence her self-esteem. A lack of sexual information, a teen pregnancy, sexual victimization, or confusion over sexual orientation can lead to self-criticism and self-condemnation that follows a young woman into her adult years.

What does it mean to be a woman? Girls bring different notions of womanhood into adolescence, notions formed with the help of various models, both positive and negative. As teenagers, their understanding of what it means to be female evolves. The value of appearance learned in early childhood takes on new power, for example, when they are asked out on a date only if boys consider them "hot."

It's also during the teen years when cultural, ethnic, and other messages about female sexuality become mixed and complicated. On one hand, teenage girls are told that women are powerful and competent, and on the other, they learn the dramatic lesson that they are in danger simply because of their gender. Women have vivid memories of their first experiences with their sexual vulnerability.

> "At 16, I remember going to a pro basketball game with friends. In the parking lot, these drunk guys wouldn't leave us alone. They harassed us, calling us 'cunt' and 'sweet ass' and words I've never heard before or since."

> "I was at the mall by myself. In a crowded elevator, this man started rubbing my bottom. I was terrified but afraid to say anything. I know it doesn't make sense, but I thought I must have done something wrong to be picked on by him."

> "I was dating this guy who got mean when he was drunk. One night he raped me. I didn't tell my parents because I was afraid they'd be mad at me for drinking, too."

There is a point in every girl or woman's life when she feels bad about having a body that is noticed in an exploitive way. For some girls, it happens very young and may include sexual abuse. Although it is not her fault, a young woman feels ashamed of herself for being noticed. She feels that she must have done something wrong to "invite" this attention. Her sexuality seems wrong because it's noticed in a way that takes away her control of her own body.

When women recall these events from their childhood, it's always with sadness. It is one of the reasons why sexuality is far more complex, at a much earlier age, for women than it is for men. An adolescent girl may be told that sex is special and wonderful, *and* that she must be on her guard against date rape and stranger rape. She may encounter adults who treat her lovingly, then turn around and slide their hands over her breasts and buttocks. It's a cruel discovery for young girls that they are vulnerable solely because of their gender. It's equally cruel that they will have to carry into their adult years a sense of vigilance and suspicion that can interfere with their capacity to love and experience life with a sense of abandon and joy.

As sex therapists, we often talk with women about their childhood memories of loss—the loss of innocence, protection, and the right to grow safely in their sexuality. These experiences are traumatic and can cast a dark shadow on sexual development. If these kinds of experiences happened to you, Chapter 10 may help you.

Gender Identity and Sexual Orientation

In recent years there has been increased public awareness of "transgendered" and "intersexed" men and women, conditions in which a person's gender identity is different from the anatomical, genetic, and hormonal composition of her or his body, or when someone is born with both female and male chromosomal, anatomic, or hormonal characteristics. For more information on these forms of gender identity, check the "Suggested Resources" under "Lesbian, Bisexual, Transgender, and Intersex."

An important part of gender identity, of course, is sexual orientation. It's during the adolescent years that lifelong sexual interests and sexual orientation emerge, although a woman may not acknowledge these interests or orientation until later in life. Many of the themes found in an adult woman's sexual fantasies originate during her teen years. It's in the adolescent's fantasies that she meets her desired sexual partner and experiences her ideal of romantic encounters. As a young woman explores her sexuality, first in fantasy and later in relationships, she becomes aware of the range and content of her sexual interests. These interests evolve over time. A woman's sexuality unfolds gradually and most often in the context of feeling connected to another person.

Interest in same-sex relationships is quite normal for young women. Even though sexual orientation usually becomes apparent during adolescence, attraction to another female, especially during the early teen years, doesn't mean that the young woman is a lesbian.

> At 12, in the seventh grade, Sophie fell in love with Stephanie. They talked nonstop about school, their crowds, and who liked whom. Occasionally they still spent an afternoon making up stories for their Barbies and acting them out. But they did this with a certain self-consciousness, aware that childhood was behind them.
>
> Sophie and Stephanie listened to music for hours. Sometimes they stood in front of a mirror and danced together. They liked practicing the steps and took turns being the "boy" for the slow dances. "Stephanie and Sophie, Sophie and Stephanie . . . Best friends," wrote Sophie along the edges of her notebooks.
>
> When they slept over at each other's houses, they talked through the night, hugging each other so close together that their voices were barely whispers between them.

"Let's pretend we're kissing," Sophie said, and closed her eyes. They pressed their mouths together, bumped noses, and giggled.

"Come on, try again," whispered Stephanie. This time, eyes open, they kissed and kissed.

The kissing practice happened many times, but they never spoke of it the next day. There was something about daylight that made Sophie feel a little vulnerable in her strong feelings for Stephanie. During the day, she would roughhouse with Stephanie, or giggle and gossip.

Years later, when Sophie was a grown woman with a husband and children, she would think back to those adolescent days and wonder what that first love had been all about.

Most adolescents and even young adult women have intense romantic feelings for other females—they quite literally fall in love with their girlfriends. The touching and hanging on each other, even the kissing, caressing, and fondling that occur, are not definitive statements about a young woman's sexual orientation. Instead, these are early forays into having strong attachments outside the family group. Usually the focus in these relationships is not on sexual activity but on the intense love and attraction one has for another person. This is normal development and an important precursor for relationships to come. These relationships usually give way to other friendships that are more boundaried.

Sometimes, the experience of first love turns out to be true love. For lesbian teens, early feelings of affection for other girls turn out not to be fleeting and experimental. Instead, these teens experience a growing and ongoing awareness that they are sexually attracted to women, not men. In a culture that is still largely intolerant of sexual diversity, this discovery often remains private. The lesbian teen may feel ashamed, embarrassed, and isolated. A young woman can talk to many friends about concerns related to her heterosexual activity, but if she is questioning her orientation, thinking she might be more attracted to women than men, she often feels that she has no one she can talk to. Support from other lesbian teens and mentoring from older lesbian women can help a young woman gain pride in who she is as a sexual person.

> "When I hear the words 'Coming out,' I think of *brief*, like it happens quickly. But for me, coming out was a long process, sometimes filled with terror about being found out alternating with terror that *I* wouldn't find out about myself. I got through it with the help of some close friends and a lot of reading that I did."

In adolescence (and continuing into adulthood), sexuality is influenced by cultural attitudes, biological development, peer influence, sexual experience, and relationships. For women, sexual orientation is a blend of biology and experience. Some women knew early in childhood that they felt "different" and didn't aspire to the male/

female relationships they saw around them. Many become much more aware of an attraction to women—or to both men and women—in adolescence, when sexual interest escalates. For most girls, at least in our experience, orientation is so straightforward and self-evident that they don't question it. They just know they're attracted to guys, and the world around them confirms what they feel inside. But for those who don't feel that way, discovering their orientation can be a long journey, one that, if you are still struggling with this issue as an adult, might be aided by the orientation exercise in the Appendix under "Ways to Know Your Sexual Story." If you feel that you may be a lesbian or bisexual and are confused or disturbed by this discovery, make a conscious choice to respect your feelings and your choices, and trust that your decisions are right for *you*. A wealth of resources are currently available for lesbians and bisexuals. We list many of these books under "Suggested Resources" at the end of the book. Websites are also plentiful, and we suggest you spend time checking them out.

> "I love being a lesbian. I'm happy in who I am and what I do. It surprises others around me when they find out I'm lesbian because there are so many stereotypes. You can't fit me in a box or under a label."

Ethnic and Cultural Identity

It is in adolescence that many girls become aware of how they are different, and how their families are different, from what they see on television or at the local mall. Ethnicity and color exert a powerful influence on our self-identity, beliefs, and values as we grow and develop. From inside your community came one set of messages about how you, as a young woman, were perceived. Outside your community, people may not have seen *you* at all, only your color or your ethnicity. From inside and out, your ethnicity and color affect your sense of sexuality.

> "Dating was always hard in high school. If I dated non-Asians, my parents weren't pleased, and I'd have to fight myths like 'all Asian women are sexually exotic.' The Asian guys I dated found me too American—because I've lived here all my life. I felt like I didn't fit anywhere."

> "We moved here from India when I was 14. I wasn't used to seeing so much female nakedness and pretend sexual passion on television. In India, there was more censorship. You might see two flowers intertwining or two birds with their beaks together to represent a sexual image. I was uncomfortable seeing so much sex here."

> "When I was growing up, seeing how women of color were portrayed in the media made a real impression on me. It seemed they were always shown as hookers or unwed mothers. It became a point of pride for me to keep my sexual urges under control—I was going to prove the stereotypes wrong. Unfortunately, I think I got too good at keeping my sexual side buried."

In some cultures, it is typical for families to exercise control, directly or indirectly, over young women's sex lives—perhaps by restricting dating or requiring a daughter to live at home until married. These forms of control may seem inconceivable to outsiders. Nevertheless, they are longstanding traditions within some groups and are not easily opposed.

"Other than church activities, I didn't do anything with guys as a teenager. In my African American family, it just wasn't allowed. Even when I graduated from high school and began to date, the weekly grilling from my relatives hardly made it worth the effort."

If you were raised in North America but your ethnic heritage included the custom of parental involvement in your dating and partner choices, you had to decide if, or how strongly, you would oppose this practice. Looking back on your adolescence, you may have wanted to honor your parents' wishes but, at the same time, were influenced by the images of dating and romantic love you saw all around you. Your sexual development occurred in the context of conflicting worldviews.

"Growing up in my ethnic community, we weren't supposed to have premarital sex. I was curious about sexual activity but thought I was wrong to have thoughts about it. I wanted to ask my older sister, but she said women in our culture discussed these things only after they were married, and then only with their husbands."

"I remember the statue of the Blessed Virgin Mary in our living room. Grandma would always point to the statue and say to me, 'Benita, you must be pure like our mother Mary.' But it wasn't very easy to be pure and popular at the same time."

In order to know your sexual story, it's important to understand and appreciate your ethnic and cultural identity. In the Appendix, we give you a chance to ask yourself questions about your color and ethnicity. The questions are designed to stimulate your thinking about your childhood and adolescence and the messages you've internalized about your sexuality.

Peer Pressure

"Don't you want to do it? Everybody is," Brenda said, smiling smugly at Kelly. "We've been doing it for a long time. Sometimes we sneak out during lunch hour to fool around in the parking lot."

Kelly giggled uncomfortably. "Aren't you worried about getting pregnant?"

"No," Brenda said. "I know when my period is. Sometimes he pulls out, too. He doesn't like condoms. We're cool about it. Besides, it makes our relationship so special to have sex, and we really love each other."

During adolescence peers often have more influence than parents on a teen's attitudes and behavior. Peer culture often condones and even encourages sexual behavior under certain conditions. In some teen groups, sexual activity verifies the boy's masculinity and the girl's femininity. A young woman may feel that she has status in the eyes of her friends if she does "sexual things" with her boyfriend. A couple may be expected to be sexual once they decide to see each other exclusively. Like exchanging class rings or clothing, sex may serve as a sign that the couple has an exclusive relationship.

Sometimes there's a fine line in teen culture between a young woman finding peer acceptance and suffering peer scorn. Despite the sexual revolution, a double standard still exists. Boys who are sexually active are almost universally applauded for their conquests. Girls who are sexually active still run the risk of being labeled "sluts," "blow job queens," or "friends with benefits." Years ago young women, regardless of age, were usually stigmatized if they were sexually active. Today, adolescent attitudes have changed so that the good girl/bad girl dichotomy more often applies only for young women in junior high and early high school. Starting around 16, sexual behavior is more tolerated and even respected among peers, as long as the young woman is monogamous and doesn't "sleep around."

Peer pressure can be a two-edged sword. It can influence a young woman to have sex before she is ready and comfortable. It can also crucify her mercilessly if she does have sex but for some reason doesn't meet the accepted parameters of the in-group. Many adult women, remembering how impossible it was to figure out the acceptable amount of sexual behavior, still carry emotional wounds inflicted by their peers during adolescence.

Sexual Experience

In adolescence, young women engage in sexual activity for many different reasons. It can be the result of curiosity, a quest for the thrill and pleasure of sex, an attempt to win or retain a boyfriend's attention, a way to prove love, or an expression of affection. Adolescents have a growing ability to love another person and feel intimate. In this context, it feels natural to become more physically involved—kissing, touching, and even having intercourse. A young woman's sexual exploration normally progresses from holding hands, to kissing and French kissing, to breast fondling, genital fondling, masturbating her partner, oral sex, and finally intercourse. The male partner often sets the pace.

There is tremendous variability in sexual interest and activity among adolescent and young adult women. Many young women are sexually active with their partners but have never themselves masturbated to orgasm. Interestingly, many young women tell us that they are happy to "go down" on their boyfriend or manually stimulate him to orgasm, but they express discomfort with his interest in giving her oral sex or masturbating her to orgasm. They tell us that they aren't into orgasm for themselves, either through masturbation or sexual activity with a partner. They like to give the sexual pleasure but aren't comfortable being on the receiving end. It appears that many young women need more time than males to feel comfortable with their bodies and their sexuality before they're really interested in, or ready for, "hot sex."

For most teens, sex takes center stage in their moral world. At home, school, church, synagogue, or mosque, they are constantly lectured on the virtues of purity and the value of abstinence. The decision to be sexually active is burdened not only by fear of being caught, becoming pregnant, or contracting a sexually transmitted disease, but by the weight of moral guilt and shame. Many young women feel caught, trying to reconcile their sexual actions with their self-image of being virtuous and moral. Many give moral lip service to one set of values while living on the wilder side.

Being sexually active involves a great deal more than just intercourse, but intercourse remains a rite of passage in most cultures. "Passage into what?" many women might add, aware that for boys, intercourse is a rite of passage into sexual maturity, whereas for girls, intercourse is a rite of passage into loss of virginity. For boys, the opportunities may open up, but for girls, the choices may shut down. In a recent national poll of teens, almost three-fourths of the young women who have had sexual intercourse acknowledged that they wished that they had waited until they were older (National Campaign to Prevent Teen Pregnancy, 2000).

Although the percentage of young women having sexual intercourse before age 15 has remained fairly steady over the last 30 years, the age at which a young woman has her first intercourse has dropped; 60% of all young women (in the United States) have had intercourse by the time they are 19, with the average age of 17 for the first occurrence, and 70% have intercourse before marriage (Laumann et al., 1994).

A young woman's first experience with sexual intercourse is often disappointing. Many women report that their first sexual experience, in retrospect, was one in which they felt either physically forced or emotionally coerced by the intimation that they would lose the love of their partner (Laumann et al., 1994). The first time rarely delivers that expected thrill and ecstasy implied by media images of sexual abandonment and passion. So many young women feel let down by their first sexual experience that the term "Peggy Lee syndrome" has been coined to describe the "is that all there is?" quality of the experience (Hyde, 2000).

Some women remember feelings of anger, doubt, guilt, and shame after their first intercourse. Although some experience physical discomfort or pain afterward, they feel they cannot ask their parents for help for fear of rejection or anger for having sex in the first place. This fear usually increases feelings of isolation and loneliness. A teenager may also experience her partner as being selfish and uncaring after sex. Even if the first intercourse is consensual, some young women report being treated violently during the experience and feel traumatized by the experience.

So, instead of pleasure and satisfaction, a young woman may feel stunned or numb after intercourse. Language captures the culture's lack of respect for women by describing a woman's first coitus as "losing her virginity" and a young man's as "scoring." Although some young women feel that their status in their social group temporarily rises as a result of having had intercourse, over time, many describe the experience ruefully as "giving up virginity" in order to gain social acceptance. The ultimate slap in the face is the way that young women are described as either "virgins" or "sluts"—as if there were no other sexual states (Wolf, 1997).

Sex Education

Many young women learn about sex in confusing ways that have no contexts and no parameters other than "Just say no" (from their parents) versus "Everybody's doing it" (from their peers). In magazine ads, young teens are made up to look like sexy, savvy women. In the media, they see images of sex and passion selling everything from rock songs to rocking chairs. The biology lessons in school aren't even remotely related to what they are feeling in their own biology.

> "When I was a teenager, I didn't know much about sex. But I would have died before I asked my parents. I was sure I knew enough to take care of myself."

Most young women have difficulty admitting that they know very little about sexual behavior. Their knowledge of birth control and STDs is often confused and misinformed. Sex slang is vague and usually holds multiple meanings, thereby rendering the terms useless. When describing sexual activity, many young women don't even know the names of their genitals, their patterns of sexual response, and sexy alternatives to having sexual intercourse with a partner. Sadly, many young women have no idea how to decide what is "right and wrong" for them in sexual relations, or how loving couples should behave toward one another. If you're reading this book as a parent, you may wonder how to talk about sex with your own daughter. In the "Suggested Resources" section, we list books and websites that are helpful in talking about sex with children and teenagers.

If an adolescent is sexually active, she most often denies the possibility of unwanted pregnancy or sexually transmitted diseases. Getting pregnant or getting herpes, let alone AIDS, is not a real possibility in her young world. The basic law of cause and effect is still being sorted out in adolescence, and it feels like life will go on as it is forever. Actions that have irreversible consequences seem as remote as old age. Bad things happen but "not to me."

Parents often participate in this denial by turning their backs on adolescent sexuality. Uncomfortable with sex themselves, they haven't a clue how to discuss sex with their daughters (or sons). They may pass along a book about sexuality but, more often than not, they shy away from a face-to-face dialogue. Or they have "the big talk," but it's a one-time event, never to be repeated. Unfortunately, no single discussion can cover all the questions and choices that will arise daily throughout their daughter's adolescence. By avoiding ongoing conversations about sex with their daughters, parents fail to share their own understanding of sexuality and their own memories of teenage excitement and confusion.

Do you remember the fairy tale of "Sleeping Beauty"? We think that is the story of young girls becoming women. In the story, the evil fairy predicts that Sleeping Beauty will prick her finger on the spindle of a spinning wheel and die before she turns 16. A less powerful but good fairy commutes the sentence from death to deep sleep.

Sleeping Beauty's parents are heartbroken. In their grief and desire to protect their daughter, they have every spindle in the kingdom removed. They want Sleeping Beauty to grow up in a world without spindles so that she will never be exposed to them, won't even know they exist.

We all know what happens. Just before her 16th birthday, Sleeping Beauty (at least in the Disney version) finds the one spindle in the entire kingdom. Because she has never seen one before, she is fascinated by it and drawn to it. Because she doesn't know that it can hurt her, because she hasn't been taught to make choices about right and wrong, the good and the bad regarding spindles, she is in big danger.

Sleeping Beauty does that which every fascinated junior scientist does: she moves toward the mystery to investigate it. She touches the spindle. The rest we leave to Disney.

Women often look back at their sexual adventures and misadventures during their teenage years and wonder, *Where were my parents? Why didn't they talk to me?* Like Sleeping Beauty, hiding the spindles didn't protect them. Ironically, a woman may repeat this silence of denial with her own daughter because that is how sex was treated in her family and she still doesn't have a clue how to talk about sex, not with her partner, not with her daughter.

A teenager needs her parents' continual input about the normalcy and pleasure of sexual feelings, and what's okay and not okay in their value system. Ideally, discussions about sexual feelings and behavior parallel and reflect a young woman's growing ability to love another person and to take responsibility for her actions. While reassuring her about the normalcy of these feelings, parents can also help their daughters rehearse how to handle different situations before they arise.

CHAPTER TWO

Adult Sexuality: A Lifelong Story

From the first days of life to the threshold of adulthood, your developing sense of who you are included what the world expected of you as a female. As you grew into your body and began to have sexual experiences, your values and your sexual interests emerged and your sexual story took shape. But your sexual story didn't end when you reached adulthood, and it doesn't close with marriage, divorce, menopause, or even old age. It is a lifelong story, made up of your ongoing discoveries about what it means to be a sexual person. No matter what your age, the ending has yet to be written.

You can spend your entire life capable of sexual response, pleasure, and enjoyment. To what extent, and in what ways, you fulfill the promise of your adult sexuality is up to you. You are the author of your sexual story, and if you are dissatisfied with any aspect of this personal narrative, you have the opportunity to revise the chapter you're living right now and supply your story with a new, more fulfilling ending. To do so, you have to review and reflect on the chapters you have already written from your childhood and the years of adulthood you have lived so far.

You may believe you know these chapters by heart—after all, you lived them. Just as reciting the words of a poem is not the same as understanding its many layers of meaning, being able to list the sexual experiences of your life isn't the same as fully understanding how they brought you to where you are today. Many women tend to take only a glancing look at their sexual past, moving on to other thoughts when their memories evoke a chiding response of "Girl, what *were* you thinking of?," or a wistful nostalgia for passion lost, or an echo of pain at trust betrayed. Looking more closely at how your experiences, sexual and otherwise, have shaped your current sexuality is an important key to guiding your sexual growth in the direction that is best for you. Looking forward, anticipating how various life events might affect your sexuality, can also help you meet challenges and opportunities with an insight that will contribute to lifelong healthy sexuality.

The discoveries that women have shared with us about the events that influence their sexual growth are as individual and unique as their faces and personalities.

> "The first time I ever had sexual intercourse, I was ready and the timing was just right for me. I felt this curious mix of being in charge and being utterly at sea. I thought everything would come naturally and that I'd be awash with wanting, but it wasn't like that. I felt self-conscious because I wasn't acting like the women I'd seen in the movies making love. Now I think that the newness and the unfamiliarity of intercourse made me self-conscious. Being lovers takes practice. I didn't know that then, but I wish I had."

> "I learned about one sexual myth the hard way. It had been fed to me with my cereal and trotted out with my Barbie dolls. It was that there would be a perfect Ken for me. He would read my mind and know exactly what I needed sexually. I married Ken all right, and then spent years withdrawing sexually and feeling resentful because he didn't make sex work for me. We went to counseling, and I was smug at first, certain the counselor would join me in putting the responsibility onto Ken. She didn't. It was hard, but I learned how to be responsible for myself. Now I grieve about the years that were lost to both of us because of my ridiculous dependency, entitlement, and resentment."

As you read this chapter, we hope you'll be moved to explore your sexuality in your present life as well as in your past. If you discover you have led your life as if sexuality were something you could shrug off like an unneeded sweater, we hope you will reconsider and find a prominent place for sexuality in your life. The women we know whose sexuality is an integral part of who they are and what they experience lead the full, vibrant lives that we wish for you.

> "Over the years I've read many books about menopause. As a result, I grew to respect my body just as it is. I walk with a confidence that I never had in my youth. I am as sexual as anyone I meet. My body is far from perfect, but I have lived and loved in it for decades, and I carry that with me wherever I am."

> "I'm a nurse. I know the healing benefits of touch. I sometimes marvel at how wonderful hands are: they comfort, connect, reassure, and sexually arouse, too. To me all of these things are connected to my sexuality as a woman."

> "It took some doing, but I got all three kids off to a sleep-over. Carlos and I had a whole night together—and it was terrific! Yes, it took planning, but so does everything else in a life as busy as ours. If we're going to have a sex life together, we have to be intentional about planning it. Wild abandon is not for a working mother with three kids—unless she schedules it!"

Unfortunately, even in our enlightened age, many women think of sexuality as a series of disconnected, discrete behaviors. Women *have* sex, they *act* sexy, and they *think* about sex at various times during any one day. But sexuality is not something that we turn on and off, like a tap. We are sexual beings all the time, and the more we understand about how this facet intertwines with all the others, the richer our lives become.

Just as sexuality is connected to all that we are at any one time, it is also an important part of us throughout life's stages. Each stage of life is comprised of interlocking experiences and biological changes that influence sexuality. The burst of hormones you felt during puberty and adolescence transformed your childhood sexual curiosity to a strong fascination and a desire to explore all that is sensual. The emancipation that you felt when you graduated from high school and moved out on your own led you to look for new relationships, including sexual ones. Your "biological clock" may have influenced your timing for having children. The physical and time demands of parenting may alter your sexual relationship with your partner. As the children grow up and move out, your relationship with your partner undergoes further changes. It may flourish, or it may break apart—either way, sexual activity and satisfaction will be affected. Divorce may impact your sexuality by depriving you of a partner or by opening you to opportunities for better relationships and better sex.

During middle age, your body undergoes changes that can affect your feelings of desirability and desire. The sense of mastery that comes from raising children successfully or succeeding in a career may infuse your sex life with new confidence and enthusiasm. Retirement may set you even freer to pursue pleasure in your body, including sexual pleasure. Failing health and widowhood each has a unique impact on your opportunities, desire for, and capacity to be sexual, but neither need derail your sexuality or sexual identity.

> "Having breast cancer has affected my body on the outside, but it has made me stronger on the inside. I have even learned to love my scars. When I look at them, I see what I have come through and conquered. In a strange way, I've opened up more to sex than at any other time in my life. I like to savor all of my senses: I've never appreciated them as I do now. Now when I'm stroking my husband's penis, I'm not just focusing on his arousal, I'm aware of the wonderful feel of the soft skin over his firm erection."

"My husband and I had a sex life that was more methodical than sensual. One night I talked him into renting a racy movie. It showed oral sex and was very arousing to me. Later in bed I really let my hair down. I got my courage up, pulled the sheets off, and started stroking and then kissing his penis. It seemed very natural to get into the rhythm of sucking him. I noticed that his diaphragm was shaking a little. I was feeling pretty shy, so I stopped and noticed he was giggling. 'What?' I asked. He said, 'Your boobs are bouncing up and down—you look like you stuck your finger in a light socket.' At that moment I knew that I'd never, ever again throw the bed sheets off with Theo. My eyes were wide open and I realized that sex was just the tip of the iceberg of our constrained relationship. I found my courage again and got out altogether. It was the most freeing thing I ever did. It took awhile, but I am in a new relationship, and the sex is a lot of fun."

Knowing your sexual story means understanding how life experiences have influenced how you accept your body, experience pleasure, and relate sexually to your partner(s). It also means knowing yourself well enough to anticipate how these experiences might affect your sexuality as they occur in your future. This is, sadly, no easy task for women today. Although, as a whole, we discuss sexual matters much more openly than did our mothers and grandmothers, we still don't share our stories and experiences with one another as freely as we could. We commiserate about menstrual difficulties, and pregnancy and childbirth seem to bring us together to share the most intimate physical details of this female experience. But when it comes to expressing worries about what are "normal" sexual feelings and activities or to sharing the joys and trials of our sexual self-discoveries, we often hold back. Women tell us, with deep sadness, how much they regret having been afraid to talk to others about themselves, including their sexuality. They cringe about their "dumb" choices when we ask them to explore their past. They seem visibly lighter when we help them to see, for example, that women learn to orgasm with a partner, and it often takes time; or that for most women arousal doesn't come automatically, like flipping on a light switch. Overall, our knowledge has become more sophisticated, but many of our worries remain the same. By resisting thinking and talking about these concerns, we deny ourselves the full opportunity to learn from other women about the common experiences that impact many of us as we move across our life span.

We hope this chapter will help fill this gap. We describe what women have told us about their experiences with major life events, and we pose questions that will challenge you to think about your own sexuality in similar situations, whether these events have already occurred in your life or still lie ahead. We also make suggestions for finding additional information about each topic, either in a later chapter or from resources listed at the end of the book.

In the Appendix, we provide exercises to help you take an even closer look at how your life events have shaped your sexuality. In addition, we include exercises to help you see how your ethnicity, sexual orientation, and the values you've learned from others have influenced your sexuality. The self-knowledge you gain from reading this chapter and doing the exercises in the Appendix will give you the springboard you need to better benefit from the rest of the book.

SEXUAL EXPERIENCES

What we call your "sexual story" is what psychologists talk about as your sexual development: the maturation of your sexual feelings, behavior, attitudes, and knowledge. As such, it is about far more than just your sex life at any one age or stage of life. Your sexual story is the product of all the events that occur at each life stage and how you respond to them. These responses, in turn, are shaped by your cognitive, emotional, moral, and social development. This perspective encourages you to explore and accept sexual feelings that might only confuse or worry you if you viewed sex and sexuality as one-dimensional and governed by one-size-fits-all rules and standards. The ever-broadening definition of what is sexually normal is liberating. Still, given how uniquely complex each woman's sexuality is, it's obvious that your sexuality not only *should* be defined by you but, really, can be defined *only* by you.

A large part of a woman's expression of her sexuality is, of course, the choices she makes about when to have sex and with whom. Years ago a woman's sexual choices were made *for* her. With certain cultural variations, she "saved herself" for marriage, giving her sexuality to her husband as part of her dowry, after which he could do with it—*her*—what he liked. A woman who was brought up to follow these rules might feel desperately bad just for *wanting* something different—much less for *doing* something differently. And a woman who didn't *feel* bad about having her own ideas and taking charge of her own sexual destiny was usually *labeled* "bad."

For many of us, all that has changed. Now we have choices about when to have sex and with whom. Unfortunately, those choices aren't always easy to make. Would you give in to desire and have sex with your boyfriend, even though your family and religious values tell you to wait until marriage? Could you explore the possibility that you are bisexual without feeling as if you were violating a taboo? How would you feel about choosing to make love to your husband when you don't feel all that loving, just because it's easier than talking through your marital problems? Would having an affair sound the death knell for your marriage, or would you consider it just a brief fling? What if it were your husband who had the affair? Is it okay for you to have casual sex with a man you just met, but not okay for your 19-year-old daughter to do the same? If you finally ended your marriage because you could no longer live the lie that you are heterosexual, would you be able to have an active and open sex life as a lesbian, or would you remain celibate out of fear of shocking your friends and family?

As with all choices we make in life, sexual choices often present us with dilemmas—conflicts between two firmly held values, fine lines between wants and needs, mores versus manners, our needs versus someone else's, the benefits of planning weighed against those of spontaneity. How we resolve these dilemmas contributes to our sexual development. Not every sexual experience you have had or will have is transformative or momentous, but each sexual experience affects your ongoing experience of your body, your sense of yourself as a woman, your self-esteem, your sense of your place in the universe, and much more. When your sexual decisions are based on the personal values and external influences most important to you, then your sexual experiences will generally feel emotionally comfortable and satisfying as well as physically pleasurable. If your sexual experiences today do not fit this description, it may not even be your current sex life that's the problem but a pattern of past sexual decisions that contradicts your most important values and needs.

Time has a way of changing everyone's perspective; you need to take the factor of time into account when you reexamine the experiences you've had. Maybe you blush at your "stupidity" when you think about that guy you fell into bed with in college when you were both drunk, but the erotic films that would have made your face flame then seem like a healthy part of a woman's sex life now—with or without a partner. For decades you might have lived by the precept that marriage is the only place for sex, but now, having finally fallen for someone five years after your husband's death, you think it might be okay to get to know each other sexually before committing to each other. We know one woman who was unashamed of the number of men she slept with during her 20s but now reports unhappily, "I tend to keep a lid on in the bedroom because it's like I'm afraid that wild woman will reappear and mess everything up." We know many, many others who avoid intimate relationships altogether, pretending they no longer care about sex, when the truth is that they can't reconcile the less-than-perfect 40-year-old bodies they now own with their memories of the physical and sexual ideal they fulfilled 20 years earlier.

Development, sexual and otherwise, means *change*. If you can examine your sexuality today and say with confidence that you have matured and are where you want to be, then clearly your past decisions played a positive role—even if, in retrospect, they seem as if they must have been made by a stranger. If not, you can probably benefit from a closer look at why you did what you did in the past and why you're doing what you're doing sexually today. As to the future, forewarned is forearmed: be prepared for the types of changes that women describe in the rest of this chapter!

Kinds of Sex: What Drives Your Choices?

In the movies, sex just happens. That's not the way it is in real life, even though our romantic notions sometimes trick us into believing that sex is just the result of two people getting carried away in the moment. Some sexual encounters do occur out of sheer abandon. Some are undertaken after a lot more conscious, deliberate thought than others. Each sexual circumstance is unique. Whatever the case, we've found that most women benefit from understanding their reasons for their sexual choices—if not beforehand, then at least upon reflection.

You made love with your best friend in an attempt to comfort each other over another close friend's death. Your best friend is married. How do you feel about the experience? How do you *think* you should feel? How will this experience affect your future decisions?

At a conference, you slept with a fellow physician you'd just met hours earlier. You're now chastising yourself for being unprofessional. Does that mean you shouldn't have enjoyed the sex?

You really liked John and hoped the relationship would go beyond friendship, but when he asked you to go to bed with him you knew it was casual—just for fun. And it *was* fun. But now you're really falling for him, and he's still just looking for fun—elsewhere. You're wondering if, for you, there is any such thing as casual sex.

All of our sexual decisions are complicated, even if they seem quite simple at the time. You may initiate sex for one reason but come out of the experience with an entirely different feeling. One partner in a sexual encounter may have an agenda, while the other is really giving in to the passion of the moment. The reason you give yourself for a sexual decision may turn out to be self-deception. The reason it's important to understand all this is to improve your capacity for self-determination in the future.

Loving Sex

A common reason for choosing to have sex with a partner is love. Loving sex is a powerful connection between two people who share a strong emotional bond; it's a way two people can say with their bodies, "I love you." It's one kind of sex that is often depicted in movies and books, and it has inspired poems and paintings throughout history. For those who are in love, sex can be a magical experience unmatched by anything else. Sex gains a new depth when motivated by love; love gains a new dimension of closeness when this profound emotion is expressed physically.

Unfortunately, loving sex does not always live up to its fairy-tale reputation. First of all, being in love is no guarantee of legendary sex. The earth does not automatically move for women just because they are having sex and not even when they are in love and having sex. Fantastic sex often takes practice; see the Appendix for ways to understand your body and create better sex with your partner.

Second, for some people, having sex imposes pressure to declare love that may not be felt. Teenagers today are just as likely as ever to use "But I love you so much" as the reason to coerce a potential partner into having sex. Some women, especially young women, may even convince themselves that they love their partner as a way to assuage guilt brought on by the clash between a cultural and/or religious prohibition against unmarried sex and their growing sexual desire. Or they may simply confuse physical desire and emotional love. However it happens, when two people mistakenly believe that their sexual encounter is based on love, the experience is bound to disappoint.

We have met many women who, years later, were guilt-ridden about a sexual experience motivated by lust not love, or by an affair they'd had when they were dragging through the final months of an unraveling marriage. In cases like these, many women are greatly relieved to learn that it was perfectly natural for them to have sex motivated by sheer desire—or by many of the other forces discussed in the following pages. What's important is to gain perspective on why they did what they did in the past and how it may be influencing them, positively and negatively, today.

Casual Sex

Sometimes the motivation to have sex is pleasure, pure and simple. This is what many people call "casual sex." Nothing seems to inspire such heated debate as this form of sex. Is sex without love immoral? Is sex with different partners safe, in this era of AIDS and STDs? Is casual sex a normal instinct for men but abnormal for women? Is *casual* the equivalent of *irresponsible*? Conventional wisdom on this subject has varied over the years, and the answers to these questions will always vary depending on the speaker's cultural and religious background, life experiences, and other personal factors.

What does the phrase *casual sex* conjure up for you? To some, it means any sex outside of an exclusive commitment like marriage. For others it may mean promiscuity. For still others, unfortunately, it may mean unthinking sex. Casual sex includes any situation where two consenting adults enjoy physical pleasure with each other and the sex is responsible, nonexploitative, and mutually respectful. Perhaps a 28-year-old woman goes to bed with a man she met earlier in the evening; both are honest with each other and take precautions to prevent pregnancy and infection. Or a 50-year-old woman chooses to have sex with a man she meets on vacation. Perhaps two residents of a nursing home visit at night so that they can be sexual. We believe the choices and direction shouldn't come from experts in such situations. Rather, they must be based on a woman's personal values, desires, and common sense. As mentioned earlier in this chapter, making the choice may involve reconciling conflicting factors. One woman told us that although she has promised herself she'll have sex only when she and a partner have made a commitment to each other, sometimes she has sex with someone "just because it feels great." Another woman notes ruefully, "It's sometimes easier to have sex with someone than to talk with them about condoms."

Casual sounds easy, but responsible casual sex is anything but. As sex therapists, we tell our clients that casual sex, practiced safely, responsibly, and respectfully, falls well within many people's value system—and for many other people, it does not. If you are going to make decisions you can live with, you have to think about which group you fall into ahead of time.

Sex as Solace

> "I was halfway around the world when I got the call that my mother had died. I was devastated. David was a colleague and good friend, but certainly not my lover. I needed to talk that night, and he listened. I needed to cry, and he held me. I needed to feel close to another human being, and we made love. I'll never forget his tenderness. I'll never forget how powerful my need was at that moment to feel alive and cared for."

There are times when two people with no permanent commitment to each other have sex, and the act is anything but casual. Intense emotions can trigger a hunger or yearning to make intimate contact with another human being, even if the shared intimacy might be fleeting and short-lived. Although some women later regret or feel embarrassed about having sex as solace, their judgment is too harsh. Sometimes sex occurs when a person's grief, isolation, fear, or shame makes her momentarily vulnerable and open to sexual decisions that she would not make otherwise. The woman connects with her body because it temporarily eases the emotional pain she is in; it feels good to be touched and to touch.

Sex as Conquest

If you are a young adult, in your twenties or thirties, you may feel close to the cultural stereotype of sexual beauty. If you're in your forties or fifties, you may want reassurance that you are still attractive. Knowing that you've attracted someone through your beauty and sexuality is a powerful feeling, no matter what the age, and many women have engaged in what could be called "sex as conquest" at some point in their lives. Some women confine their power-seeking to flirting, while others choose to have sex with the men or women who become their conquests.

Is there anything wrong with this? Not necessarily, as long as you know what you're doing and how it makes you feel afterward. Sex that is motivated by power-seeking alone turns both you and your partner into objects in a power play, no longer real people seeking real contact with each other. Most women we have counseled say that the thrill wears off in time—or they lose their taste for sex as conquest once they have been the conquered as often as they've been the conqueror. One woman put it succinctly as "fun but limiting." Sex as conquest is the epitome of other-oriented sex. Eventually, sexuality has to be about what you like about yourself. For an expanded discussion of this topic, check out "Desirable versus Desiring" in Chapter 6.

Agenda Sex

Like the sirens of Greek legend, women have always known that sex can be the route to any other goal or objective. Sex can be offered as some sort of unspoken barter, or it can simply instill the euphoria that makes a partner more amenable to giving a woman what she wants. This dubious feminine wile is rooted in the perception that women (as opposed to men) have little to offer besides their sexual favors. We call sex that is undertaken to manipulate someone "agenda sex." In general, it's problematic because it fosters uncertainty, resentment, and/or anger.

Possible agendas for sex include proving something, bolstering the ego, feeling in control, manipulation, bartering, making up for some offense, and avoiding boredom. Some agendas are even well-meaning. It's not uncommon for women to have sex with a partner to make him or her "feel better"—more loved, more attractive, more virile, and so forth. As an occasional gesture made out of love and compassion, this kind of agenda sex is not necessarily problematic. It's when sex is habitually undertaken without desire or love that agenda sex usually backfires in distrust and resentment.

"I don't really like sex with my partner," said one woman we know, "but he expects it at least once a week. He gets off, then rolls over and goes to sleep. I don't think sex with him could ever improve, so I just have it to keep him from bugging me." She is so busy keeping the peace that she may lose touch with her own sexual needs to make the sex better for *herself*. In the long run, satisfying a partner because a woman doesn't want to deal with the challenge of honesty will result in resentment and yearning; she'll resent her partner for his demands and oblivion, and she'll secretly yearn for a better lover who would be sensitive to her needs. Agenda sex always has a goal *other than* honest connection and intimacy.

Sex to Dispel Loneliness

One example of agenda sex that is so common and important that it warrants separate consideration is sex that serves as an antidote for loneliness. Young women away from their childhood home for the first time, or older women out of the security of a long-term relationship may find living on their own lonely. A relationship soothes you when you're lonely or scared. Many women say that they put up with sex in a relationship because it is the price they pay for being with someone—and it's the *being with* that is important, not the *someone*.

> "I never think about masturbating. I know about masturbation, but when I do it, I feel lonely and kind of empty. I like sex with someone because I like cuddling

and sleeping together at night. It's not about sex, it's more about knowing someone is there."

If you always need to be in a relationship with someone, perhaps you use sexual connection to relieve loneliness or anxiety about being alone. If you are having sex primarily to avoid being alone, we suggest that you may not be ready to have a sexual relationship at this time. Your work lies in learning to soothe yourself, learning how to be in charge of you, and yes, even learning how to be alone. This is not to imply that loneliness is not a painful circumstance for many people or that you "should" never feel lonely. But if you are bargaining with sex to avoid confronting your apprehensions about loneliness or being alone, mastering the aloneness is the better solution.

> "I couldn't stand to be in my apartment alone. I would find excuses to crash at a friend's house. I invited Roy to live with me two weeks after we met. I knew we didn't have a chance of making it together, but I had sex with him almost without thinking about it, because I knew he would stay then, and I wouldn't have to be afraid to be alone."

Experimental Sex

For many women (and men), sexuality is the most fascinating laboratory to which we have access. Because sex offers the possibility of seemingly boundless pleasure and limitless potential for human connection, some women engage in what we call "experimental sex." This may mean exploring the boundaries of erotica (see "Suggested Resources") or experimenting with heterosexual sex (for lesbians) or with lesbianism or bisexuality (for heterosexuals). Not everyone needs to explore their orientation or the boundaries of what's considered "conventional" or "acceptable," but for some women this exploration is vital to their identity. They don't want to be constrained by narrow definitions or locked into one orientation. Still other women find the thrill of the exotic or forbidden a compelling aspect of sex and enjoy experimenting.

Celibacy

Some women choose to remain celibate. Celibacy may be permanent or temporary; it may include masturbation or not. It may be a lifelong religious commitment, or it may be a choice to avoid sexual activity while not permanently partnered. Some women view it as a means of increasing nonsexual intimacy in relationships, others as a way of avoiding exposure to STDs. Celibacy doesn't obliterate a woman's sexuality; she is sexual whether or not she's having sex. Celibacy is part of a woman's sexual choices and sexual identity. A woman might choose celibacy in order to develop nonsexual relationships, to learn more about her own feelings, or to concentrate on a goal that she must attain in her work or personal life. Listen to what these women say:

> "Being celibate is a conscious decision. You still feel all your sexual feelings. You make decisions about celibacy continually; you work at it. Sometimes people say the most stupid things to me. They'll remark that because I'm celibate, it must be so much easier because I never have 'those feelings.' What a flat, dull, two-dimensional view they have of me. I struggle with my celibacy, but I see what I gain by not seeking sexual connection with another. I feel that I am trying to deepen intimacy with others through nonsexual means—through friendship and honest dialogue."

> "Because I'm a nun, people don't think I have sexual feelings. How wrong they are! There are days when I get turned on watching the mailman walk by. You know, you just don't fall out of bed one day and become a nun. It's taken me years of prayer, work, and spiritual reflection to understand my spiritual path. But I do love to touch and hug others; this is vital to my life. And I know that, for me, the only real way I can show my love for God is by what I show in my love for others."

Sexual experiences are an important part of your sexual story. To better understand how they have impacted your life, reflect on the following questions:

- Do my past sexual experiences feel the same to me now as I felt about them then? If not, what could I have changed?
- How would I categorize my most fulfilling sexual experiences of the past: as loving sex, casual sex, sex as conquest, agenda sex, sex to dispel loneliness, or experimental sex?
- How would I categorize my most negative sexual experiences of the past: as loving sex, casual sex, sex as conquest, agenda sex, sex to dispel loneliness, or experimental sex?
- Is there one kind of sexual experience that predominates in my current sex life? Is it the same kind as in the past?
- How have I expressed my sexuality during a period of celibacy or abstinence?
- When I make a decision to have sex, what do I think of first: my own desires right now, the other person's desires, how I might feel later, how my best friend will react, or some combination?
- Do I usually plan my sexual experiences ahead of time or just let the moment dictate?
- Are any of my past sexual experiences still a source of embarrassment, shame,

or guilt? If so, what are some possible reasons? Do these reactions impact my sexual experiences today?
- If I devised a set of rules for making sexual decisions, what would they be? Are these the rules I tend to follow? If not, why?

Decisions you have made in the past are just that—in the past. Appreciate the decisions that have brought you joy or helped you to grow in sexual wisdom. Learn from the decisions that you now regret, and try to move on. If you find it difficult accepting some of your past choices, refer to the techniques in Chapter 13 under "The Solution, Not the Problem, May Be in Your Head." In that chapter, you will find techniques to help you better understand and modify unfair and self-defeating thoughts and beliefs that can haunt you with feelings of guilt and shame.

Sexual decision-making is as complex as any other set of life decisions. Some women wait to have sex until they're with their life partner. Other women have sex with someone they're with for the evening. You are always in the process of exploring your sexuality, because it is ever fluid. We encourage you to ask questions, make mistakes, take risks, and, above all else, be passionate about caring for your sexual self.

WHEN BEING SEXUAL HURTS YOU

We've been describing sexual experiences as choices—either ones you have made or ones you may make in the future. In reality, not all sexual experiences are choices, and some are hurtful. Sexual trauma can be so devastating that we've devoted a whole chapter to it; see Chapter 10. But even when a sexual experience seems positive, it can still have a bad outcome, like getting an STD or having an unwanted pregnancy. Then there are those many experiences that leave women feeling guilty, ashamed, or confused. There is a big difference between the lasting effects of abuse or exploitation and the uncomfortable feeling that can follow a less-than-ideal sexual encounter, but all negative experiences call for self-care and reflection.

"We're all supposed to be so well-informed these days that when I met Ian, I thought he'd be like other guys I'd had sex with: up front about it if he had an STD. We cared about each other, and so I made assumptions I shouldn't have. I never thought about getting an STD from him, but now that I have herpes, I can't think about anything else. Whenever I even consider having sex with anyone, I think about herpes."

"I thought sexual harassment was something that happened only to dumb, naive, women. In fact, I thought it was only dumb men who tried it. After all, there've been enough widely publicized negative consequences for it that I figured you'd have to be an idiot to try to get away with that today. Well, let me tell you, there are all kinds of harassment. I thought my coworker Matt was just being helpful when I started my new job. But his helpfulness was very controlling: for weeks no one else got near me, and he blocked my attempts to get to know others, especially guys. That's when I realized that I was being harassed."

"When is a choice to have sex not really a choice? I'd like to tell my daughter just to say no loudly and clearly when that's what she means. But I remember once in college when I said no and no again, ended up sort of wrestling with the guy, and then just let it happen. After all, I'd slept with this guy before, it was the era of 'free love,' and it seemed silly to make a big deal of it. When it was over—which was pretty quickly—I didn't make anything out of it at all, but over the years I've felt vaguely ashamed. Why did I just give in if it was something I really didn't want? Maybe because it was uncool to make a big deal out of sex in those days, or maybe because I didn't even want to consider the other possibility—that this friend of mine had essentially raped me. Did I make a choice or was the right to make the choice taken away from me? I don't really know, and that still bothers me."

As you look back on your sexual explorations, you may remember lonely, scary moments when you had to face sexual dilemmas like an unwanted pregnancy or discovering you had an STD. Perhaps there was a period in your life when you had to get drunk to have sex. Perhaps you entered a sexual relationship thinking that you were making an informed choice, only to discover later that you had been manipulated or exploited. You may remember being forced to have sex or being sexually assaulted. These are examples of when being sexual can truly hurt you.

There's an old phrase, "You play, you pay." Although being sexual can sometimes hurt you, it's not because sexuality itself is wrong, dangerous, or harmful. It's because of a lack of information and a culture that too often tolerates exploitation, coercion, and absence of choices.

As you read about the sexual misfortunes described below, take time to reflect on the following questions:

- Have I experienced this problem?
- If I have, has it impacted my sexuality?
- Have I taken steps, such as confiding in a friend, reading a self-help book, or seeking counseling, to deal with the hurt?

Sexual Assault

In any situation where you had sex because you were forced, drugged, drunk, or assaulted, you were sexually vulnerable and you were hurt. Sex wasn't lovely or fun; it was used to dominate and control. In fact, one of every four women report being forced to have sex at some time in their lives (Laumann et al., 1994). A woman's reactions to forced sex can range from teariness and distress to trying to deny it happened or treating it like it was no big deal. Because the range of reactions to forced sex is so varied, and because denying the event can lead to later problems with depression, low self-esteem, anxiety, or posttraumatic stress disorder, we encourage all women who have been sexually assaulted to speak to a mental health professional. Your nurse, physician, pastor, or community mental health clinic can help you arrange counseling.

Some types of sexual assault cause a trauma reaction of terror or deep shame and humiliation. Women can feel cut off from others, convinced that no one would accept them if they knew what had happened. If you have these feelings, we encourage you to read Chapter 10 to help you cope with the loss you've experienced.

Sexual Exploitation

> "After I graduated, I started to sleep with my high school teacher. I was 18 and he was 30. I thought I was cool at the time—until he brushed me off for another woman. I felt ashamed then, but now I'm appalled at *his* behavior. How could he do that?"

At some point in your life you might have made what we call "sexually vulnerable decisions." Perhaps you had sex with a much older person or much more powerful person, like a boss. You thought it was consensual, two equal people at the time, but now you know you weren't in a position to make an informed choice. Your situation and sexual curiosity were exploited. Perhaps you remember having sex while drunk or high, and now you feel you were exploited even though you consented at the time. Feeling exploited takes away pleasure and pride in sexuality, just as do rape and sexual harassment. It can also erode your ability to trust others with whom you enter into a sexual relationship. Perhaps even worse, it can cause you to lose trust in yourself and your ability to make wise decisions.

Women cannot and should not take sole responsibility for having been exploited, but in many cases their decision-making *did* play a role, and this may be a difficult fact to face. If you feel you have been exploited sexually, it's important to try to understand to what extent any decisions you made played a role. And it's paramount to find out how you can reverse the pattern if you have been exploited repeatedly. By completing the exercises in the Appendix, you'll be able to see whether you have a pattern of being exploited and how this pattern of exploitation impacts your sexuality. If you discover that there is a pattern, we recommend that you seek counseling to better understand your decisions and then avoid further exploitation.

STDs, UTIs, and Yeast

> "I say I don't like to have sex on the first few dates . . . and then I make sure there are no later dates. Or I say I have my period and we'll have to wait. Or I just stay home and watch TV. The truth is, I have genital warts and don't know how to

talk to men about the problem, so I just avoid sex. It looks like I'm going to end up spending the rest of my life alone."

Sexually active women are exposed to STDs. Physiologically, women are more vulnerable to these health risks during their early adult years than at any other time of their lives. In a woman's late teens and early 20s, her cervical cells go through accelerated changes toward physical maturation, which dramatically increases susceptibility to STDs (Greenspan & Nakashima, 1994; Kenney, Reinholtz, & Angelini, 1998). It's a sad irony but true that the riskiest time in a woman's life for contracting STDs coincides with the stage in which she is most apt to be sexually active in many different relationships. This is the ultimate double standard; there is no equivalent in male physical development.

A woman may also experience chronic yeast infections or chronic urinary tract infections (UTIs). These recurrent medical problems are often so painful and irritating that the woman loses sexual desire.

STDs and infections can cause a lot of unnecessary shame. Contracting an STD does not rob you of the right to have sex for the rest of your life, though you'll certainly want to take steps to protect yourself in the future. For more information on coping with these problems, see Chapter 8 for information about pain, Chapter 9 for a discussion of the impact of STDs, and Chapter 14 for suggestions about overcoming low sexual desire.

Unwanted Pregnancy

"They say that no birth control method is 100% effective, and I'm living proof of that. I'm not even interested in this guy anymore, and I just found out I'm pregnant with his child. I can't believe I have to decide whether to have this baby or have an abortion."

Despite education, available birth control, and firm resolve, unplanned pregnancies occur. A woman's life is thrown into turmoil as she sorts out relationship issues with her partner and makes a decision whether or not to terminate the pregnancy. Regardless of the decision made, sexuality and passion from that point forward may never feel the same. If this experience has happened to you, you may have difficulty enjoying sex. Sex may no longer feel carefree and liberating—memories of the emotional roller coaster that followed discovery of the pregnancy can cast a shadow on future sexual experiences. If you can't enjoy sex, you may find it helpful to read Chapter 13.

Sex and Alcohol

"I used to get drunk before having sex, then I didn't have to take any responsibility for it. My self-esteem got lower and lower, and the more I drank, the deeper the despair. I finally got counseling to sober up and help myself dig out of that pit."

If you have sexual inhibitions, alcohol and drugs can make it easier for you to have sex with a partner. The problem is that, if you come to rely on substances to produce the desired state of arousal, you're denied the opportunity to learn about your own sexual desire and arousal. Early on in your sexually active life with partners, even if you do not have a full-blown addiction problem but *do* have a pattern of relying on alcohol, you are holding back your sexual development by escaping (or so it seems) the social dilemmas and sexual decisions that you face. You let alcohol do it for you. Let us assure you: it doesn't get easier to go it alone (without mood-altering substances) later.

Some women with a past history of sexual abuse or trauma tell us they will intentionally use alcohol to dissociate and disconnect from the experience. Other women tell us that they'll use alcohol to "pump" themselves up for sex if they're anxious or depressed. Unfortunately, no amount of alcohol or drugs will make the underlying conflict go away or produce long-term sexual satisfaction.

Being in recovery from alcohol or drug addiction also requires new sexual awareness, since you may never have had a sexual experience without being high. In the sexual arena you will need to "begin at the beginning," taking time to explore your values, your history, your relationship to your body. Many professionals in the recovery movement observe that a person's sexual and interpersonal development stopped at the point where chemical usage began. If this is true, then you will need to have patience as you begin sobriety and the journey of knowing yourself. Hopefully, the sexual exercises outlined in this book will provide you with tools to help you reconnect with your sexuality.

In our culture, most women have either had some bad experience with sex or know of a woman who has. If your sexual experiences have not been entirely positive, ask yourself the following questions:

- Do I feel shame, guilt, or embarrassment about any of my past sexual experiences?
- If I were giving advice on sexual choices and decisions to someone I care about, such as a son or daughter or young friend, would my advice gibe with the way I've made my own choices?
- Does recalling certain sexual experiences evoke different thoughts and feelings now than I had at the time?
- [If you had a negative sexual experience:] Have I gotten help from my healthcare provider with any physical problems it caused?
- Does having sex today bring to mind negative memories of past experiences?
- Does it take a lot of time and effort for me to trust my sexual partner?

- Do I tend to think of sexual activity as merely a means of physical release, unconnected to emotional attachment?
- Do I have a problem with low sexual desire and arousal?
- Do I have difficulty achieving orgasm?
- Do I associate sex with immorality?

If answering these questions makes you aware that you may have had a negative sexual experience that is still harming you, consider reading Chapter 10 ("Trauma") and Part V ("Overcoming Sexual Difficulties"). If these do not provide sufficient help, be sure to talk to your healthcare provider or consider seeing a therapist.

WHEN ONE BECOMES TWO

Most women enter into partnerships that include sex. Falling in love is a time when the world of one person suddenly becomes a world of two. In the early days of a partnership, romantic love unfolds. Most couples experience a wonderful preoccupation with each other, accompanied by intense physical feelings of attraction and arousal. A partner's strong points become exaggerated and weak points are nonexistent. Sexual passion is high, sexual activity frequent, and for a brief time, life can seem like a remarkable state of existence. But in all couples—heterosexual or gay/lesbian—that euphoric state gives way to the reality of day-to-day living. In Chapter 12 we discuss the challenges that couples face as they make the inevitable transition from a sex life that seems effortless to one that needs attention.

"You've Lost That Lovin' Feeling"

> "Something changed between us. When did fantasies inch him out of my dreams? We're happy together and we've got a million interests in common, but I just don't lust after him like I used to. He thinks I've got a sexual problem, but I think my feelings are normal—that after being married for a while, you just lose the passion. I don't think he really tries to be sexual with me either—he just wants to fall into sex before rolling over into sleep. I don't know where the urgency went. I miss it, but it's too hard to figure out how to fix it."

Most couples experience a decrease in passionate feelings after the first or second year of partnership. You no longer exaggerate your partner's strengths and you're left with a life-size lover. Sex can take a nosedive. Couples who live together before marriage experience this deflation even before the wedding ceremony.

The drop in sexual frequency can occur for many reasons. When a couple is together over time, the sense of urgency about sex drops. The novelty wears off and passion gives way to affection. Although boredom may be part of the problem, there is also the reality that new relationships allow fewer distractions and often rely on sex to cement the partnership. Once you feel secure in a relationship, other demands—household tasks, career, family, and friends—require attention and create fatigue.

Women often tell us how unsatisfying their sex lives have become. They wish their partners were better lovers or that they had more time for foreplay and getting turned on. They feel that if they weighed less, slept more, and had another three hours in the day, there would be time for sex and the sex would be better. Women tell us they feel more powerful and competent in managing their careers and household schedules than their love lives. Women claim they have bad sex because of a busy life, no life, or a lifeless partner.

Sexual problems like low sexual desire, sexual pain, anorgasmia, or sexual boredom can develop in any relationship. These problems can be the result of life stressors, tension in the relationship, or old fears and inhibitions reappearing once the intense passion and feelings of "new love" have subsided.

Every couple needs to take care of their sexual relationship by devoting time to creating fulfilling sexual experiences. Because sex is fun and pleasurable, we mistakenly believe we don't need to work at it. Women who have had satisfying sex lives with one partner over decades report that they conscientiously make a place for sex in their lives, not only by making time for sexual activity with their partner but also by masturbating. If you feel you've "lost that lovin' feeling" with your partner, Parts IV ("Creating a Better Sexual Relationship") and V ("Overcoming Sexual Difficulties") will help you take positive steps in your relationship.

> "I was beginning to trash my partner to my girlfriends, complaining that all he wanted was sex and all I wanted was chocolate. Then I realized how crummy this was, as if I'd decided to have fun by dumping on sex rather than being sexual. So I decided to turn things around. I told my partner that Thursday nights were just for us—no phone calls, no e-mails. Because we won't have sex unless we get to bed at a decent time, I make an early meal. While he cleans up the dishes, I get in the mood for sex with a hot bath and some erotica. By the time he joins me in the bedroom, chocolate is the last thing on my mind!"

Arranged Marriages: Unique Challenges

In some cultures, forming a partnership presents unique challenges, especially in regard to establishing a comfortable sexual relationship. Arranged marriages are common in Indian as well as some Asian and Middle Eastern cultures. Women from these cultures may have their husbands chosen for them by their families. As adolescents, their exposure to sex education will be controlled and their knowledge of their future partner will often be limited. In an arranged marriage, sexual difficulties can emerge early in the relationship. The first sexual experience doesn't occur until the wedding night, and there may be family pressure to prove the marriage has been consummated. A lack of sex education and experience and not knowing each other can lead to problems with rapid ejaculation for men and painful intercourse and difficulty with arousal for women.

Many couples brought together through family arrangements report that, in time, they come to know, respect, and love each other deeply. As their relationship grows, so does their ability to explore and enjoy their shared sexuality. Some couples enhance their sexual relationship by openly discussing sex during their engagement and marriage. If they encounter problems, they seek advice, read self-help books, or work with a counselor.

> "I wanted to respect my family's wishes in an arranged marriage, but having grown up in North America, I was scared about marrying a complete stranger. My parents and I made an agreement: they would make a suitable match for me, but then I would date the person until I got to know him. I needed time to become friends and grow to love him."

Growing Together

Relationships go through different stages. At times sexual difficulties or disinterest will correspond to a particularly difficult or challenging period of life. Yet many women also tell us that sex improved after getting through an especially trying time. Some women experience a stronger interest in sex in their 30s, others after their kids are born, and still others when the children leave home and the house, once again, is theirs. The sex you have in your relationship will be unique to the two of you, but certainly work, having children, aging, and illnesses will influence your sexual life together. The greatest asset to a good sex life is to remain curious and committed to growing together sexually.

If you are in a partnership, ask yourself these questions:

- Do I care about being sexual with my partner? [If yes] How have I demonstrated this through words and actions? [If no] Is it because there are problems in the relationship, or am I feeling turned off by sex in general? (Part V, "Overcoming Sexual Difficulties," provides valuable information and suggestions.)
- When was the last time I made specific plans to be with my partner sexually? Did I follow through? (If you can't remember making any such plans, or you've made them but never followed through, check Chapter 12 for helpful suggestions.)
- Which one of us tends to be the prime mover in our sexual time together?
- How do I picture my sex life with my partner 10 years from now? Twenty years? Thirty years?

If you're not currently in a partnership, take some time to reflect on the following questions:

- How do I picture a long-term relationship altering my sex life? Would it be freeing or limiting?
- How do I maintain my feeling of being a sexual person even though I'm not in a sexual relationship?
- Would I like my future sexual relationships to be like any I have had in the past? If not, why not?
- What would my ideal sexual relationship with a spouse look like?

AND BABY MAKES THREE

Couples who partner during childbearing years face the decision about whether to have children. Answering in the affirmative will have a dramatic impact on a couple's sexual relationship because even in the process of trying to conceive, the focus can shift from passion to pregnancy tests. Other couples find the decision thrust upon them with an unplanned pregnancy. Either way, the drama intensifies as couples cope with coitus interruptus during pregnancy and childbirth or coitus interminable with the pain of infertility. These challenges are discussed in detail in Chapter 5.

When women with children recall their lives prepregnancy and prebaby, they often feel they were unaware of some important questions regarding their sex lives. If you are childless or considering having a baby, ask yourself the following questions:

- How do I picture my sex life changing after having kids?
- Do I know any women who are mothers and with whom I can talk about the physical changes they felt during pregnancy and after childbirth?

"Baby, Baby, Where Did Our Love Go?"

Kids bring life, quite literally, to a partnership, but they can bring death to sex. With babies, priorities don't just shift; they go through major upheavals. Some women fall so in love with their babies that their partners cease to exist. Their passion turns to nurturing their children.

> "I could go through the motions of having sex, even fake it like Meg Ryan when she does the orgasm bit in *When Harry Met Sally*. But if you really wanted to see me show passion, it was when my baby Jake clapped his hands and said, 'Mama.' "

Most women find that child-rearing increases demands on both parents but primarily on themselves. There is less privacy, less (if any) time to be intimate, far more demands to meet, and far greater fatigue to bear. Current books on women, work, parenting, and homemaking document the grueling pace that has become characteristic of modern-day motherhood. A woman can be up until 1:00 A.M. every night doing housework after homework, then sorting laundry, prepping for the next day at the job, and finally firing up the crock-pot because tomorrow is another day of carpooling the kids after work.

> "Sometimes I look over at my husband, Chris, when we're all sitting in church together, and I think, *What a great guy he is.* I'll feel this surge of love that is sexual, too. The trouble is—the timing's *all* wrong. When we're alone together, I'm tired or busy with other tasks. If we're just hanging out, there are five of us, and I have to attend to getting three of us ready for bed and the next day of school. Chris says I need to put that stuff on hold and just come to bed so that we can enjoy each other. Why can't I do that? How come I only put us first if someone else is taking care of the kids?"

On those rare occasions when women get together as friends, much of the conversation is about how busy and tired they are, as if fatigue were the primary bond that women share. So much for those sexy Saturday mornings in bed that they so enjoyed when they were childless. Some couples may even think, "So much for sex, period!"

Women with children may feel overwhelmed by the extent of their responsibilities. They may also have ambivalent feelings about the changes in their post-pregnancy bodies and may resist being seen naked by their partners. They may feel resentment toward their partners, seeing them as unappreciative, uninvolved, and too demanding. It's not surprising that many women during this stage in their lives announce that they don't like sex and can live without it.

Because of the demands of raising children, sex often loses its place in the life of a couple. Some women simply resign themselves to becoming asexual; others refuse to relinquish this core part of who they are as sexual human beings but do little more than complain about their predicaments. Whether you have children or are thinking about having them, ask yourself these questions:

- Am I getting together with women friends to dump on sex and my partner? Have I thought about what I get out of these gripe sessions with other women?
- Is sex important enough for me to work on? If not, when will it be important enough?
- Do I complain about sex with my partner because I secretly fantasize that I could have a better sex life with some other partner?
- Do I believe that women have the power to create better sex lives for themselves, or are they helpless to make changes in themselves and in their relationships?

If you don't want your sex life to end just because you're a mom, read Parts IV ("Creating a Better Sexual Relationship") and V ("Overcoming Sexual Difficulties") to identify strategies that will help you keep sex alive in your relationship, and more importantly, in *you*. In addition, the exercises in the Appendix will help you better understand the origins of your feelings of helplessness and anger.

> "We figured out that the house just wasn't a sexy place for us anymore; there's baby paraphernalia in every room. Some nights we have what we call 'takeout sex.' When the babysitter arrives, I'm out the door. First I stop for Chinese takeout, then I head to Don's office. We lock the office door and make love on the floor. I'm lobbying for a thicker carpet pad next time he redecorates the office!"

Being Single with a Baby

For a number of reasons, a woman may have a baby without a partner. Women who do so remark that their sex life is dramatically altered and that being single *and* a mother presents challenges.

> "It seemed that after I had the baby, I could only meet two kinds of guys. There were the ones who would run for the door as soon as they found out I had a kid, and the ones who came on hot and heavy—figuring I must be an easy lay. After a while, I pretty much gave up on sex and relationships."

This "giving up on sex" is not unusual. For a variety of reasons, women go through periods of their lives when they're not having sex. However, your sexuality is still part of you and "giving up on sex"—meaning, sex with a partner—does not have to mean giving up on the pleasure you can feel sexually. Find a place for sex through masturbation, fantasy, reading erotica, and taking time to be good to yourself. If you are considering involvement with someone, read "Endings and Beginnings" later in this chapter.

Whether partnered or single, children will occupy a big part of your life, but they don't have to take your whole life. The pleasure you feel in your own sexuality can bring you a deeper and fulfilling sense of all of who you are.

LOOKING 50 IN THE FACE

The greatest barrier to a woman's sexuality in midlife is the socially transmitted disease of *ageism*. The vibrant sexuality of women in their middle years is often socially invisible, obscured by our dominant culture's preoccupation with equating sexiness with youth. Nevertheless, women in their 40s and 50s continue to be sexually robust. Yes, your body changes; in life, change is certain. But by the time you are coping with the physical changes associated with menopause and aging, you are doing so with the advantage of lifelong experience with meeting and overcoming challenges.

> "We were heading out the door when my 16-year-old daughter turned to her friend Abby and said, 'Guess what! My parents are going out to celebrate my mom's 50th birthday.' Abby looked at me and exclaimed, 'Gee, that's great. And you don't look 50—in the face!' "

Our clients have taught us that women are sexual because they want to be and choose to be, not because they are young, in perfect shape, or gorgeous. Some of our stereotypically beautiful clients are the unhappiest because they have spent so much time obsessively striving to replicate the cultural standard that their view of themselves has shrunk to the single dimension of body appearance. They experience no inner peace or freedom in their sexuality. Conversely, many of our older clients describe an intimacy with their partners not possible in youth and a comfort with themselves unmatched in more youthful times.

> "I love sex in my 50s. During sex when I was younger, I tried to hide my thighs with my hands or insist on having the lights off. Now I don't care if my body's not perfect. I leave the lights on because every little detail of our lovemaking is erotic to me, and I don't want to miss a thing."

Passion That Isn't Skin Deep

Aging can actually be sexually freeing. Many older women report that the increased confidence of age and experience gives them the courage to be more passionate in their identity and in their sexuality. A passionate woman wears the clothes she wants to wear and looks men straight in the eye and smiles. Passionate women develop an attitude that says, *I'm delighted with this age and this body of mine.* Passionate women think talking about sex is important. Passionate women take time to have sex with their partners or masturbate regularly.

Perhaps you've noticed that you don't get the "looks" you got as a younger woman. You may be upset by the physical changes of aging and lament wrinkles in your face or increased thickness in your waist. Your hair may be thinning, to your dismay. If you are in perimenopause, the years before you stop having periods there will be changes in your menstrual cycle, your metabolism, and possibly your energy level. You may find that your skin is dryer and your muscles need more regular workouts to stay toned. Hormonal changes occur. Your sexual response may change. Read Chapters 4 and 5 for a discussion of the hormonal, physical, and sexual changes associated with aging.

Yes, these changes can be a challenge. You may judge your body's new shape and state as sexually unappealing, causing you to withdraw from your sexuality. This is a choice-point in your life. Will you continue to be sexual by finding a place for your sexuality and loving your body in all the shapes it will assume over your lifetime? In Part III, "Making Peace with Your Body," we discuss body image, pain, illness, disability, and trauma and suggest ways to continue to be in touch with your body's remarkable ability to be sexual throughout your life, even in the face of change and challenge. Ask yourself these questions:

- If I'm physically uncomfortable, am I seeing a healthcare practitioner, reading books, and talking with other women about adjusting to perimenopause?
- Have I spent time masturbating and enjoying my own physical sensations?
- If I'm feeling more depressed or anxious, or not sleeping well, have I considered this might be related to perimenopause? (Discuss this with your healthcare provider.)
- Do I continue to recognize myself as a sexual person? If not, am I prepared to take responsibility to change my negative thinking?

Looking 50 in the Face Together

If you are in midlife and in a healthy relationship, sex with your partner isn't skin deep. You're likely aroused by your partner's personality and your shared experiences. You may be less afraid of making sexual mistakes and more interested in making the most of your connection. Many times the early years of a couple's sexual experience involve intense, explosive, genitally focused sex. Sex in your middle years tends to incorporate the luxury of exploration, taking your time, and expanding the sexual act far beyond the scope of the fast and furious genital rubbing and penis-pushing of earlier times. For those who have worked to achieve it—be they straight or lesbian couples—sex and intimacy may be intertwined in ways that are possible only through time and trial in a relationship.

> "We took yoga lessons together. At first we felt awkward, but then I started getting turned on by watching him stretch. So one day he says, 'Why don't we try tantra, spiritual sexuality?' We started going to workshops, learning about breathing, energy, and spirituality. Where have we been? This has fired up our sex life by teaching us new ways to be sexually alive."

Of course there is the possibility that your sex life with your long-term partner has become stagnant, predictable, and boring. Or perhaps a sexual problem has developed decades into your relationship. Maybe old preferred patterns of lovemaking don't "work" anymore. Sometimes the type of stimulation that used to feel wonderful now feels irritating or even painful. Perhaps you were always more passive to your partner's active, but now your partner needs more initiation and physical stimulation from you to achieve and sustain the same level of arousal as in earlier years. Some couples have taken their sexual life together for granted. They have no language or experience for solving problems when they occur. One or both partners withdraw from the problem. Weeks drift into months or years, and sex is avoided altogether. Sleeping in the same bed with physical distance between you and your partner "graduates" to separate bedrooms, usually under the guise of other reasons ("he snores," "she gets up too much during the night").

If you recognize yourself here, read Parts IV ("Creating a Better Sexual Relationship") and V ("Overcoming Sexual Difficulties"). Ask yourself these questions:

- Have we "checked out" sexually, settling for shopping and eating out as substitutes for passion?
- How sexually interested and supportive is my partner?
- Am I more turned on by fantasy—chick flicks, erotic novels, and the younger trainer at the health club—than by reality with my partner? If yes, am I ready to stop escaping and address what's wrong with our sex life?
- Do I expect my partner to fix our sexual problems?
- Does my partner have an unaddressed sexual difficulty (such as erectile dysfunction)? If yes, are we avoiding the subject or even sleeping separately?

Empty Nest

Looking 50 in the face often means also looking at a suddenly empty household. When children grow and go, it is often a mixed experience. At first your living space may feel different. Your relationship may feel different. You may feel different.

Elsewhere in the book we refer to *other-oriented* sex. This is sexual activity based not on what *you* feel, want, or desire, but on what the *other person* expresses, indicates, or desires. Life with children is certainly other-oriented, so your daily activities and sexual activities can mimic each other in ways that aren't particularly focused on you. By the time the children move out, some women turn their backs on sexuality because they have lived with other-oriented sex for too long, and they don't know how to be self-oriented in their sexuality (or perhaps in their empty nest). But many more women take a deep breath and relax, ready to embark on the adventure of sexuality (and time) for themselves.

Once children are grown, many times (hopefully) the child-rearing dramas go with them. Perhaps menopause and major work insecurities are behind you as well. You may have privacy for the first time in years. Although every stage of life presents us with unique and varied challenges, this stage, at least, may be freer of burdening responsibilities and time demands.

> "The first year or so after our youngest went to college, I felt torn when he would come home and leave again. I'd miss how the vitality of him and his friends

would fill up the house. Then I began to notice a shift. After a while I'd enjoy his time at home, but my partner and I were getting used to our freedom and privacy, and we'd really miss that when he was back. Sometimes we'd wave him off as he left again, with a tear in our eyes, but then we'd make a beeline for the bedroom."

Looking 50 in the face is tough, but it is a wonderful tough. The "gift" of time beyond reproductive years is something our ancestors couldn't even have imagined. In fact, as we indicated earlier, as life expectancy continues to expand, you can look forward to having as many adult years post-menopause as you had during your adult reproductive years. You have been exposed to the myth—and it *is* a myth—that sex and sexual allure are for the young. Not so. That is true only if you allow it to be. Passion and sexuality come from the inside, and the secure sense of personal empowerment you may feel now that you are freed from the insecurities and uncertainties of youth can be the strongest aphrodisiac of all.

ENDINGS AND BEGINNINGS

In life one thing is certain: there will be losses. A woman's sexual life is inevitably affected by loss, whether it's in the form of her partner having an affair, the death of her partner, or divorce. Relationships tend to end either abruptly or slowly and painfully. In the case of an affair, the relationship may not necessarily come to an end, but the fantasy of unending love and total commitment does. In this section, we explore common *endings* that women experience in their adult sexual lives and the important *beginnings* that can, and often do, follow.

Ending a Fantasy: Affairs

In as many as 40% of marriages in the United States, one or both partners have sought sex outside the relationship (Reinisch, 1991). There are many possible reasons for this pervasive pattern. People may be looking for what they think is missing in their marriage—be it passion, respect, or intimacy. They may be angry with their partner and want to "get even." The affair may be the product of a moment of vulnerability—an evening of too much alcohol or a time of inconsolable sadness. An affair may be an attempt to repair an old hurt of being ignored and unloved as a child. In recent years, a new phenomenon has emerged—technical infidelity or "virtual affairs." A growing number of women and men are turning to online relationships for emotional intimacy and eroticism.

Affairs can signal the presence of a wound that will fester and tear the marriage apart unless it is healed. Affairs are often experienced as a violation of highly personal space, leaving the partner feeling a loss of pride and self-esteem. Trust may not easily be restored. Sex in the relationship can become strained or nonexistent because it serves as a poignant reminder of the hurt and feelings of betrayal. Perhaps what is most difficult is that an affair destroys the fantasy that the couple will enjoy a storybook life together—that they will "live happily ever after."

When an affair occurs, the question to be asked by the injured partner is not "How could you do this to me?" but "How could you do this to *yourself*?" For any chance of reconciliation, the person who has had the affair must grapple with this question. The partner has to ask similar questions: "What value does monogamy hold for me? What will be necessary to keep me in this relationship?" A couple who are committed to answering these questions honestly can best determine either how to repair what is broken or whether to bring the relationship to an end. They will make a commitment not to save the marriage at all costs but to be honest with themselves and each other about their goals and values. If promises are to be made, we recommend the partners make them to themselves and include these three:

"I won't tolerate [or have] an affair again."
"I won't be silent about my needs or disappointments."
"I won't settle for the kind of communication, sex, and intimacy we've had in the past."

Even when wounds heal well, they leave scars that will always be noticed. But scar tissue is tougher and stronger than skin.

> "After the affair, we went through such turmoil. We argued, talked, and grieved. We each questioned whether we'd stay together. We went to counseling and began to look at the differences we had. We got very specific about the kind of marriage we wanted. It was a painful but important process."

We cannot do justice here to describing the complexities of affairs and the ways in which people address and overcome these problems. If you are coping with an ongoing affair or the aftermath of one, we encourage you to seek counseling. You might also read the books on couples communication and intimacy noted in the "Suggested Resources" at the end of the book.

If you have had, or are having, an affair, reflect on the following questions:

- What was I looking for by going outside of the relationship?
- Did I find it, or was it a mirage?
- Was I trying to hurt or get even with my partner?

If your partner has had an affair, you may find answering the following questions helpful:

- Did I assume there must be something wrong with me?
- [If you entered counseling after the affair] Was my goal to bash my partner? Myself?
- [If you chose to stay in the relationship] Why did I stay with [him or her]?
- [If you stayed in the relationship] Have I been able to let go of my anger and hurt, or does it continue to cast a shadow on us?
- [If you and your partner have resumed sexual activity] Has our lovemaking been out of a desire to reconnect or out of fear of losing [him or her]?
- Have my sexual feelings and responses changed since learning of the affair?

Ending in Divorce

One out of every two or three women who marry will get divorced. The number of women facing life after the breakup of a relationship is even higher when you include women who have ended civil unions or live-together relationships. Despite jokes about the wild sexual life of single women, being divorced is not the sexiest time in a woman's life. Most newly divorced women admit that they don't like casual sex and are looking for partnerships involving intimacy and mutual caring.

The months after the breakup of your partnership can bring depression, a drop in self-esteem, and a sexual shutdown. These feelings can prompt you to idealize your former partner and fantasize about reconnection. You may periodically have sex with your relocated partner and wonder if the two of you should reunite. You may even find that the sex is better now that you're not in daily conflict.

The more ambiguous and ambivalent you were about the divorce or breakup, the more difficult it will be for you to grieve the loss of the relationship and make sense of your current life. Eventually, however, you will most likely realize that you can't "turn back the clock," and you will move ahead. If you find you can't move on, consider getting counseling and support to make sense of your feelings.

Looking ahead, you may fear that you'll re-create past problems or may not trust your judgment about future partners. It makes sense to take time to know yourself better before rushing into a new relationship. This includes knowing about your own sexuality.

Sex may have been great in your former partnership or it may have been awful. Now is the time to decide, on your own terms, what sex is going to be like for you in the future. Remember that being single doesn't mean anything negative about your sexuality. You're sexual regardless of your partnership status. Masturbation, fantasy, reading erotica, buying a vibrator, even checking out sexy websites are all safe and friendly ways to continue to be sexual. They don't involve a partner, require a babysitter, or commit you to meeting someone's first-cousin from Toledo.

But don't stop here! Think about the ways that physical activity, friendship, and being in charge of your life can work for you.

Ending in Widowhood

Forty-five percent of women 65 or older are widows (Administration on Aging, 2000). Widowed women face unique challenges when trying to take care of their sexual selves. In most cultures, they are not viewed as sexual persons. They face double indemnity because neither do most cultures view older women as sexual. Although widows, young or older, often report that they don't feel sexual interest immediately following the death of their spouse, over time, interest in sex usually returns. But not only do widows face cultural stereotypes that negate their sexuality, they also may have to contend with strong internal ambivalence.

> "It had been two years since Henry died, and I was becoming very fond of Murray. One night we began necking like young kids, and I was really excited. But all of a sudden it hit me that this was the first time in 45 years that someone other than Henry had touched me this way, and I immediately froze up. I felt like I had just gotten caught cheating on my husband."

Grieving the death of a spouse requires considerable time and work. You'll never forget your partner—he'll always be an important part of your life. But, in time, the grieving process will allow you to reposition your partner to another place in your life, one that is less central, less exclusive, less dominating. The grieving process will eventually free you emotionally to seek new relationships.

This process can take time—two, three, even four years is not an unusual amount of time before a widow is ready emotionally to pursue an intimate relationship without awkwardness or guilt. During the interim, while doing the work of grief, it is important to remember that your sexuality didn't expire just because your partner died.

> "In my loneliness, sometimes I would try masturbating, but it reminded me I was alone in my empty bed. Instead of being a sexual turn-on, my crying faucets would turn on, and I'd lie there, my hands rubbing my vulva while tears streamed down my face. Then I realized that this was just how my life felt. I'd have good days and still want to weep. I began to allow sex back into my life the same way I did with other things, a little bit at a time—inching ahead. Sex reminded me that I was alive and what I was still capable of. I began to treasure my sexuality and see it as one of the parts of me that had been there before and was here with me now."

Beginning to Venture Out

Widowed, divorced, or single due to other reasons, you may feel awkward when reentering the dating scene. If you decide to have sex with a new partner it can be intimidating and downright scary.

> "When I was 22, it was hard enough the first time a partner would see me naked. Even though I had a pretty good sex life with my ex-husband, I haven't had sex with someone in a long time and don't know how it will work out."

Beginning a new sexual relationship is even more complex and challenging if you have children living at home.

> "Being single with kids meant making a lot of decisions with no 'road map' to follow. I learned to be honest with myself, recognizing my vulnerability about wanting passion and sex in a life full of responsibility and work."

When a single mom decides she's interested in a sexual relationship, she has to consider the effect this will have on her children. She'll have to take into account how old they are, how much time she has to spend with them, and their likely reactions to a new adult on the scene. She'll have to decide whether to bring home the person she's dating to meet the children, whether to have the new partner spend the night with her, and how and when to arrange time to be sexual.

If you are a single mom, many questions specific to your own situation will need to be answered now or in the future. The following questions may help jump start your thinking about being a single parent and having sex:

- At what point in a relationship should I introduce a new partner to my kids?
- Would I have sex with a friend or only someone I'm in love with? At what point in the relationship would I have sex?
- Would I engage in public displays of affection in front of the kids? If so, how far would I go?
- Would I ever have a new partner spend the night at my home—with or without the children at home?
- Would I spend the night at my partner's place?
- Would I feel comfortable renting a motel room for "quickies"?
- Am I staying aware of my children's emerging sexuality and their needs for privacy, predictable routine, and the ability to "go about the business of being a family" without dealing with a sexually charged environment?
- Do I explain to my kids my need to have friends and love, while assuring them of my continued commitment to them as a top priority in my life?
- Parent or not, when the bedroom door closes, how do I feel about my sex life?

Remarriage: When One Becomes Two Again

New partner, fresh start. That's the hope you bring to a new partnership. Some women report being surprised that sexual problems experienced before can re-emerge in this new relationship. If you've put off addressing a concern, now is the time to tackle it. Review Part V, especially Chapter 13, to gain insight into your sexual difficulties and learn ways to overcome them.

All remarriages or new partnerships begin in loss. If you were widowed, you may experience a normal resurgence of grief when entering a new partnership, even though you're happy to be with this person. If you have been divorced, you are likely to be "sadder but wiser" about partnerships, and it may take several years before you trust that this relationship isn't going to break up.

When it comes to sex in a remarriage, the most important question is: who else is in the house? If you and your partner are home alone, your sexual activity may be easy to establish, but in many remarriages, kids and exes present formidable challenges. If you and your partner have teenagers, they may be uncomfortable with your sexuality and make comments like "You're so gross when you hug each other." This is not going to enliven your relationship with each other. One set of parents coordinating the activities of one set of kids is exhausting enough; imagine the complications when you have up to three sets of parents and two sets of kids requiring coordination and accommodation. You can feel like you're trapped in an endless cycle of figuring out whose kids are staying with which parents on what weekends. This, too, affects your sex life—big time.

> "It was hard to keep my desires in check. After such a long dry spell, I wanted sex when I wanted it, but there were the kids, their activities, our jobs, constant juggling. I wanted this to be simple, but that's not realistic."

Women with children often report that sex in a remarriage can fade quickly if they try to make this new relationship mimic the early days of their first marriage. In a remarriage, you don't have the same control over your freedom, time, or privacy as you probably had when you entered your first marriage. And your children certainly will not go out of their way to make your sex life easier!

Your sexual relationship with your partner will be most successful if you first take care of some basic rules for outside the bedroom. Research indicates that when you remarry, you and your partner need to give up your fantasies about a perfect unified family. You'll need to address conflicts, tolerate stress, and normalize the need for flexibility in the new family structure (Walsh, 1991). You'll need to recognize and combat unrealistic expectations that you may place on yourself. For example, as a mother, you may feel pressure to make the family "successful." If the kids are unhappy in the remarried family, you may feel guilty about taking private time for you and your partner or having any sexual pleasure. Chapter 13 provides helpful suggestions for combating such guilt by identifying and fighting the underlying irrational or self-defeating beliefs and assumptions.

The answers to the following questions will help you build a positive sex life with your new partner while, at the same time, respecting the needs of your family.

- Have I resolved any emotional baggage from my previous relationship? Should I consider counseling if I haven't?
- Have we established a stable household with predictable schedules, and clear rules and expectations for everybody?
- Have we explained to the children that we sometimes need to be alone in our own bedroom?
- Do they know to knock before walking in? Do we have a lock on the door so we won't be accidentally "surprised" when having sex?
- Have we discussed the importance of flexible planning for issues such as custody arrangements?
- If our kids are grown, have we discussed how they may find our sexuality uncomfortable when they visit?
- Have we discussed how we're going to handle our frustration if sex gets interrupted repeatedly, or if we have to scrap a weekend away, or if we have to go weeks before we're alone?
- Have we discussed that it will take time to create this new family and that we're going to have periods of ambivalence and differences of opinion?
- Is sex a glue to help us through these times, or do we use sex to avoid discussion?
- Do I treat my partner's requests for sex as one more demand on me?
- Are we willing to schedule sex so that we are sure to have special time together?

As you read through these questions, you may recognize problem areas. Chapter 12 provides you with helpful suggestions for enriching your sexual relationship.

Being Single Is Not an Ending

The end of one relationship is not always followed by the beginning of a new relationship. Still, the end of a relationship does not mean the end of your sexuality. Some single women who were previously partnered can honestly predict that there is little likelihood that they will find a new sexual partner. Their sexual response to this status is as varied as their circumstances. Some choose not to be sexual at all, others continue to masturbate and explore sensuality, and some even choose to have occasional sexual experiences. These sexual experiences, as we discussed earlier in the chapter, may be driven by passion, neediness, adventure, or desperation.

As singlehood stretches out over the years, a woman redefines herself, including her sexuality, from being partner-oriented to self-oriented. Unlike a woman's young adulthood, later in life her single "sexual self" may not be highly valued by the culture. Women often remark that they have to encourage themselves to stay sexually vibrant. They work to keep sex as part of their life even as they refocus attention and passion to other aspects of life, like family, friends, and meaningful activities.

If you are single, ask yourself these questions.

- Do I value myself as a sexual person?
- Am I willing to continue to explore my sexuality?
- Do I regularly allow myself to fantasize, read erotica, masturbate, and enjoy my sexuality in other meaningful ways?
- If I'm uncomfortable with my body and with touching myself, am I interested in doing the exercises in this book to help me grow sexually comfortable? (The exercises in the Appendix and Part V will help you.)
- If I am in a period without physical intimacy, can I get regular massages or facials to treat myself to being touched in nonsexual ways? Do I initiate hugs with my family and friends, ask for and give back rubs, or hold hands when we walk together?
- Should I consider some form of bodywork or exercise by taking a course in Feldenkreis body awareness, martial arts, dance, swimming, or any other kind of movement?
- Do I foster my sensuality in the ways that I dress, decorate my home, or the activities I choose?
- Do I intentionally think of myself as a sexual person? Do I allow myself to have sex with myself, be curious about sex, and enjoy this deeply important part of me?

THE LATER YEARS: "THEY SAY THERE'S BEEN A REVOLUTION"

"What amazed me was sex in my 60s. No one told me how much I'd get turned on and how fun it would be. I'm more adventurous than I thought I'd be, trying a vibrator and getting my partner to try Viagra."

"Sexy grandmother" is *not* an oxymoron. The best-kept secret is sex in one's 60s—that's where the real sexual revolution is embodied. It's a time when the expectation of sexual freedom and comfort is most likely to be a reality. Sex in a woman's 60s is free of time demands. Not only do women make time for themselves to exercise and pursue personal interests, but they also spend time masturbating and increasing their erotic focus.

Relationships also change. Characteristics of personal strength and assertiveness are valued, and sexual attraction develops from the relationship rather than appearance. This pattern is in contrast to what younger people experience, where superficial physical attraction is often the initial basis of coupling and affirmation.

And this sexual revolution isn't confined just to women in their 60s. Used to being ignored as too old or asexual, women in their 70s and beyond have gone about taking charge of their sexuality and proving just how sensual and erotic they can be with themselves and their partners. If they're in long-term partnerships, they find that sex and intimacy can deepen in ways that are possible only for relationships that have been tempered by time, shared trials, and honest communication.

Physical illness, disability, and stress over financial security and retirement can complicate sex during the later years, however. Widowhood also becomes a significant factor during this stage in life. But healthy or not, partnered or not, women in their later years continue to be sexual people capable of responding to sensual pleasure.

> "What irritates me most in my 70s is the way that people write me off as a sexual has-been. We've always had a good sex life, but we didn't talk about our sex life with anyone else. Then I had a hip replacement, and before I left the hospital the physician suggested that I avoid the missionary position so that I didn't stress my new hip. 'Make love on top,' she said. At first I was embarrassed, but my partner encouraged me to ask questions. The doctor suggested that I go on the web to look at resources and to buy a vibrator. Now we're open to new ideas from anyone! We've been reading erotica out loud to each other, especially on days when my hip or his bad knee is acting up. To be honest, I think you have to be at least 65 to be erotic."

Confusing Aging with Poor Health

A common mistake is to confuse aging and poor health. Being depressed, overly anxious, or irritable isn't part of growing old—it's an offshoot of poor health. Disrupted sleep patterns can also be a sign of depression. Just as cartilage around joints wears away as we age, so does our neurochemical resilience; we just don't "bounce back" as quickly as we face challenges and stressors. Depression can cause you to withdraw from sexual activities you used to enjoy.

As you age, you may experience chronic medical conditions (like diabetes), mechanical difficulties (like joint or back problems), memory difficulties (like dementia or depression), or fatigue. Remember that your healthcare provider should be part of the solution, not part of the problem, so find medical help that is consistently supportive of you. There may be medications, physical therapy, or a medical procedure that can help you. Use the suggestions for finding a healthcare provider that we give in Chapter 13. Practitioners trained in gerontology will usually be the most knowledgeable.

Accommodate, Don't Capitulate

Sexually active women in their later years observe that issues of physical pain, mobility, and urinary incontinence are the greatest barriers to partnered sex. They find that healthcare providers may not be knowledgeable about their sexual difficulties or are uncomfortable discussing sex with women in their later years. Rather than giving up and giving in to social stereotypes that sex is reserved for the young, these women find ways to make accommodations. When engaging in intercourse, some position changes may be necessary to accommodate more fragile bones. Women report that they work on their mind–body connection, increasing their ability to fantasize, focus erotically, and tune in on those parts of their bodies that feel good. Chapters 7 and 8 may help you make the physical accommodations you need.

Urinary incontinence is to a woman in her 70s what yeast infections are to a woman in her twenties—one big hassle! To cope with wetness and odor, some women spread dark-colored absorbent towels on the bed before having sex, use lots of slippery lubricant to get wet before getting sexual (so additional wetness isn't noticed as much), and use lightly scented candles or incense and body fragrances or perfume. Other women, not comfortable with "wet," skip intercourse and engage in other sex play. Kegel exercises, explained in Chapter 8, may also help maintain your muscle tone.

> "Let's be honest. I didn't feel comfortable leaking pee when Frank and I were having sex. It just wasn't me, and I wasn't going to change that much at the age of 86. So I wore panties with a bladder control pad during sex. First I made the mistake of trying to use menstrual pads, but they just don't absorb urine. Frank placed the vibrator on the outside of my panties and the stimulation reached my clitoris. When I orgasmed, the urine leakage went straight onto the pad."

As a sexual woman in your later years, ask yourself these questions.

- Am I addressing my physical difficulties and willing to consider new ideas for medical care, even if these include medications, physical therapy, learning to use a walker, hearing aid, or other prosthesis?
- Am I exercising regularly, including my pelvic floor muscles (Kegels)?
- Would I consider an antidepressant medication to improve my mood, sleep, or memory?
- Am I avoiding sex because of urinary incontinence?

Privacy in Assisted Living Facilities

Some women discover that their interest in partnered sex makes their grown children uncomfortable, and unfortunately many senior housing and care facilities often try to prevent sexual activity between residents and aren't comfortable providing privacy for masturbation either. The lack of freedom and privacy to enjoy sex is a great loss for many residents. Continue to remind your facility managers that older adults have a right to sexual privacy. If senior years are still ahead of you, advocate for the privacy of the seniors in your life who are in assisted living facilities.

Going the Distance: Your Lifelong Sexuality

Inevitably, all relationships will end, and the majority of married women who live past 70 will be widowed. In youth the possibility of facing this loss seems obscure and unlikely. Most couples who pledge "till death do us part" in their younger years have no concept of what they are promising. Women respond to this loss in different ways. Some may seek a new partner. Other women who are widowed or divorced in older age may choose not to seek new partners but continue masturbating regularly. They report learning new ways to self-pleasure by using sexual fantasy, vibrators, and dildos. Many cope with loss by learning to refocus their attention and passion on other aspects of their life, like family and social activities.

However they cope, women of age do not appear to meet this challenge by withering and withdrawing. It may seem a paradox, but older single women do not describe their lives as lonely or empty, despite the blatant fact that the majority of them do not have a sexual partner. In fact, they describe less loneliness than at other periods in their life (Friedan, 1994).

Why do women describe less loneliness at an older age? We may be tempted to conclude that sex is not important for women at this stage. That would be erroneous. Sex, intimacy, and touch remain important, but at this stage intimacy has been established in a much broader context.

Women have always been known for their enduring ability to form and nurture meaningful relationships. Whether in the quiet companionship of women quilting together or two friends exchanging voice messages in the midst of a hectic day, women tend to weave their lives around relationships.

Women of age have developed a capacity to experience closeness in many deep and abiding forms. This frequently translates into intimacy that does not depend upon, or define itself through, genital sex or intercourse. This does not mean that what is lost or missing is not grieved, but emotionally healthy older women do not seem to waste away or pine for what they do not have. Instead, they draw upon their remarkable abilities of connection to experience intimacy in ways that transcend narrow definitions. Ask yourself:

- Do I continue to fantasize, masturbate, and enjoy touch?
- Do I draw pleasure in remembering positive sexual experiences? (If memories of sex are traumatic, you may find it helpful to read Chapter 10.)
- Do I continue to develop myself by being social and nurturing my friendships?

PART II

Understanding Your Body

Sex research routinely points out how little most women know about their anatomy and sexual function. Our clinical experiences confirm this. In fact, we are constantly surprised by how many of our clients would probably agree with a statement from one client that we've never forgotten: "I really don't know much about sex. I just do it."

Our bodies are central to our sexuality. If sex, in the broadest sense, refers to experiencing pleasure, it is a pleasure we experience in our bodies. If we consider sex in the context of relating to another person, it's through our bodies that we connect and share pleasure. Even love, which we usually consider more emotional than physical, yearns for physical touch and connection. When a woman doesn't know her body, she doesn't know the pleasure she can feel in her body.

Understanding your body and how it functions is an important way of taking care of your sexual self. This knowledge helps to demystify sex and makes it easier to learn ways to increase your sexual comfort and pleasure. Just as loving someone requires knowing that person, the ability to accept and love our bodies requires us to know and understand them. It's a factor that is critical to healthy sexuality.

In the next three chapters, we offer straight talk about anatomy, hormones, and sexual function. Corresponding exercises to help you become more familiar with your sexual anatomy and more comfortable with your body are in the Appendix. In this section we hope to answer the questions so often asked in our offices:

- Is there really a G spot, and if so, how do I find mine?
- Why do women have both male and female hormones?
- Are all women capable of having multiple orgasms?
- Why does it seem so easy to orgasm from stimulation of the clitoris but so hard with intercourse alone?
- Am I more likely to get pregnant when I orgasm?
- How do I choose the best birth control method for me?
- Is it true that women often get pregnant when they stop trying so hard?
- Does intercourse cause premature labor?
- Is menopause the beginning of the end of my sex life?
- What kind of menstrual changes should I be worried about?

CHAPTER THREE

Your Body

In their earliest weeks of existence, tiny, developing embryos—biologically determined to be a boy or a girl—are already forming their future reproductive organs. The entire embryo at this point is no bigger than a pea. Imagine the tiny genitals and reproductive organs—small, even for Thumbelina. The egg and sperm-producing glands would be impossible to tell apart during early fetal development. Similarly, until about the fourth month of fetal growth, genital development of developing boys and girls appears almost identical. Actually, the human prototype, embryologically speaking, is female.

At about seven weeks after conception, developing males and females have the same external genitals. There isn't much differentiation at this point: both boys and girls have an "outie," or a small bump that's called a genital tubercle, and an "innie," which is an opening called the urogenital slit. There are folds of tissue and swellings that will develop into labia or a scrotum. It takes hormones called androgens to make the genital tubercle become a penis. As the genitals develop more fully, the clitoris and the tip of the penis (glans) will both have many nerve endings, making them highly sensitive to stimulation. The penis and the clitoris, as well as other parts of the vulva, will have erectile tissue that is capable of swelling up or engorging with blood. Males will develop testicles, which will produce sperm, and females will develop ovaries, which contain ova, or eggs. The developing embryo already "knows" if it will be a boy or a girl. This is determined by the chromosomes—XX for girls and XY for boys—which keep development on track. Genes will help the process along by releasing the appropriate hormones at the appropriate times, so that a boy develops a penis and a girl a clitoris.

As babies grow into toddlers, parents of sons have it easy when it comes to teaching genital names: penis. No confusion about what they are naming—it's right out there and they can teach the rest later. No toddler is running around talking about his *vas deferens*. Parents of daughters have a greater challenge. A girl's genitalia require more names for more parts, and they aren't all that visible. We suspect your parents did what most do—they taught you one name: *vagina*. It's the girl's analogous body part to the boy's penis. He has his; she has hers. But a boy urinates out of his penis, and a girl from her urethra, so there's one difference that isn't covered with the anatomical name of vagina. A little girl has a vulva that is immature. It encases her vagina, urethra, and clitoris, but most little girls have no idea they have a vulva at all.

Why don't girls (and women) know the names of their genital parts? Besides the relatively greater complexity of female genitalia, we suspect it is partly due to parents' apprehension about saying "the clitoris is a part of your genitals that feels good," and the parents' anticipation of their small daughters' responses: "How?" Sticking to the generations-old habit of labeling little girl parts "vagina" has simplified things.

The terms used to describe female genitals and reproductive organs are either Greek or Latin terms or words made from the names of the male physicians who "discovered" the organ. Popular slang terms for female genitalia do not offer a suitable substitute for the Greek and Latin ones because they aren't consistent or necessarily accurate—they can mean different things to different people. The Latin and Greek words have meanings that are standardized, objectively accurate, and adopted for anatomical description by the World Health Organization. If, at a young age, we were taught what these Latin and Greek terms mean, we would probably establish a better, more knowledgeable relationship with our own bodies. As you are reading this material, if you have any questions about your own physical development or the development of an infant or child that you care for, seek the advice of a medical practitioner. (See Chapter 1 for further discussion about genital names and adult responses to girls' awareness of their sexual parts.)

> "I'm embarrassed to say that, although I am college-educated, I didn't know what a vulva was or how to care for my own. It wasn't until I had a daughter, and her pediatrician showed me how to separate the folds of her labia to clean her appropriately—because I hadn't been doing it—that I realized how little I knew. My ignorance hurt her, and I became determined I would teach her what I never learned."

THE VULVA

Take a mirror and position yourself so you can see your genitals (see Figure 3.1). The visible part of female genitals is called the *vulva*, which means "covering" in

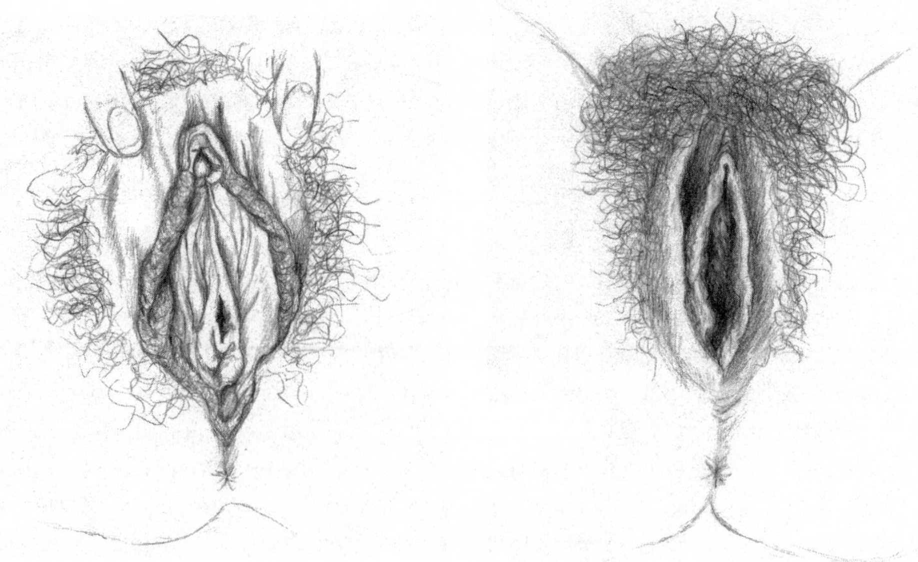

FIGURE 3.1. The vulva. Vulvas differ in appearance woman to woman, as depicted here.

Latin. As noted, many people mistakenly refer to a woman's external genitals as her "vagina," but the vagina is actually part of the internal sex organs. Only the vaginal opening is considered part of the vulva, because it's visible from outside the body. The vulva is comprised of the venus mound (mons), labia majora and minora, clitoris, and clitoral hood, the opening of the urethra, and the introitus.

The Venus Mound

The Venus mound is an easier term to relate to than *mons veneris*, its Latin name, which means mount or mountain of Venus, the Roman goddess of love. This is the fatty, cushiony mound directly over the front pelvic bone. It is an area rich with nerve endings that make it sensitive to touch and pressure. In adults, it is covered with pubic hair. This mound, with the triangle of pubic hair covering it, is the only part of a woman's sexual anatomy that is generally visible when she's nude and upright. Pubic hair has as much variety as hair on women's heads—it can be short or long, wiry or soft, thick or sparse. It may be the same color as the hair on one's head or a contrasting color. Pubic hair thins at menopause, a change that a woman may scarcely notice or over which she may experience some feelings of loss.

Labia Majora

The *labia majora* (Latin: larger lips) are also called the outer lips. Referring to the labia majora as "outer lips" is somewhat confusing, because they don't look at all like the inner lips (*labia minora*). The outside of the labia majora consists of fleshy, skin colored folds, covered with pubic hair. The inside portion of the labia majora, the part closest to the inner lips, does not have any pubic hair. The labia majora (outer lips) form a full, rounded oval around the inner lips, the clitoris, the urethra, and the vagina (see Figure 3.2).

Labia Minora

The labia minora (Latin: smaller lips) are the inner lips. The formation of the labia varies from woman to woman, much like penis size and shape vary for men. The shape of the labia tends to be irregular, with less symmetry, say, than eyebrows. Labia vary in thickness, length, and form. The labia have been referred to as the petals of a flower. The upper portion of the labia minora forms a hood over the clitoris. The interior skin of the labia minora is pink and often moist. During sexual arousal, blood flows into the labia and the inner lips may more than double in size. The engorgement of the labia during sexual excitement contributes to a woman's sexual pleasure. The labia are rich in nerve endings, making them most sensitive to stimulation. The labia protect the opening, also known as the *introitus*, of the vagina. They are also useful for helping to direct a stream of urine.

The Clitoris

The term clitoris comes from the Greek word *kleitoris*. How the name originated and what it means is uncertain. The best guess is that it means to titillate, to seek plea-

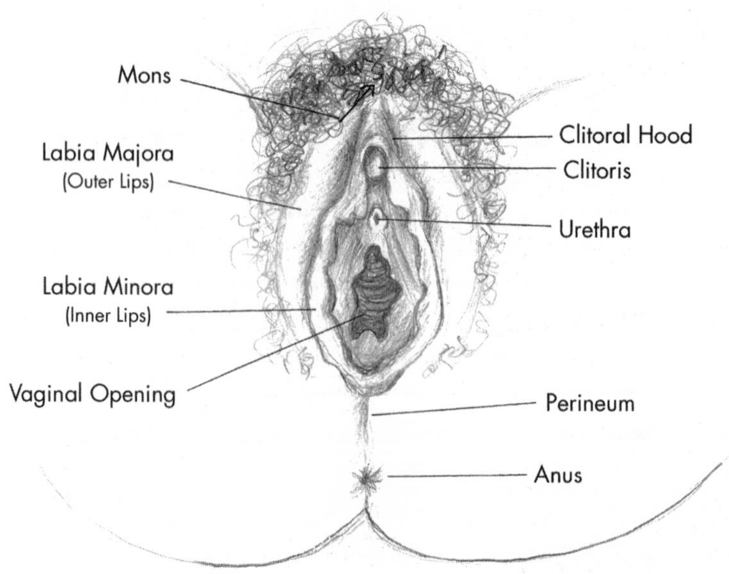

FIGURE 3.2. The visible part of female genitals.

sure (Angier, 1999). The clitoris has only one purpose and function: pleasure and sexual excitement. It is covered and protected by the labia minora. The clitoris is a small, rounded organ composed of erectile tissue. Similar to a man's penis, this spongy erectile tissue can become engorged with blood and increase in size during sexual arousal. The *glans*, or visible part of the clitoris, has thickly clustered nerve endings, even more than the head of a penis, making it an organ often described as "exquisitely sensitive." The root of the clitoris runs below the surface and is also extremely sensitive. The shaft of the clitoris separates into two parts, wishbone fashion, where the shaft is anchored to the pelvic bone. The clitoris, including the parts that can't be seen, becomes engorged with blood during sexual stimulation and is important in sexual arousal and orgasm. The clitoris is protected by a clitoral hood, or *prepuce* (Latin: foreskin), which is part of the labia minora. This hood of protective tissue can be manipulated to expose more of the clitoris. Women can masturbate by rubbing the exposed portion of their clitoris or by stroking the shaft of the clitoris below the clitoral hood. Thrusting during penetration may cause a tugging on the clitoral hood, which can affect clitoral stimulation and thus become one of the major sources of pleasurable sensation.

The Urethra

The labia also enclose the small opening from which urine is eliminated, the *urethra* (Latin and Greek: to urinate). The urethral opening is above the vagina and below the clitoris.

The Introitus

The *introitus* (Latin: going inside) is the name of the vaginal opening. You cannot see the introitus unless the lips of the labia are spread open. This would be a little like stretching the tissues of your cheek to get a look at the inside of your mouth. A ring of muscles, called the *bulbocavernosus muscles*, surrounds the introitus. The muscles are sphincter muscles, which means you can voluntarily squeeze them. The introitus has many nerve endings, making it a very sensitive area. Technically, the introitus belongs to the group of external sexual parts, the vulva, because it can be seen from the outside.

INTERNAL REPRODUCTIVE SEXUAL ORGANS

The Vagina

The *vagina* (Latin: sheath) is the organ that gets all the publicity as a female genital part. Perhaps that is because of the vagina's function. The vagina envelops and contains the penis during heterosexual intercourse, and it becomes the birth path-

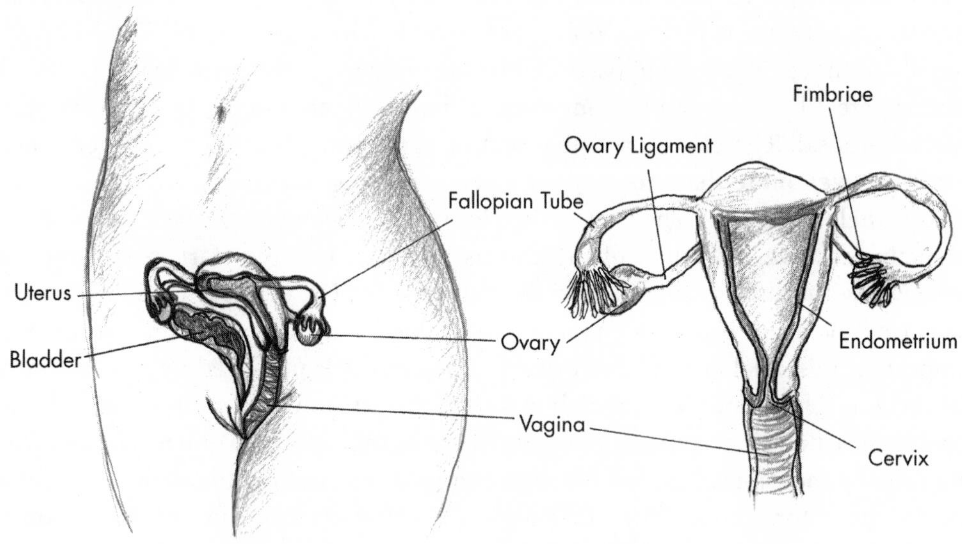

FIGURE 3.3. Internal reproductive sexual organs of a woman.

way to the world for the newborn. The vagina also is a passageway and connection from the uterus to the outside of the body (see Figure 3.3). Menstrual blood leaves the body through this passageway. The vagina is a closed muscular tube, three to five inches in length, but expandable. It's a little bit like the inside of an empty mouth. A penis, tampon, finger, or newborn inside the vagina will cause it to expand.

The vagina is a closed passageway; objects inside the vagina can't wander to other areas of the body. The only connection to the rest of the body is through a very small opening of the cervix called the *os* (Latin: mouth, opening). The os opens enough to allow menstrual blood to exit and semen to enter. If a woman has surgery in which her cervix and uterus are removed, the top of the vagina is stitched so that there is no opening from the vagina to any other body part.

The vagina is moist because there are glands in its lining that keep it wet and slippery—and just how wet depends upon many factors. During sexual arousal, the vagina can become very wet, indeed. The spongy tissue that lines the walls of the vagina engorges with blood. As the tissues swell, they push tiny beads of fluid, called vaginal mucus, through the glands in the walls of the vagina. The upper portion of the vagina is lined with more spongy tissue, so that most of the lubrication is produced closest to the cervix. The color and type of secretion from the vagina can change both throughout a woman's monthly menstrual cycle and throughout the day. For example, during sexual arousal there may be a great deal of clear, slippery mucus. At other times the secretions may be moderate and creamy in color and consistency. Hormonal changes or medication side effects can also reduce secretions, causing vaginal dryness.

The vagina is pinkish in color and has a rippled texture that a woman can feel if she explores with her fingers. The portion of the vagina closest to the opening, or introitus, is sensitive to touch and sexual stimulation, but the upper portion of the vagina, closest to the uterus, has fewer nerve endings. During sexual arousal, this upper portion of the vagina either lengthens and balloons out or compresses, depending on the type of stimulation. We describe this and other physiological reactions of the genitals in Chapter 4.

The Hymen

Most baby girls are born with a thin membrane called the *hymen* (Latin: membrane; also Greek: god of marriage), which partially covers the opening to the vagina. We aren't sure why the hymen exists; it's just there. The hymen can be tough and thick in some women and practically transparent in others. The absence of a hymen is not proof that a woman or girl has had sexual intercourse. As you can see from the definition, the term refers not only to the membrane but also to marriage. In fact, in many cultures the intact state of the hymen is important evidence that a bride is virginal, and penetrating the hymen on the wedding night is necessary to secure the dowry, the price of the bride, and/or the woman's reputation (Brumberg, 1997). In some countries, engaged women seek operations to replace their hymens so that they won't bring shame on themselves or their families.

After puberty, the hymenal tissue is usually elastic and easily stretched to accommodate penetration of a tampon, finger, or penis. Prior to puberty the vaginal and hymenal tissues can be easily hurt or torn. Some girls will have no evidence of a hymen by the time they reach adolescence. Participation in sports or other vigorous activity as well as even minor accidents, such as falling on the crossbar of a bicycle, can injure or break the hymen. Some girls lose their hymens while experimenting with masturbation by inserting fingers into their vaginas. Others have lost their hymens to the intrusion of sexual abuse.

A hymen may have one, two, several, or no openings. An *annular* hymen has one opening in the membrane. A *septate* hymen has two distinct openings. A *cribriform* hymen has numerous openings, almost honeycomb in appearance. An *imperforate* hymen means no opening is evident. If a hymen is both imperforate and thick, a minor surgical procedure may be needed to open the hymen later on. This is rare.

The Grafenberg Spot

Ernst Grafenberg was a German gynecologist who described an area within the vagina on the anterior (upper) wall, between the opening (introitus) and the cervix, that is particularly sensitive to stimulation. In the 1970s and 1980s Drs. Beverly Whipple and John Perry collaborated on research studying the patterns of orgasmic response in women by focusing on what they called the G spot after Grafenberg (Ladas, Whipple, & Perry, 1983; Perry & Whipple, 1981). They reported what many women and couples already knew from experience—the G spot responds and swells when stimulated, often resulting in orgasm for many women. The spot is described as a small area of tissue, possibly erectile tissue similar to the nipples or the clitoris, that appears to enlarge in size during sexual arousal. This spot isn't typically detected during a pelvic examination because the tissue isn't in an aroused state during such an exam.

During orgasm, stimulation of the G spot may cause some women to expel a clear fluid from the urethra, an ejaculation, which is a different composition from urine (although some women may also expel a small amount of urine). This "female ejaculation" is not confined to an orgasmic response from stimulation of the G spot, although that is how it came to the attention of the researchers. On the basis of the research of Dr. Whipple and others, it appears that the expulsion of fluid during a state of high sexual arousal is an absolutely normal phenomenon, though it doesn't happen for all, or perhaps most, women. For those women who have this experience, the amount of fluid they expel and the circumstances under which this happens can vary dramatically.

Uterus

The *uterus* (Latin: belly, paunch, womb) is about the size and shape of an upside-down pear. The walls of the uterus are very powerful muscles, about half an inch thick, which cover and surround a central area. Every month the uterus prepares for the possibility of nurturing a developing fetus. The lining of the uterus is called the *endometrium* (Greek: within the womb). Each month the lining becomes soft and thick. During menstruation the endometrium is sloughed away, then renewed again the next month unless implantation of a fertilized ovum (egg) occurs. Numerous strong, stringy tissue ligaments support the uterus and tie it to the bony structures of the pelvis—which is a good thing, since a 40-week-pregnant uterus expands to about watermelon size. There is also a rich blood supply to the uterus.

Women often experience a pleasurable contraction of the uterus as part of their orgasmic response. A hysterectomy (removal of the uterus) will affect the sensations experienced during orgasm. This may be a loss to a woman who has experienced her uterus as an organ of sexual responsiveness.

The Cervix

The *cervix* (Latin: neck) is located at the bottom of the uterus. The narrowed neck of the bottom of the cervix protrudes into the vagina and can be seen easily during a pelvic exam. You can probably locate your own cervix by probing with your fingers; it feels something like the rounded part of your ear or the tip of your nose, at times a bit softer. The opening to the cervix, the os, is the only passage into the uterus. The cervix functions as a protective barrier to the uterus, constantly producing mucus to keep out unwanted bacteria. This self-cleansing operation works so well that healthcare providers have concluded that douching should not be recommended for routine vaginal care.

The opening of the cervix changes very little after a woman has had a baby. Although labor contractions lead to a complete dilation of the cervix at the time of birth, afterward the body adjusts and the cervical opening contracts.

Some women report that they experience a pleasurable sensation from thrusting during sexual intercourse derived from stimulation of, or pressure against, the cervix. Other women may experience this sensation as unpleasant or even painful.

Fallopian Tubes

Droopy and delicate, the *fallopian tubes* (named for Gabriele Fallopio, an Italian anatomist) extend from either side of the uterus. The *infundibula* (Latin: funnel), the flared ends of the fallopian tubes, are fringed with microscopic strands called *fimbria* (Latin: fringe). The tubes, infundibula, and fimbria are constantly in motion, swaying back and forth, ready to capture the egg released from one of the ovaries and to draw it into the adjacent fallopian tube. The tiny passageway of the tube is about the size of a daisy stem.

Eggs aren't mobile by themselves, so they are propelled along the fallopian tubes toward the uterus by muscle contractions. If pregnancy is going to occur in any given cycle, fertilization of the egg by sperm happens when the egg is about a third of the way to the uterus. Within a few days the fertilized egg reaches the uterus, where it implants in the endometrium. The fallopian tubes also sweep the sperm toward the egg.

Ovaries

The *ovaries* (Latin: *ovum*, egg) have two jobs. One is to produce the powerful message-senders—hormones—which regulate the menstrual cycle as well as provide other functions that are discussed in Chapter 5. The ovaries also produce eggs (*ova*) for reproduction. A girl baby starts out with about two million ova, but by the time she is prepubescent, the number has dropped to about 300,000, the rest having been reabsorbed into the body (Strong & Devault, 1988). Despite this dramatic drop in the number of ova, she will have more than enough for the years ahead. She will actually cycle only a few hundred eggs in her reproductive lifetime. Although ovaries hold eggs numbering in the millions, they are the size of a small nut, and each egg is no bigger than a fine pencil dot. The ovaries do not float free in the abdomen—they are anchored by ligaments to the abdominal walls.

PELVIC FLOOR MUSCLES

The pelvic floor muscles, or *pubococcygeus* (PC) muscles, make up the largest muscle group in the body. Located around the vagina and the anus, the pelvic muscles are responsible for urinary control, assistance in maintaining posture, and keeping the internal organs in place (see Figure 3.4). They are also very important in sexual response. The opening of the vagina is ringed by strong muscles that create the physical tension that sheaths and stimulates a penis during intercourse. The nerve source for the pelvic floor muscles is the same as for the clitoris, vagina, and vulva, so contraction of the muscles can produce sexual pleasure. These muscles also contract during orgasm—at least, during the orgasms that are triggered by the clitoris.

Like other muscle groups, the pelvic floor muscles can lose their tone. If the muscles are weak or overly tense, or if a woman has no sense of voluntary control over these muscles, the quality of her sexual response—including orgasm—can be greatly diminished. The tone of the pelvic floor muscles affects whether or not there is "stress incontinence" (an involuntary dribbling of urine that can occur, for example, when a woman sneezes).

Pelvic floor muscle exercises—tightening and then relaxing the pelvic muscles—can improve a woman's voluntary control over these muscles, intensify her sexual pleasure (especially during orgasm), improve urinary control, and help tone the vaginal opening after childbirth. A description of these exercises, called Kegels,

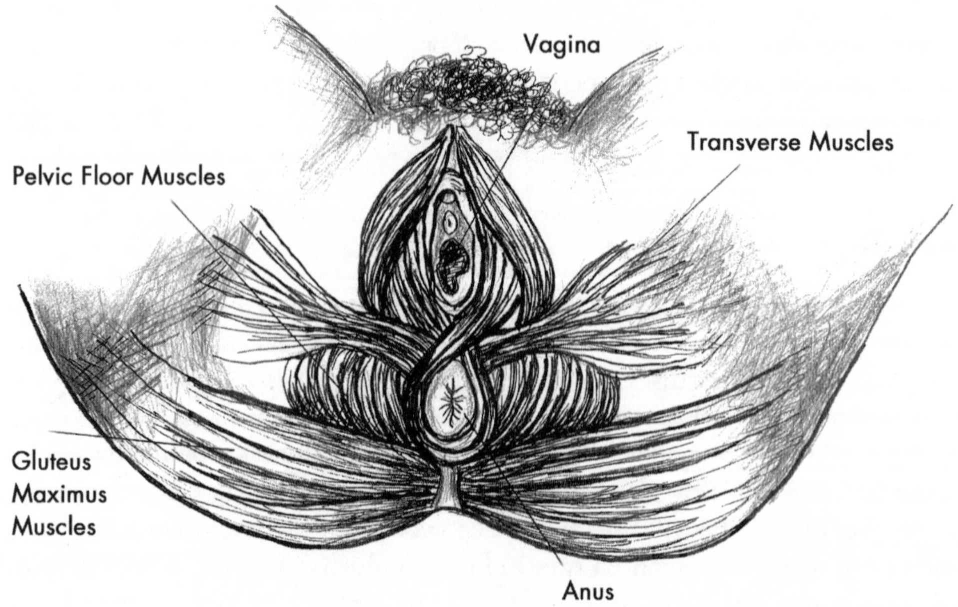

FIGURE 3.4. The pelvic floor muscles.

can be found in Chapter 8. (You may be aware of sexually pleasurable feelings in your pelvis when you practice these exercises.)

Some women experience painful muscle spasms in the pelvic muscles. These spasms, or cramps, can feel like a charley horse and make penetration painful or impossible. The large pelvic muscles are the only muscles in the body to have muscular tone when they're at rest. Even physically fit women who are very aware of the presence or absence of muscle tone may be unaware of muscle tension in the pelvis, which can contribute to muscle fatigue and chronic pelvic tension. Muscle spasms are involuntary, much like blinking is reflexive if there is a threat of something hitting the eye. Sometimes the pelvic muscle spasms occur for unknown reasons that may be psychological in origin. We think that some women carry psychological stress in their pelvic region, similar to neck and back muscle tension that other people experience.

Women who have had uncomfortable sexual experiences—for whatever reason (vaginal irritation, infection, sexual abuse, or other reasons)—may involuntarily tense their pelvic muscles, as a learned defense against pain or discomfort, when intercourse is attempted. The cycle of attempted penetration and muscle pain can be frustrating for a woman and her partner. The good news is, treatment is effective. We encourage any woman who is experiencing vaginal, vulvar, or pelvic muscle pain to seek help. Chapter 8 offers many suggestions for dealing with pain while maintaining your sexual relationship.

THE NERVES OF SEXUAL RESPONSE

The *pudendal nerve* is the primary nerve group responsible for a woman's experience of sexual response. Originating in the spinal cord, the pudendal nerve carries much of the sensory information—the physical feelings—of the clitoris and other areas of the genitals and is responsible for the muscle contractions of orgasm. The same nerve activates the vaginal secretions during the excitement phase and signals the tissues to engorge with blood. Other nerve pathways important in sexual responsiveness are the *hypogastric*, *pelvic*, and *vagus nerves*. The physical sensation that results from stimulation of the vagina, cervix, and some of the pelvic floor muscles is due to the response of these nerves. In fact, there apparently is no direct neural pathway linking the pudendal nerve and the uterus, so the sensations and contractions of the uterus during orgasm come from another neural pathway. The same is true for the G spot.

BREASTS

A woman's breasts have two primary functions: sexual pleasure and nourishment for babies. Breasts consist of fatty tissue that protects its many milk-producing glands. A system of ducts funnels the milk to the nipple, where it is let down by a hormonal signal triggered by a sucking infant. As glandular organs breasts are a part of a woman's genital and reproductive system. Breasts are sensitive to hormonal changes. For example, during sexual stimulation, breasts in women who have not yet been pregnant may enlarge. Breasts can also undergo changes in size during certain times of the menstrual cycle and become enlarged and feel tender just prior to a menstrual period. During pregnancy, breasts typically become larger, and the nipple and areola may darken in color.

Nipples are made of erectile tissue that is responsive to stimulation. Nipple stimulation causes the release of hormones—the same hormones that cause uterine contractions during orgasm or during nursing. With sexual arousal and orgasm, nipples are typically erect. As all women know, being cold can also stimulate nipple erection, as can other tactile sensations.

Numerous medical conditions can cause breast problems or changes. Evaluation of breasts and nipples should be a normal part of health maintenance. Your healthcare provider can teach you how to perform breast exams, which should be done monthly. Some women pick a specific day of the month, such as the first, or the date corresponding with their birthday, to remember to perform the breast exams regularly. Breast examination is a routine part of good gynecologic care; self-care exams should not take the place of regular medical exams.

If the media is an accurate barometer of our culture's attitude toward women's breasts, then clearly they exist primarily for display purposes. Carefully selected models; provocatively airbrushed, enhanced photography and filming; and clothing designed to reveal breasts are hallmarks of American graphics, be they print, film, or live. No wonder that women often express dissatisfaction with their breast size and/or shape, and breast alteration is a frequent medical request. In fact, normal breasts—breasts on real women—don't typically look like Barbie-doll breasts. Normal size includes large and small, droopy and firm.

Typically one breast is larger and/or a different shape from the other. Nipples and areolas (the darker-colored area around the nipple) vary just as much in size and shape, from one woman to another. Depending upon the pattern of a woman's hair distribution, she may also have hairs growing at the outer edge of the areola. We believe that so much media attention is focused on an exaggerated idea of beautiful breasts that many women are needlessly self-conscious about their breast or nipple size or shape and therefore are unable to experience their breasts as a full sexual part of themselves.

CHAPTER FOUR

Sexual Response

Sex wasn't studied in people until after the United States had the hydrogen bomb, television, the Salk polio vaccine, and space travel. It wasn't that clinicians were not interested in how women and men worked sexually but that study required observation in a clinical setting—which was simply deemed inappropriate. Instead, scientists made extrapolations about people based on the information they amassed by studying animal sexual behavior. In the 1950s Dr. Alfred Kinsey provided the medical community with access to the first comprehensive scientific data on human sexual behavior—not through observation but through a large survey that revealed what people said they did sexually.

During the same decade Dr. William Masters was curious and bold enough to undertake studies with human subjects in a controlled setting, observing their sexual activity and charting and filming their responses. The studies that he and Virginia Johnson conducted in the later 1950s provided the most information ever gained, to that point, about sex and people. Sex was now acknowledged to be a part of the human experience, not just a by-product of reproduction. The work of Masters and Johnson was particularly important in its exploration of women's sexual responsiveness. They specifically focused on clitoral stimulation and its relationship to orgasm, concluding that there is nothing immature about a clitoral orgasm, thereby disputing Sigmund Freud's earlier assertions that a woman attained sexual maturity when she experienced vaginal rather than clitoral orgasms.

In 1980 Dr. Beverly Whipple and Dr. John Perry challenged Masters and Johnson's contention that female orgasm comes solely from the clitoris. As noted they provided significant scientific support for the fact that there is another site for orgasm in women, which they termed the G spot (Ladas, Whipple, & Perry, 1983; Perry & Whipple, 1981).

Typically, sexual response is discussed in terms of a triphasic model comprised of desire, arousal, and orgasm. This model accurately describes biological responses of men and women, but it implies that each phase leads to the next, with orgasm being the normally anticipated end point. Following this line of thinking, a person could easily, and incorrectly, conclude that anything less than passion, physical arousal, and orgasm is an inferior sexual experience. This is not at all the case. Lovemaking and self-pleasuring can be fulfilling and satisfying without an orgasm. The triphasic model, in fact, has been criticized for more accurately charting male than female sexual experience and expectations. Two contradictory myths about women and sex have endured for years: (1) For women, great sex means orgasm, preferably *multiple* orgasm; and (2) women care most about cuddling and emotional closeness, and orgasm doesn't matter. The fact that these myths contradict each other shows some of the confusion still exists about women and sex.

Discussing sexual experience as a series of physical reactions runs the additional risk of overemphasizing the importance of biological factors for a satisfying sexual response. As we point out throughout this book, sex is also an intimate relationship that a woman has with her own body. This relationship is not dependent on hormones, blood flow, or the G spot but on a woman's history, self-concept, and comfort with her body.

The human sexual response is an intricate and unique mind–body experience that is not confined to "phases." Talking about sex in specific sections—desire, arousal, and orgasm—is useful, however, for organizing information about how the body, regardless of gender, responds to sexual cues. This model is helpful in highlighting the distinction between wanting sex, physically responding to sexual stimulation, and having an orgasm. Any of these experiences can occur alone or in combination with one or more of the other experiences. By understanding how each of these experiences is distinct and is influenced by physical and psychological factors, we are in a better position to understand how we respond sexually and how we can enhance that sexual response. It is also helpful in deciphering problems that can occur in each of the areas. In Part V we discuss strategies for overcoming problems of low desire, lack of arousal, and inability to orgasm. As therapists we have seen that, despite the presence of sexual information on the Internet, in magazines, and on talk shows, women do not know what goes on in their bodies when they are responding sexually.

SEXUAL DESIRE

Sexual desire: the phrase itself seems to burn and flame. Societies organize around regulating it and at the same time revel in it. The social agent in the United States to which we're all constantly exposed—advertising—would be hard pressed to exist without it. Well, for that matter, we wouldn't exist without it.

Sexual desire is referred to in academic literature as libido, drive, passion, sexual instinct, and sexual motivation. The words *turned on*, *horny*, *hot*, and other slang that refer to an innate biological drive toward sexual activity are also used in writing about sex. Because desire is now accepted as a normal and healthy drive in people, sex therapists and scientists conclude that, without influences that thwart this normal drive, people will regularly act on opportunities for sexual expression, including sex with a partner or masturbation.

There are many powerful social and physical factors that influence sexual desire: emotions, circumstance, upbringing, expectation, attitude, and general health (including, in particular, hormones, the brain, muscles, the vascular system, and the breathing system). Sexual desire is important to sexual activity, of course. While it is possible for you to engage in sex with no desire present, this is not a context that will typically produce pleasure or joy. Sex without desire brings to mind a Victorian approach to sex where nice girls have sex only to fulfill a societally designated marital responsibility.

Behind the Scenes of Sexual Desire

Recall a sexy scene in a movie. The fact that your memory searches and selects a particular scene to remember suggests that a lot went into the production of that scene. If it was graphic and riveting, it may have been the director's intention to jolt the viewer. If it was warm and romantic, the lighting may have been deliberately muted and softened to create this mood. If the scene was intense and pulsing, it may have been accompanied by the sound of rhythmic crashing and receding waves, replicating the thrusts and withdrawal of sexual intercourse. What you didn't see in the scene, and thus can't recall, is what went into creating the ambiance that makes a scene memorable. You didn't see the cameraman zooming in and controlling the scope and focus of the lens; the director orchestrating the scene; the sound technicians, the props and lighting; and how all of this came together to support the actors in convincingly portraying that part of the movie. Your body has every bit as much going on behind the scenes in its process of producing sexual desire and arousal as any movie.

Cues or Signals for Sexual Feelings

Why do you respond to sexual cues sometimes and not other times? Think of the movie scene analogy for a moment. The director may want to shoot a scene near the ocean with a couple holding each other as the sun is setting. To some extent the director can control this scene, but if it is pouring rain on the evening of the shoot, the action will have to be postponed. Though many parts come together—the script is set, the actors are in place, and the crew is assembled—the scene can't be completed as planned. Since sexual response is equally complex, you can see how all the parts of the scene can be in readiness, but something physical or emotional might arise to override the sexual cues. For example, the distressing symptoms of a head cold might well preoccupy an individual and blow away the neurological and hormonal processes that are also going on (pun intended).

We caution against the tendency to see sexual drive as an "itch that needs a scratch." This implies that if the desire and drive are present, the rest will naturally take care of itself. It's odd that sex is about the only area in which we apply such logic.

> Sharon is sitting on her couch distractedly watching television. She thinks about her partner Mark and feels the familiar disappointment that he doesn't seem to know how to "turn her on" anymore. Sex isn't that exciting; in fact, she can scarcely remember feeling "that old magic." Mark is expected back any minute from his business trip, but she doesn't feel motivated to think, even briefly, about creating some of the romance for which she yearns.
>
> Curling the afghan around her knees, Sharon becomes mesmerized by the beauty and grace of a figure-skating champion on television. During a slow-motion replay, Sharon marvels at the astounding three and a half revolutions the elfin skater seems to accomplish with little more effort than a feather floating on a breeze.
>
> Sharon yearns to be skimming across that ice, but she doesn't really think she could rummage through her basement closet, find her old ice skates, hurry to her local rink, and leap into the air to flawlessly execute a spinning jump. Sharon knows perfectly well that if she wants to command the ice, she will have to practice with dedication. But she cannot see that sexual desire demands anything more from her than showing up.

We see desire as a crucial part of sexual response, indeed, as the foundation on which the rest of the sexual experience builds. Experiencing desire as merely an urge does no more to define the quality of a sexual experience than experiencing physical hunger ensures a balanced diet or an exquisitely prepared dinner. One of the most common myths that we've seen women carry into their sexual relationships is that sex should be natural and spontaneous. An extension of this faulty reasoning is: if my partner really loved me, he or she would know exactly what I need sexually. In reality, desire for sex means little unless you are willing to take responsibility for your sexual satisfaction and pleasure.

How the Body Works in Sexual Desire

Brain Activity

Actually, when things are working normally, researchers have a difficult or impossible time sorting out what affects what and in what order. This speaks to the astonishingly effective ways our bodies function in sexual situations. The sensory centers in the brain receive and interpret messages from various stimuli and, in turn, cue the body to respond in certain ways. As with other body functions, the central nervous system must be working, perhaps as a kind of director coordinating all the other responding parts, if sexual desire is to be experienced in any meaningful way. The temporal and frontal lobes of the cerebral cortex appear to be the areas of the brain that are the most active in the start-up of sexual activity.

If a technician had access to the workings of the brain (in the way that a computer whiz has to the hard drive of a computer via the keyboard), the technician could stimulate a sexual response. It would be possible to produce an engorgement of the tissues of the clitoris in a woman or an erection in a man, for example. Without the brain to organize and interpret these responses, however, the erection or blood-engorged clitoris would not be experienced as a sexual feeling. Returning to our movie scene for a moment, it would be like one of the actors having a script and reading his or her part alone. Without the other parts—not to mention the camera, set, background music, and so on—the words would be a monologue without much meaning.

Hormones

Hormones are essential to the rhythms and cycles of female sexuality. Hormones are chemicals secreted by endocrine glands that signal the start-up and shut-down of activities in all parts of the body. The discussion of hormones in this chapter is confined to those connected with sexual responsiveness. How the menstrual cycle and reproductive hormones work is covered in Chapter 5.

Androgens are the hormones associated with sexual desire for both sexes. They're produced in the ovaries and the adrenal glands (about 50% of the androgens in the bloodstream come from adrenal glands). The androgen we are the most familiar with is testosterone, generally known as a "male hormone." Testosterone is as important to male sexual development and maturity as estrogen is for women. Men have 2 to 20 times more testosterone than women but this does not mean that men have 20 times the sex drive. A higher level of androgen is required for male sexual desire than for female desire, so normal is different for men and women.

For women, other hormonal action going on during different phases of their menstrual cycles will affect how much testosterone will be blocked. Think of a powerful sunscreen that blocks the ultraviolet rays of the sun and thus prevents sunburn or overexposure. Without the sunscreen, more rays of the sun penetrate the skin, which is susceptible to skin damage and an increased risk of skin cancer. Certain female hormones, such as progesterone, can act like a sunscreen to block the body's testosterone receptors. Women are more sensitive to androgens than are men. An intricate hormonal system protects women from overexposure to androgens, which could have a masculinizing effect on the distribution of body fat, muscular development, and hair growth—and, even more serious, the potential for the development of ovarian cancer.

If androgens in the form of testosterone are associated with sexual desire, could women take testosterone as a supplement, sort of like a "sexual vitamin," and thereby increase sexual desire and activity? An increasing amount of research is being conducted on this question, and the findings are promising. It appears that, in cases where androgen levels are low, taking testosterone *can* enhance a woman's sexual desire. But this is one of those cases where just because a little of something is good doesn't mean more of it is better. Taking a testosterone supplement when androgen levels are already normal will not only fail to increase sexual desire but also can increase the risk of harmful side effects, including masculinization, liver damage, and heart disease. Many women with low sexual desire have normal testosterone levels. We need to be careful not to reduce our understanding of sexual desire and behavior to biological factors alone. It's important to remember that nonbiological factors, such as upbringing, relationship issues, and body image, exert an important influence over sexual behavior.

Although sexual desire can be influenced by the dramatic hormonal fluctuations that occur during the menstrual cycle, it is not regulated or controlled by the menstrual cycle. In most animal species sexual activity is directly connected to the reproductive/hormonal cycle, so that sex occurs only during the fertile time of the female. Humans are different from other animals. Researchers have concluded that our sexual functioning and responsiveness does not follow a pattern that can be tracked readily by cyclical hormonal changes. Unlike animals, we can desire sex and be highly responsive regardless of where the woman is in her menstrual cycle.

In terms of sexual function, estrogen enhances sensitivity to sexual activity and creates a physical climate conducive to sexual behavior. It helps the vaginal tissue remain elastic and contributes to lubrication. Despite all of the research that has been done on the hormone estrogen, its role in sexual desire remains unclear.

There is another set of chemicals, called *pheromones*, that are linked to sexual attraction for both men and women. That is, you are attracted to others and they are attracted to you partially due to the pheromones you and they secrete. Although there is scientific evidence that pheromones exist, little is known about them. A major difference between pheromones and hormones (about which much more is known) is that hormones are secreted and circulated inside the body through the bloodstream, and pheromones are secreted outside the body through the sweat glands, skin, and urine. Interestingly, although we do not consciously detect pheromones by the sense of smell, the olfactory function must be working in order for pheromones to be effective; no sense of smell, no pheromone-related attraction. We don't have to be aware of pheromones for them to have an effect.

It appears that pheromones play a far more significant role in animal mating behavior than they do in human sexual behavior. Because human behavior and preservation aren't dictated by a sense of smell, pheromones probably influence us in subtle rather than compelling ways.

SEXUAL EXCITEMENT

Sexual excitement involves the narrowing of concentration so that other things are tuned out as sexual responsiveness is tuned in. There are intricate body responses and intense emotional responses as well. If sexual excitement involves a partner, then the interaction with that partner, including his or her pleasure, the scope of the relationship, the context of the sexual action that is taking place, and the feelings behind the sex will all contribute to the experience. If, for example, your partner is breathing heavily and nibbling, nuzzling, and stroking your earlobe, you may respond with a welcoming arching of your body and an intense excitement that matches your partner's. This section will explore what is happening in your body as sex becomes increasingly exciting. Although each woman's response will differ and may even vary widely from one sexual experience to another, sexual arousal includes some specific physiological changes common to most women. See Part V for advice on dealing with sexual arousal difficulties.

Blood Flow Changes

The excitement phase of sexual response can last minutes or much longer. During this time your blood pressure rises, breathing becomes more rapid, and pulse rate increases. As sexual excitement intensifies, blood flow to the vagina and vulva increases, resulting in vasocongestion: the process by which vaginal tissue becomes plump and swollen with an increased volume of blood. Blood flows in, and the hydraulics of sexual arousal temporarily keep the blood from flowing back out. If you squeeze the base of one of your fingers, you can cause congestion of blood into that finger. You can even see it change color. The most receptive parts of the vulva, particularly the labia minora, may also change color to a deep pink or burgundy. The primary source of blood for vasocongestion during sexual arousal is the pudendal artery. (Anatomical sexual parts are described in Chapter 3.)

Vasocongestion also contributes significantly to sexual sensitivity. The labia majora become engorged and retract, similar to how the petals of a flower open. In most women the clitoris will become erect, but this does not happen for everyone. Some women develop a skin mottling, resembling a rosy skin rash, that begins on the trunk of the body around the upper abdomen and can spread to the breasts, buttocks, back, and even the arms, legs, and face. This is called a sex flush. Blood engorges the nipples as well, causing them to become erect.

Lubrication

The presence of lubrication is an important feature of sexual excitement for women. Lubrication is the product of a process that happens within the tissues of the vagina: *transudation*. Facilitated by estrogen, the vaginal walls "sweat" with lubrication, which is a clear, slick fluid we've heard described as "an engineer's dream" because it's a non-oily lubricant. As the spongy tissue of the walls of the vagina engorge with blood, the swelling pushes tiny beads of this lubrication through the glands in the walls of the vagina. The composition, odor, and amount of this vaginal secretion vary from woman to woman, as it can vary for you as an individual at different times of your life.

Internal Evidence of Sexual Arousal

During sexual arousal, you will generally not be aware of the physiological changes that are going on inside of your body. This is partly because there are fewer nerve endings in the inner parts of the vagina. Also, the external organs, especially the clitoris, become acutely sensitive during arousal and their responses can easily overshadow the more subtle sensations coming from further inside your body. There are exceptions. Changes near the vaginal opening are more noticeable than those in the inner vagina because of the rich supply of nerve endings near the entrance. In addition, sexual play and direct stimulation are often concentrated in the area around the clitoris and the opening to the vagina, which will draw your attention there. Another exception is the G spot. When stimulation is focused on this portion of the sexual anatomy, the spongy tissue swells and becomes quite distinct. The focused stimulation of the G spot can lead to intense sensations inside the body.

When the primary sexual stimulation is focused on, and originates from, the clitoris, the innermost portion of the vagina, nearest to the uterus, begins to expand. Think of a strawberry. As the pale fruit ripens, it becomes plump and red. During sexual excitement, as blood engorges the vagina, it, too, becomes plump and "ripe." As the strawberry rounds out in its ripeness, its flesh pulls away from the center, creating a space. The voluptuous, sexually aroused vagina also rounds, and its expansion creates a space. In contrast to the deepest part of the vaginal ballooning, the opening of the vagina swells, giving it the capacity to grip a finger or penis.

During arousal, the uterus also changes size due to blood engorgement. As the inner part of the vagina expands, the uterus is elevated and pulled forward, which changes the position of the cervix. As noted, some women enjoy the physical sensation of feeling their partner's penis push against the cervix, a sensation that is enhanced by the body's arousal.

When sexual stimulation is focused more internally, on stimulation of the G spot, the physical changes are different. Even though there is blood engorgement and considerable swelling of the tissue, the muscles around the entrance of the vagina tend to open rather than grip. The innermost part of the vagina expands less than it does during intense clitoral stimulation. The uterus and cervix press against the upper portion of the vagina, actually compressing it a bit. During the height of arousal coming from G spot stimulation, you may experience a bearing-down pressure, as if you were pushing against or expelling the stimulating hand, penis, or vibrator. It is unlikely that your partner will notice these subtle physical differences in how you respond to clitoral and G spot stimulation.

You may question how these different changes affect your chance of getting pregnant. An old myth still finds its way to our offices: female orgasm increases one's chance of getting pregnant. In fact, for conception to happen, sperm must come into contact with an ovum (egg). Because the ovum isn't in the vagina or cervix, conception doesn't generally happen at the moment of high arousal but after the sexual contact is over and the genitals have returned to their quiescent, prearoused state. If you're trying to get pregnant, therefore, it makes sense to lie still for a brief time after intercourse so that the ejaculate fluid remains in the vaginal canal.

Other Physiological Changes during Female Sexual Arousal

Along with rapid breathing, increased heart rate, vasocongestion of the internal and external genitals, and heightened concentration tuning other stimuli out, you will likely experience a generalized tension throughout your body. This makes sense. For a few moments try to breathe rapidly, and you will find that at least your upper body muscles meet this "stress" almost automatically, by tensing and focusing. (When sex therapists work with women who are tense during sexual activity due to fear, first they help these women distinguish the physical responses of fear from the normal physical tension of sexual arousal.)

Changes also occur in the clitoris. As noted, a fold of skin called the prepuce, or clitoral hood, covers the clitoris. The skin of the clitoral hood is normally loose, not taut like the skin that covers your fingers, for example. It is connected to the labia minora, as explained in Chapter 3. During intense sexual arousal, the clitoris is retracted up against the pubic bone. Ironically, it becomes much less visible and prominent when excitement is the highest and the labia the most swollen. The clitoris is thus protected against direct stimulation, which may feel far too intense to be pleasurable.

Breasts also change during intense sexual arousal. Women's breasts may swell as much as 25%, especially in women who have never breast-fed. The nipples typically become erect during arousal, and as arousal increases, the areola—the darkened circle around the nipple—begins to swell. Indeed, the areola can swell so much during arousal that it can look like the nipple has retracted. These breast changes recede as soon as sexual arousal diminishes.

"Plateau" of High Sexual Arousal before Orgasm

Sexual arousal often reaches a plateau that is a highly erotic, focused period of intense sexual tension. This phase lasts moments or many minutes depending upon the individual woman, the circumstances, her health status, and how relaxed or anxious she is. Masters and Johnson (1966) delineated and named this phase of sexual response and described it as being the sustained height of sexual tension. A state of protracted, intense sexual pleasure can be supremely gratifying and complete in itself.

ORGASM

Orgasm is the briefest phase of sexual response, lasting only seconds. Often called "climaxing," "coming," or "getting off," orgasm is the rhythmic pulsing that occurs as the body releases sexual tension, Orgasm is often depicted in the media by thrashing, moaning, gasping, writhing, and fascinating gyrating behavior. Such portrayal may be entertaining but is woefully noninstructive or worse. We believe it perpetuates the myth that a woman's orgasm is a spontaneously occurring event, happening as she is swept away in a consuming tidal wave of unbridled passion. Instead, we have come to know that a woman's orgasmic response is learned through experience, experimentation, and self-awareness. There might be writhing and moaning, but not always. And we certainly don't expect to see an intense, spontaneous orgasm "just happening" for a woman who is sexually inexperienced and unaware of her body's responses, no matter how skilled her lover may be. Let's look at this more closely.

When boys hit adolescence, there is a direct connection between pubertal development and ejaculation. For girls, however, there is no connection between the beginning of puberty—such as the appearance of pubic hair—and orgasm. In studies of boys the findings are consistent and clear: hormonal factors much more than social factors determine sexual response, including orgasm. For girls, social factors appear to be a much stronger determinant than sex hormones for becoming orgasmic. "Social factors" were not consistently defined in these studies. Our own clinical work and the work of other sex therapists support our strong view that orgasm for women is more learned than spontaneous. It is important to note, however, that for many girls orgasm can precede pubertal development or sexual activity with any partner.

This learning process is most likely ongoing, perhaps beginning during childhood when a girl explores her vulva, vagina, and clitoris, and continuing on through her adult life as she communicates with her partner about her body's sense of pleasure and sensitivity. In other words, a woman's orgasmic response, including the overly acclaimed multiple orgasm, depends first upon a woman's curiosity about, knowledge of, and experimentation with her body and how it responds. One abiding myth is that if a woman masturbates, she "uses up" sexual energy that could go to her partner and therefore should give up masturbation once she's in a partnership. There is no research to support this myth, and in fact we find that self-pleasure enhances sexual pleasure in a partnership.

Physical Response of Orgasm

When orgasm happens, a woman's body is generally in a state of high sexual arousal. We say "generally" because it is very possible for a woman to have a "quickie" orgasm, bypassing some of the signs of sexual excitement. For example, some women describe feeling the pelvic contractions of orgasm almost immediately when using a highly stimulating vibrator on the clitoris. But despite the fact that these contractions are present and perhaps powerfully felt, women often describe these orgasms as different from orgasms reached by progressing incrementally and more slowly in sexual arousal.

> "I come almost right away when I put a vibrator against my clit. It's almost too intense. Afterwards I often feel an odd combination of numbness and overstimulation. I feel like I got there too fast and my body is in a state of suspension for a while, like I've missed out on something and I'm still waiting."

The G Spot

As explained in Chapter 3, the G spot is a small area of erectile tissue in the front wall of the vagina that becomes engorged during sexual arousal and is especially sensitive to stimulation. The sensations of an orgasm generated through stimulation of the G spot are described by women as being different from the orgasms generated primarily through the clitoris. They say that the G spot orgasms feel like they occur deeper inside the body with fewer pelvic floor muscle contractions. When orgasms are evaluated in laboratories by technical measurements, this is borne out. The G-spot-stimulated orgasms result in less activity in the pelvic floor muscles and more activity in the uterus and cervix. It should be kept in mind that because more than one nerve group can be stimulated at the same time, simultaneous G spot stimulation and clitoral stimulation are mutually enhancing.

Pelvic Floor Muscles

As we discussed in Chapter 3, the pelvic floor muscles are very important to a woman's sexual pleasure. During orgasm, these strong muscles contract, involuntarily, in intervals of 0.8 second. Sometimes they are felt very strongly and, at other times, more like a gentle ripple. A woman may experience three to 10 of these contractions during an orgasm.

The muscles have different names and locations. Some of them form a figure-eight shape around the anus and vaginal opening (see Figure 3.4 in Chapter 3). Others actually circle the vagina in a way similar to how two hands wrap around a can of soda. As the muscles contract during orgasm, so do the vagina, urethra, and anus, together producing a highly pleasurable sensation. A woman can enhance her sexual pleasure by gaining more voluntary control over her pelvic muscles—getting them in shape by exercising them just as she does with other muscles in her body. We describe this more fully in Chapter 8. It's interesting to note that men, too, have 0.8-second rhythmic contractions of similar pelvic floor muscles, so both sexes probably feel similar sensations during orgasm.

Uterine Contractions

The uterus also contracts during orgasm. Some women describe this sensation as intensely pleasurable and satisfying. Other women are barely aware of when it happens. If a woman has consistently experienced pleasurable uterine and deep vaginal contractions, having her uterus and cervix removed for medical reasons can represent a great loss for her. Removing the cervix and uterus does not involve removal of the G spot, so the pleasure a woman can feel from stimulation of the G spot can continue to be very intense even following a hysterectomy.

Uterine contractions are not always pleasurable. Very low or widely fluctuating estrogen levels may make the uterine contractions painful. This could be associated with childbirth, menopause, or the blocked ovarian production of estrogen, and should be discussed with your healthcare provider.

The Clitoris and Orgasm

The clitoris exists for sexual pleasure alone. Its only function is to trigger a common form of orgasm—a clitoral orgasm. This doesn't mean that orgasm happens in the clitoris. Think of turning a warm shower on. You manipulate the knobs that control the water to achieve the flow and temperature of water that is pleasurable. The clitoris is the source of some orgasms, just like the G spot is the source of other orgasms. Either way, the orgasms are felt not only in the clitoris but also in the pelvis and entire genital region. The pleasure of the orgasmic pulses isn't confined to these body areas: most women describe orgasm as an intense, entire-body experience.

It's important to keep all of this within some context. Let's use our movie metaphor again. Say you are caught up in watching a comedy in which an intricate scene becomes hilarious and you laugh spontaneously, without restraint. Your eyes water, your chest convulses, your diaphragm moves, and you may even have trouble catching your breath. If your laughing jag was carefully evaluated in a laboratory setting, the intricate involvement of muscles and nerves and other body responses would be studied. The researchers could describe in great detail exactly how the body responded during laughter, but they would not be able to pinpoint which physiological response primarily defines laughter. Furthermore, no laboratory in the world could define the experience you were having while laughing, what was the most pleasurable aspect of the laughter, or even what was funny. Orgasm is like that. It might allow infinite definition, but each experience is uniquely yours and is made up of far more than its various sensations and responses.

All sexologists agree that many women—perhaps, most women—do not experience orgasm regularly from sexual intercourse alone. We can't give you the exact percentage, because the research on women and orgasm does not always include information about how a woman is having her orgasm—whether by intercourse alone or by intercourse combined with additional stimulation. We aren't so interested in percentages. What we want to stress is that not experiencing an orgasm with sexual intercourse alone is not a sexual dysfunction. It is normal. Refer to Part V, "Overcoming Sexual Difficulties," for questions about orgasm difficulties.

Multiple Orgasms

Women have the physical capacity to have more than one orgasm during the same session of sexual activity, whether through masturbation or with a partner. Men usually require a "cool-down" period after an orgasm; women usually do not.

Multiple orgasms have been given a lot of sensational attention in the media, but they are not achievable for all women and certainly not essential for sexual pleasure and satisfaction. Some women find they are so physically sensitive after an orgasm that further stimulation can be uncomfortable rather than pleasurable. Many women find that their first orgasm is highly satisfying and that a second orgasm doesn't necessarily enhance the sexual experience. We have found that women and their partners may feel pressured to achieve multiple orgasms, as if this were a superior accomplishment. Some couples strive to achieve multiple orgasms with a "we'll-get-this-or-die" approach, which is not particularly conducive to increased pleasure or satisfaction. We realize that we are debunking the glamour of multiple orgasms. Think about it. We also have the physical capacity to eat four doughnuts instead of one, but proving or exercising that capacity is certainly not essential for enjoyable dining, and pushing oneself to do so could actually detract from the experience.

SEXUAL RESPONSE AT MENOPAUSE AND LATER

Sexually, a woman's body "works" fine during menopause and the later years. She remains robustly capable of functioning in all aspects of sexual response: desire, arousal, and orgasm. Yes, a woman might say that she would prefer to have her body of younger years, but the preference is usually qualified; "I want my body then but my mind now." Because it doesn't work that way, we need to deal with menopause and changes in our bodies—including any sexual changes—adaptively. We'll say it again: one of the most pernicious myths about female sexuality is that sex is for the young. Not so: *sex is a part of every woman her entire life.*

Desire

Sexual desire seems to decline with aging, although some studies show that after age 65, sexual interest and activity increase. This may be due to a newfound freedom and sense of control over one's time and environment. The hormonal changes of menopause can dampen desire because of the discomfort of dealing with the symptoms and because of reduced estrogen and androgen. Adding androgen to estrogen therapy may provide a boost in sexual interest for some women in menopause.

Medications and medical treatment can affect all aspects of sexual response, and as we age, the chances naturally increase that we will undergo medical treatment for some illness or condition. See Part V for an overview of medically induced sexual difficulties.

For older women, sexual desire will need prioritizing. If sex is going to be important, we recommend that you take time for sexual fantasy and masturbation. You'll find information on learning to fantasize in Chapter 14 and learning to masturbate in Chapter 15.

Arousal

Sexual changes following menopause are often most obvious during the arousal phase. The mucous membrane tissue of the vagina and part of the vulva may have become thin and prone to irritation and minor injury. Lubrication diminishes during and after menopause, so the sensitive tissues are more susceptible to damage from vigorous sexual activity, especially heterosexual intercourse and other penetrating sexual activities such as the use of dildos or vibrators. The cushiony thickness of the vaginal walls and the Venus mound has decreased, so some of the insulation against active sexual play is diminished, particularly sex involving penetration or lengthy periods of direct stimulation. Using a non-petroleum-based lubricant can be very helpful to protect against irritation and dryness. We often recommend Astroglide or K-Y Jelly.

Estrogen cream applied directly to the vagina can have beneficial effects that offset some of the problems caused by thin tissue and vaginal dryness. Risks associated with estrogen replacement are not totally escaped when using a topical cream. Although the amount of estrogen will be less than when using a patch or oral or injectable hormone replacement therapy options, estrogen from the cream will be absorbed into the bloodstream. A man's penis may also absorb topical estrogen during intercourse, so male partners may want to use condoms to minimize any inadvertent absorption. Estrogen cream should not be used as a lubricant! As with any replacement hormone, the use of estrogen cream should be discussed with your healthcare provider, because the use of the cream may require the addition of progestin to protect the uterus.

Another form of estrogen is the vaginal ring, which is inserted into the vagina and emits a small, steady dose of estrogen. This is considered a relatively safe option for women who experience vaginal dryness, pain or itching, but who are sensitive to the larger doses of estrogen found in hormone replacement therapy (HRT).

Orgasm

We know that regular sexual activity and orgasm help maintain a woman's sexual health. Women who masturbate or have regular sex with a partner actually continue to lubricate more rapidly and have more estrogen circulating in the body, even if they show signs of vaginal atrophy (thinning of the vagina). In fact, "use it or lose it" may be truer for women than for men. Because vaginal tissue tends to atrophy and lose elasticity not only due to lowered estrogen levels but also to lack of stimulation and stretching, we recommend masturbation with a penetrating, dildo-shaped vibrator. Using lubrication, a deep penetrating vibrator can create a satisfying sense of fullness and can help maintain healthy tissue, promote lubrication, and minimize shrinking of the vagina. The same results can be obtained through regular sexual intercourse (approximately once a week), but this latter method is not always an option or an interest for some women as they grow older.

Pelvic muscles are integral to orgasm for women and men. As noted, Kegel exercises—squeezing and relaxing the pelvic muscles—can promote strength in these muscles, which are prone to lose elasticity. See Chapter 8 for specific instructions regarding Kegel exercises.

Uterine contractions that occur as part of orgasm can change in intensity and sensation as a result of menopause. Some women find that the contractions, which they may have previously felt as pleasurable, now become uncomfortable or even painful. In some cases hormone therapy may help. Your healthcare provider may recommend an antispasmodic medication. It is important that uterine pain be evaluated because pain can be a signal of a medical problem. Any bleeding that you can't account for should be promptly reported to your healthcare provider.

Some studies suggest that, with aging, the clitoris becomes less sensitive because of decreased blood flow and engorgement during sexual arousal. Other studies report that the clitoris becomes more sensitive because of the changes in the clitoral hood and supporting tissues around the clitoris, which diminish and leave the clitoris more exposed. If you notice a change in sensitivity, adjust the intensity of clitoral stimulation during sex to a level that is pleasurable to you. Decreased sensation in the clitoris, vagina, or labia may indicate damage to the blood vessels or nerves, which can occur with diabetes and some neurological diseases. Many physicians have been trained only to recognize the possibility of neurological or vascular disease in their male patients with erectile dysfunction, and may not be sensitive to women's concerns. As with all aspects of your health, be persistent in getting the medical attention for your symptoms that you deserve.

STAY TUNED

We are only beginning to understand the rich complexity of a woman's sexual response. We know that it spans a lifetime and that women who live in cultures that honor older women are less likely to become sexually inactive. Their continued sexual activity points to a fundamental truth: *sexual response is one of the most enduring and pleasurable parts of our humanity.*

CHAPTER FIVE

Reproduction and Beyond

From the first period of menarche to the last period of menopause, from puberty to sexual activity in your 90s, your sexuality evolves with the cycles of your body. Although sexuality in our modern world is viewed broadly, exceeding reproductive concerns, from a rudimentary standpoint reproduction remains a primary purpose of sexual behavior. While it's possible to write a book about male sexuality and spend very little—if any—time on reproductive function, that's not so for female sexuality. Your sexuality is experienced through the lens of your reproductive potential. For example, if your body is functioning normally, you will have menstrual periods every month for a very long time, and your sexual choices will be made, in part, around those cycles. Your decisions and experiences regarding pregnancy will have an impact not only on your sexual activity but also your sexual self-image. For these reasons, women bring us questions like the following:

- "I want to have sex during my period. Is this weird?"
- "Is PMS all in my head? My sister says she never has it."
- "Now that I'm pregnant, I'm more interested in sex than ever, but for the first time in our relationship, my husband doesn't want it. What can I do?"
- "How do I know what birth control method to pick? And when do I start?"
- "My doctor says we can have sex again now that the baby is two months old, but I just don't want to. Why not?"
- "We've been trying for almost two years without a pregnancy. My friends keep telling me stories about women who got pregnant the minute they gave up. Does stress have something to do with conceiving?"

- "Infertility has taken all the fun and romance out of our sex life. It's all sex-on-demand and failure. Will sex ever be what it used to be?"
- "Is there any way to prevent our sex life from changing when I reach menopause?"

In this chapter we discuss the physiological cycles of women's bodies and how these cycles impact sex, beginning with a discussion of hormones and their powerful impact on women's cycles and continuing with menstruation, pregnancy, infertility, menopause, and beyond. Because Chapter 4 introduced the sex hormones that are most prominent in sexual pleasure, we'll touch on them only briefly in this chapter.

HORMONES: THE AMAZING MESSENGERS

Even when viewed in this age of technological marvels, our bodies contain a communication system that is astonishingly complex. Along with the central nervous system, invisible chemicals called hormones communicate with every part of the body—every cell, in fact—providing operating instructions. Hormones are produced by glands: in women, the adrenal glands, the thyroid gland, and the ovaries. When the hormones have a job to do, they are released into the bloodstream. Every process the body goes through, like menstruation, gets its start-up and shut-down instructions from hormones, often in combination with signals from the central nervous system.

Sometimes even a tiny amount of a hormone can cause a big effect, depending on how sensitive the receiver is to that particular chemical. Some receiving organs have very alert receptors and they respond strongly. Think about the sensitivity of your fingertips. Nerve endings in fingers are distributed in such a way as to be very sensitive to texture. If we want to experience the smooth feel of satin, for example, we use our fingers rather than our elbows to examine the cloth. In the same way, organs and cells vary in their degree of sensitivity to certain hormones, as can each individual woman.

Hormones operate by changing the chemical process within a cell: the cell or organ reacts when the hormone enters it. If we add baking soda to vinegar, we see an instant foaming action that happens only when the ingredients are combined. (Of course, the endocrine system that regulates hormonal action is much more complex than this culinary analogy.)

Hormones that regulate the changes of the menstrual cycle are part of a governmental system that is headed by the hypothalamus, an organ found deep in the skull at the base of the brain. We can think of the hypothalamus as having an office in the basement of the Pentagon. In this office, the hypothalamus is bombarded with information from the outside world, while at the same time it has the job of keeping things running smoothly within its domain: the body. The hypothalamus keeps track of reproductive status by monitoring different body signals, including the levels of hormones (estrogen and progesterone) being released by the ovaries. Hormone output from the ovaries can vary greatly during the menstrual cycle. To regulate the menstrual cycle, the hypothalamus communicates with the nearby pituitary gland by producing a chemical called gonadotropin-releasing hormone, or GnRH for short. The hypothalamus releases GnRH a little at a time to signal the pituitary gland when and by how much to respond. Think of it as e-mail instructions, sent every hour or so. Based on instructions received from the hypothalamus, the pituitary gland releases one of two regulating hormones: FSH or LH. *FSH* (follicle stimulating hormone) stimulates the growth of ovarian follicles for the production of a mature egg, and *LH* (luteinizing hormone) stimulates the release of that mature egg from the ovary. Later in this chapter, we discuss how these hormones regulate the menstrual cycle.

Hormones are difficult to pin down in medical parameters. A blood test can show the healthcare provider the level of different hormones at a certain time on a certain day, but these levels change continuously, so that the same test several days later would probably produce very different results. Each active hormone is changing at a different rate as well. It's like an orchestra production of a symphony: the trumpet players may sit with their instruments in their laps for most of the piece, but when it comes time for their part in the musical production, they will be heard and appreciated. Because of this complexity, it's not surprising that precisely how some of these hormones function is not yet fully known or appreciated.

Estrogen

Estrogen signals an embryo to develop as a female and then stimulates her body at puberty to develop breasts and fully mature her vulva, vagina, clitoris, and internal reproductive organs. Somewhere between the ages of eight and 12 or 13, hormonal changes cause a girl's nipple area to swell and small breast buds to develop, a process that will take years. At times this will be uncomfortable for her. Estrogen will also determine the way in which her body shape and body fat distribution will differ from a boy's. Estrogen will provide the vagina and vaginal opening with strength and elasticity. The pelvic girdle bones will widen an inch or two at puberty, preparing her body for the future possibility of giving birth.

Estrogen affects a young woman's skin and complexion and helps determine when the growth of her long bones, like arms and legs, will stop. In concert with genetic factors, it will determine the distribution of her body hair. Very importantly, estrogen is active almost in every cell in the body. For example, it will protect against the loss of bone density as a woman ages, and it can be a preventive factor for some cardiovascular diseases as well. The longer life span of women, relative to men, may well be due to their hormonal make-up.

Estrogen (as well as a number of other hormones) is the AT&T or MCI of the body. Just as a long-distance carrier allows you to make phone contact with a distant friend or relative, estrogen levels help communicate to the hypothalamus where you are in your menstrual cycle. This information influences what instructions are sent from the hypothalamus to the pituitary gland and, ultimately, to the ovaries.

Estrogen comes mostly from the ovaries, but fatty tissue in the body also produces estrogen. When a woman reaches menopause and her ovaries no longer produce very much estrogen, fatty tissue will continue to make estrogen by converting other hormones present in the body.

Androgens

Androgens are produced in small amounts by the ovaries and the adrenal glands. This hormone is incorrectly referred to as the male hormone. Although a form of androgen called testosterone is extremely important in the fetal and pubertal development of boys' sexual characteristics, androgens are important for women's health and sexuality as well. The role of androgens in a woman's sexual response is discussed in Chapter 4.

Progesterone

Progesterone means "pro" (for) "pregnancy" (gestation), reflecting the fact that pregnant women have very high levels of progesterone. This hormone is produced by the ovaries and, in small amounts, by the adrenal glands. It is barely present in the first part of a woman's menstrual cycle but is made by the ovary after ovulation each month. Man-made or synthetic progesterones are called "progestins" and are a primary ingredient in birth control pills. Progesterone is a very important hormone for the menstrual cycle and pregnancy. It helps create a mature uterine lining, keeps the uterus from contracting too much, and helps the body allow a fetus to attach and grow.

Pheromones

Pheromones, as explained in Chapter 4, are chemicals that we may secrete for the purpose of attracting others. Interestingly, pheromones may also be involved in "menstrual synchrony," which is a tendency for women who live together to have menstrual cycles at the same time or very close together.

THE MENSTRUAL CYCLE

The menstrual cycle for a woman has been compared with the moon, because the typical menstrual cycle mimics the lunar cycle of 28 days. It is important to note that variations are normal. Some women have very predictable menstrual cycles of 28 days, while other women have shorter or longer cycles. Cycles of 24 to 38 days are considered within the normal range. Deviations from this "normal" pattern, such as having a period at a predictable interval for three months in a row and then having a cycle that goes 32 days instead of 25 days, sometimes occur.

Menarche, or the first menstrual period, is often a developmentally defining moment for young girls. You will likely remember when and where you started your first period and the emotions and experiences you had around this event. A girl can expect to begin her period between the ages of 9 and 15, usually anywhere from a few months to a few years after she has begun breast development. Prior to her first period, she may have some months in which she notices a nonirritating clear or whitish vaginal discharge on her underpants.

Phases of the Menstrual Cycle

On the first day of your period, lowered estrogen and progesterone levels have signaled your body to let the blood and tissue from the lining of the uterus (endometrium) slough off and leave the body through the cervix and vagina in the form of menstrual blood. Over the next three to seven days you will shed about four tablespoons of menstrual discharge.

Follicular Phase

The follicular phase is the first half of the monthly cycle, and it includes the days of menstruation. It also is the time for an egg to begin maturing. For this to happen, the hypothalamus "notices" the low levels of estrogen and progesterone and communicates to the pituitary about what will be needed for an egg to mature properly so that it is prepared for the important phase of ovulation (see Figure 5.1). The pituitary sends FSH (follicle stimulating hormone) for this part of the job. Actually, the pituitary is zealous about its job and stimulates many follicles. Follicles are extremely tiny sacs inside the ovary, and each follicle holds one ovum (egg). All these follicles become revved up by their own production of estrogen, which causes the endometrium to thicken. Soon the follicles unite, sending the hypothalamus, via the messenger estrogen, the message to stop the pituitary gland from sending additional FSH and to start sending LH (luteinizing hormone). The pituitary complies and sends LH back to the follicles, where things now become selective. LH suppresses the activity of all of the follicles but one, which is groomed for complete maturity. As the follicle matures, it swells a bit and can resemble a tiny blister as the egg it contains ripens. This phase takes about two weeks.

Ovulation

Ovulation is the shortest part of the menstrual cycle, lasting only a day or so. The ripened egg (ovum) bursts through the sac (follicle) that contains it. Sometimes a woman will notice a little cramping at the time of ovulation on one side in her lower abdomen.

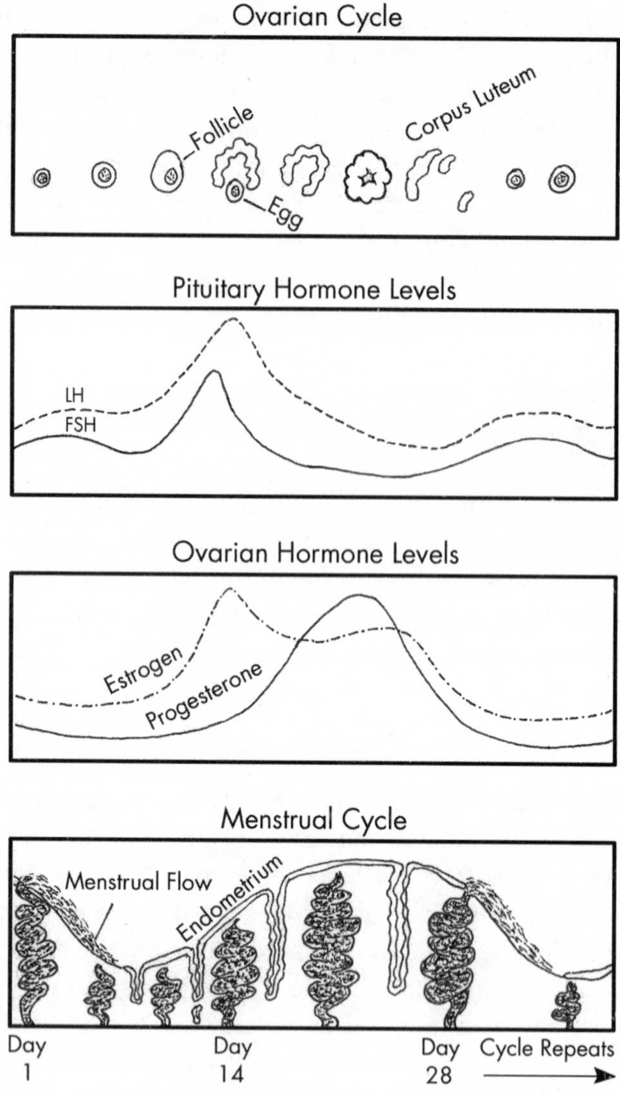

FIGURE 5.1. Phases of the menstrual cycle.

This cramping is called *mittelschmerz*, a German word for pain in the middle of a cycle. The fallopian tubes become active at this point. The fimbria, or graceful, fringelike ends of the tubes, curl and close around the transient egg, encouraging it into the fallopian tube. As soon as the egg is released, the menstrual cycle enters its last phase.

Luteal Phase

Let's go back to our empty follicle, which has been abandoned by its adventuresome ripened egg. Now the follicle undergoes a dramatic transformation. It doesn't remain an empty sac for very long. LH changes activities inside the follicle. Where there had been fluid, the cells change in composition and color, becoming the *corpus luteum* (Latin: yellowish body). Under new management, the follicle—now called the corpus luteum—again produces estrogen. The corpus luteum plans for the future and starts producing the "pro-pregnancy" hormone, progesterone. The estrogen and progesterone stimulate an increased blood supply in the lining of the uterus, just in case a fertilized ovum implants itself during the next week or so. Meanwhile the prodigal egg, conveyed by muscular contractions in the fallopian tube, stays for a few days before moving along to the uterus.

Of course, big things could happen to the little egg. If the egg becomes fertilized by sperm and attaches to the uterine lining, the corpus luteum keeps up the campaign for progesterone, which takes on the regulating function of maintaining a pregnancy. Progesterone aids in the development of the fetus and prevents contractions from beginning too early. If fertilization does not occur, after a few days the pituitary gets the message that all the progesterone that is needed has been produced, and it stops sending LH. On about day 24 of the cycle, without a pregnancy, the corpus luteum collapses and begins to deteriorate. The drop in progesterone and estrogen output signals the body to begin the menstrual period. Very soon, however, the low levels of hormones alert the hypothalamus to remedy the situation, and the cycle begins again.

MENSTRUATION

Menstruation has been the subject of more mythology than any other biological function, and most of it has been vastly negative. Through the course of history it has been difficult for people to understand a biological imperative to bleed monthly, and because of this, the forefathers of medicine (such as Aristotle) posed several theories based on their rudimentary understanding of the woman's body—all of them noxious—like, menstrual blood is fermented with impurities men are able to eliminate through sweat but women are not (Angier, 1999).

Have we come very far in our thinking? True, we are more informed, and yet we are still likely to assume that menstruation at least somewhat impairs a woman's performance of intellectually demanding, athletically demanding, or intricate problem-solving activities. Although this attitude has come a long way from the belief that women are putrid at the core, it is, in fact, inaccurate: research finds no fluctuations in performance over the course of the menstrual cycle.

If you are experiencing problems with menstruation from abnormal bleeding, cramps, or PMS, your healthcare provider is the first place to start. We recommend that you see a gynecologist or a nurse practitioner who specializes in gynecology. Also, check our resource list at the back of the book for excellent books that cover all concerns about menstruation.

Sex during Menstruation

It is important to know that having sexual intercourse, including ejaculation, is quite normal during menstruation. You can also use a vibrator or have oral sex, if you choose. Whether or not to have sex during a menstrual period, however, is a personal choice to be made by you and your partner. All aspects of sexual response "work" during your period, including desire, arousal, and orgasm. You probably won't be aware of lubrication, because menstrual flow will keep the vagina moist. And, of course, having sex during your period is messier than at other times.

Some sexual partners will specifically state that they do not want to be sexually active during menstruation, but often we have found that a partner is more focused on what the woman wants and will follow her lead.

> "I love having sex when I'm on my period. I already have a 'full' feeling in my pelvic area, and I get really turned on. It's a bit embarrassing, but we both even enjoy the mess of it. We take a shower afterwards, so, so what!"

> "I was absolutely certain you couldn't get pregnant during your period, so I felt 'safe' then. But my nurse practitioner told me to be sure to use condoms, because some women ovulate near the beginning of their period, or might even spike ovulation during their period."

> "The only partner I'm interested in during my period is my heating pad."

Menstrual Blood Flow Abnormalities

> "I'd never had any problems with my periods, but one month, days after my period had stopped, there was blood when I went to the bathroom. I was pretty nervous—seeing blood when you aren't supposed to is scary! My doc was really good. She checked things out and decided that I just had some bleeding with ovulation that month."

We find that women who experience changes in their menstruation patterns tend to experience this as more worrisome than temporary changes in other bodily functions. Perhaps this is because blood, aside from menstruation or giving birth, is normally a cue to us that something is wrong. Many times there are innocuous causes for irregularities in cycles, but nothing can replace the security of being "in charge" of your sense of well-being—so call your healthcare provider if you're concerned.

Amenorrhea (No Menstrual Periods)

If you are sexually active and miss a period, the first thing you and your healthcare provider think of is pregnancy. There are, however, other reasons for menstrual periods not occurring, ranging from minor to serious problems. If you are in your 40s, you may be in perimenopause—the period when the body undergoes changes leading up to menopause.

Hypermenorrhea (Heavy Periods)

Heavy bleeding can have many causes. This is not a time for self-diagnosis: call your healthcare provider. If you have twice the volume of bleeding that is normal for you during your period, or if you bleed for more than a week, call. If you are coping with a chronic medical problem that has heavy bleeding as a symptom, check Chapter 7.

Spotting

The cause of spotty bleeding in between periods also needs medical evaluation or attention. Causes may range from a normal response to ovulation to a signal of a serious medical problem. Some women have spotting following sexual intercourse. This should be discussed with your healthcare provider. A physical injury, such as a minor abrasion, can also cause spotting. Be persistent in seeking a cause for your spotting.

Cramps

Cramps with menstrual periods were once thought to be "in a woman's head." In the late 1970s, however, the presence of too much of a hormone called prostaglandin was discovered to be the main reason why women have cramps during their periods. The accumulation of prostaglandins during the second two weeks of the menstrual cycle can cause a strong cramping of the muscles of the uterus, similar to the aches that occur when one engages in exercise and has sore muscles the next day. This cramp, or spasm, can reduce blood flow to the uterine muscles. When there isn't enough blood, there isn't enough oxygen, which can cause pain. Cramps are also caused by pelvic congestion of fluids (creating the bloating sensation many women experience).

The good news is that many women can find ways to relieve menstrual cramps. Eighty percent of women can find relief from their cramps by taking antiprostaglandin medications. These medications include aspirin, ibuprofen, fenoprofen calcium, mefenamic acid, naproxen sodium, and naproxen. Cramps can certainly "cramp" your interest in sex, but clinicians actually recommend orgasm as a remedy for cramps! Masturbation or partner activity leading to orgasm (if you are up to it) can help. As we discussed in Chapter 4, sexual arousal involves the congestion of blood in the pelvic region, and orgasm dissipates this congestion.

Premenstrual Syndrome (PMS)

PMS became a popular term in the 1980s when an article appeared in the widely read *Family Circle* magazine that described it as a cyclical cluster of symptoms affecting numerous women (Northrup, 1994). To diagnose PMS properly, two factors must be present. First, PMS can occur only in a woman who is regularly menstruating and ovulating; the term relates to the *cycle* rather than the symptoms. This means that women who are pregnant, are taking birth control pills, haven't started periods yet, don't ovulate for some reason, or are postmenopausal do not experience PMS, even though they may experience some of the same symptoms. Second, for the diagnosis of PMS to be accurate, a woman must have several consecutive days when the symptoms are absent.

Up to a hundred physical symptoms have been associated with PMS. Among the more distressing physical symptoms women complain of include weight gain of several pounds, bloating and fluid retention, cramps, change in appetite (food cravings or nausea), backaches/joint/muscle pain, sleep problems, fatigue, and headaches.

Emotional symptoms include crying, irritability, anxiety, depression, impatience, mood swings, difficulty concentrating, and feeling emotionally withdrawn. A more severe form of PMS is called premenstrual dysphoric disorder (PDD) and can be helped with medication during the luteal phase of your period. You can ask your healthcare provider about PDD. We want to stress that PMS is characterized by several symptom-free days, so if you are experiencing these physical or emotional symptoms *without relief*, you could have an undiagnosed depression or another medical illness and should talk with your healthcare provider.

PMS can cause havoc in a woman's sex life. Because the symptoms include emotional fluctuations as well as physical discomfort, neither the woman nor her partner knows what to expect. Some women find that their energy goes into symptom management, and they become self-absorbed. They tune in to their bodies but tune out their sexual feelings and, many times, their partners too.

> "My husband joked that he wanted me to put a sign on the refrigerator telling him whether it was okay or not for him to touch me. I realized I was being unfair to him. He's a really good guy, and he couldn't predict what kind of response he would get from me! When I realized this, I went on-line and found some really helpful advice."

> "We never had sex. I mean never. I was getting so preoccupied with either my symptoms of PMS or my period that I shut Terry out completely. She finally got fed up. She said either I fix this or she would be out of here!"

If you have PMS, there are a number of things you can do to get help and to help yourself. The following suggestions have been helpful to many women.

Medical Evaluation

An evaluation should take into account other medical conditions that may be present. For example, we know that although PMS is not depression, women who already have depression or anxiety will be more likely to experience PMS. A medical evaluation can determine whether the use of antidepressant medication may be helpful, or whether hormonal treatment, diuretics, or over-the-counter medications may be indicated.

Relaxation Techniques and Stress Management

The most current treatments for PMS all include a combination of mind and body approaches. They encourage the woman to seek medical help and to manage the challenges of daily life through relaxation and stress management techniques. Yoga, guided imagery, progressive muscle relaxing techniques, relaxation tapes, meditation, and other techniques have proven to be useful in managing PMS.

Nutrition

Keeping blood sugar fairly even throughout the day is one way to use diet to help control PMS symptoms. Reducing salt and drinking plenty of water can help reduce bloating and water retention. Eliminating or reducing caffeine and alcohol is recommended because both can trigger irritability, anxiety, and other problems associated with PMS.

Exercise

A regular, moderate regimen of exercise is a reliable way to help manage PMS. Exercise promotes cardiovascular health, an overall sense of well-being, regulation of fluid retention, brain production of endorphins (chemicals that make you feel good), weight management, elimination of toxins in the body, and a natural alleviation of depression.

Planning for Sex

Sex and PMS aren't mutually exclusive. When you are taking care of the physical symptoms of PMS, you may feel that you are doing all the planning you can tolerate. But, as we say throughout this book, sex is a quality-of-life issue. You have a right to its pleasures. Because stress can increase the symptoms of PMS, relaxing, enjoyable sex can be quite therapeutic. Pick a time when you can dedicate an hour to sexual activity, time when you won't be exhausted. Make a plan that is reasonable—don't try to create the sexual atmosphere of a lifetime with expectations that are far too grand. Assess your bedroom plan: it should be an opportunity for pleasure without adding so many extra pressures that it undoes what you are striving to create.

CONTRACEPTION

At the dawning of the 21st century, we enjoy a sexual freedom that was not reliably available to our foremothers: birth control. A woman's ability to choose the timing of pregnancy has had a tremendous social impact, especially on women's health, careers, and relationships.

This book, which stresses self-responsibility and awareness in regard to female sexuality, would not be complete without a brief discussion of birth control. Being heterosexually active is inextricably connected with biological reproduction and the potential for pregnancy. No matter what your religious convictions or cultural mores are about pregnancy and sex, the consequences of regular heterosexual activity, including not only pregnancy but also sexually transmitted diseases, need to be considered carefully, in consultation with your healthcare provider, before you choose to be sexually active. Consider the following issues in making your choice:

1. Make your decision about which birth control method is right for you before you have sexual activity that involves—or may lead to—contact of a penis with (in or near) your vagina.
2. When reviewing the birth control methods, consider their potential effectiveness not just for birth control but also for protection from exposure to STDs. Read the section in Chapter 9 titled "One More Time: Safer Sex."
3. Determine whether any of the methods are unacceptable to you for cultural or religious reasons.
4. Decide whether you want exclusive or shared control over, and responsibility for, the birth control method. For example, oral contraceptives would provide you with a high protection against pregnancy (although no protection against STDs) and are entirely within your control, whereas using condoms is a shared responsibility (and provides the most protection, other than abstinence, against STDs).
5. If you are in a committed relationship, include your partner in the decision-making process, incorporating his values and preferences.
6. Factor in any medical limitations. For example, if you are a smoker, you may not be able to use an oral contraceptive method.
7. Consider when you may want to become pregnant in the future, and include this concern in your discussion with your healthcare provider.
8. When you have made an informed choice of a birth control method, stand back and seriously assess whether there are any reasons why you would not consistently use this method, then address these concerns.

With the exception of abstinence and the use of a condom with spermicide, the birth control methods discussed here do not prevent sexually transmitted diseases, although diaphragms and hormonal methods may reduce the risk of pelvic inflammatory disease. All effective methods of birth control reduce anxiety about unwanted (or "pre-wanted") pregnancy and therefore have a beneficial impact on sexual activity. When we refer to the advantages and disadvantages of each method, we mean primarily in regard to its impact on sex.

Avoiding Sexual Intercourse

Avoiding intercourse is a reliable way of avoiding pregnancy. For abstinence to be effective, it must include the prevention of any ejaculate from coming into contact with the vaginal introitus. Sperm are motile (they swim), so couples should be cautious even if their sexual activity does not include intercourse. Avoiding intercourse is a choice many women make for periods of time in their life. It is a choice that should be respected fully. In no way is it a reflection on how "sexy" a woman is.

Natural Family Planning

In natural family planning, you abstain from sexual intercourse during fertile periods of your menstrual cycle. Generally this is determined by charting basal body temperature, which is the lowest body temperature reached during waking hours. Your body temperature rises during the phase of your cycle after ovulation, when progesterone is higher. You can also chart your cervical mucus and vaginal discharge because there are changes in the consistency of the mucus near ovulation.

Natural family planning is the most effective if sexual intercourse is avoided during the first half of the cycle. The accidental pregnancy rate is high, but this method can be fairly reliable for women who have a regular menstrual cycle and follow the procedure carefully and consistently. It is important to note that women with irregular menstrual cycles are often unable to use natural family planning.

The disadvantages of this method include the fear of accidental conception, which may impact sexual responsiveness, and a feeling of pressure, in one or both partners, to have intercourse during the "safe" times because the number of these days is limited. The advantages are that both partners participate in this decision and assume mutual responsibility.

Preventing the Egg from Maturing

Hormonal control—using synthetic hormones in various combinations—works to suppress ovulation. The hormonal effects vary according to the composition of the medication used. Some hormonal contraceptives, like birth control pills, are a combination of synthetic estrogen and progestin. The effect of estrogen is to stop ovulation by inhibiting the FSH. The effect of progestin is to reduce fertility by preventing the secretion of LH and altering the cervical mucus so that sperm can't penetrate.

The primary advantage to hormonal control is its effectiveness and simplicity. A woman using this method doesn't have to think about birth control during lovemaking or chart body changes during her menstrual cycle; she only needs to remember to take pills or get the injections or the hormonal implant.

Birth Control Pills (Oral Contraceptives)

Birth control pills are very popular. The lower dosage of today's oral contraceptives compared to the dosages used when the pill first was used decades ago, results in generally minimal side effects. There are some strong medical contraindications to using the pill, such as smoking, high blood pressure, or a history of blood clots, which is why birth control pills need to be prescribed and monitored by a medical practitioner. The birth control pill offers some women benefits beyond contraception, including less pain during menstrual periods and lighter periods with less iron loss. Disadvantages of using the pill are the possible medical problems that can arise. For most women, the risk of developing a medical problem is low, but each woman should discuss this issue with her healthcare provider.

A new form of hormonal birth control, similar to the pill in function, is an injection of hormones time-released over a one-month period. But you'll need to see your healthcare practitioner on a monthly basis, because this injection cannot be self-administered.

Norplant

Norplant is an effective progestin contraceptive implant. During an office visit a healthcare provider uses a local anesthetic to numb the upper arm, and the Norplant System—six matchstick-sized flexible synthetic implants—is placed under the skin. It is permanent, effective for up to five years (although it can be removed at any time) and its effects are fairly quickly reversible. You don't have to worry about remembering to take pills or to be concerned about the "safe" days of your cycle. Issues discussed under oral contraceptives apply for both Norplant and the next method, Depo-Provera.

Depo-Provera

With this method, ovulation is prevented by an injection of progestin, which is effective for about three months. (Actually, ovulation sometimes occurs with progestin-only methods, but the other effects of progestin prevent pregnancy.) Most women have irregular spotting at first with Depo-Provera, and about 50% experience the complete cessation of their periods if they use this method of birth control for a year or so. Depo-Provera is used worldwide. Progestin can also be administered in pill form.

Keeping Sperm from Doing Its Job

Spermicides

Spermicides are topical creams or gels, foams, and suppositories that are designed to kill sperm. Most condoms contain a spermicide, but you should check the packet to make sure; otherwise a separate spermicide should be obtained. Furthermore, spermicidally lubricated condoms do not provide as much protection as a condom plus spermicide. To be effective, spermicides should be used with condoms or other barrier methods such as a diaphragm. The disadvantage is that sexual activity will be interrupted briefly to apply the spermicide. With creativity, however, this disruption can be minimized by making the application of the spermicide part of the lovemaking, as opposed to treating it as a temporary time-out.

Intrauterine Device (IUD)

There are currently only two IUDs available for use in the United States: one, a copper-wrapped device and the other, a progestin-releasing device. An IUD is inserted into the uterus by a healthcare provider under careful conditions and only after a thorough evaluation of the appropriateness of this contraceptive for the woman requesting the device. There are important considerations to choosing this method, which your healthcare provider will review with you.

The uterus responds to the insertion of an IUD by producing inflammatory cells and white blood cells in the uterine lining, preventing sperm from surviving in the uterus or reaching the fallopian tubes. The hormonal IUD alters the cervical mucus so that sperm cannot easily penetrate. It was once believed that IUDs allowed fertilization to take place but prevented the fertilized egg from implanting in the uterus. Recent studies indicate, however, that modern IUDs prevent pregnancy by preconception mechanisms, especially by thickening the cervical mucus so that it is impenetrable to the sperm. The progesterone IUD has many of the same effects as Norplant or Depo-Provera.

Contrary to popular belief, IUDs do not cause infections. However, they can enable sexually transmitted disease organisms to more easily enter the fallopian tubes. Only women who are in permanent, stable, and monogamous relationships should use IUDs. Multiple sex partners increase the risk of pelvic inflammatory disease. The presence of an IUD does not affect sexual response or activity, except by enabling spontaneity.

Keeping Egg and Sperm Apart

Withdrawal Method

Some couples rely on the male withdrawing his penis from the vagina when he experiences ejaculatory inevitability—the feeling that ejaculation is about to happen at any moment. This method has serious drawbacks, including a high rate of undesired pregnancy and the interruption of sexual activity at a moment when both partners are at a heightened point of arousal. We do not endorse this as an effective birth control method.

Condoms

Condoms can be very effective—but not if they are sitting in a jacket pocket or on a bedside table. Aside from abstinence, condoms with a spermicide are the only effective (although not perfect) protection against sexually transmitted diseases. Condoms are thin latex "rubbers" that, ideally, are rolled onto the erect penis before there is any contact between penis and vagina.

For condoms to be most effective, proper use is essential. Condoms should be used only once and then discarded. Room should be left at the tip of the condom for the semen to collect following ejaculation. Using a "retain" double latex ring in addition to the condom can prevent slippage of the condom. These rings are available at most condom shops or sex paraphernalia shops and at some pharmacies. They can also be purchased at several of the "sex store" websites we list in the "Suggested Resources" section. Condoms should not be lubricated with petroleum jelly or any other oil-based substance because these can break down the thin latex coating. If additional lubrication is needed, a water-based lubricant can be used.

A drawback to using condoms is that sexual activity can be interrupted when the time comes to put on the condom. With imagination and creativity, however, putting on a condom can be quite erotic and happily incorporated into the lovemaking.

Vasectomy

A vasectomy surgically alters the *vas deferens* (the tube that connects the testicle to the penis) so that sperm cannot unite with the fluid expelled during ejaculation. This procedure is permanent and has the advantage that birth control does not have to be considered during sexual activity. Although a vasectomy can sometimes be reversed, there are no guarantees that the surgical repair will be effective.

Diaphragm or Cervical Cap

Both the diaphragm and cervical cap are made of flexible latex and are fitted specifically to a woman's body by a healthcare practitioner. It is important that you have the opportunity to insert the diaphragm/cap and check its position while you are in your clinician's office. The purpose of the diaphragm/cap is to prevent semen from entering the cervix. A spermicide must be used in conjunction with these methods. Interrupting sexual activity to put in a diaphragm/cap is a drawback to its use. It is difficult to eroticize the insertion of a diaphragm/cap because it has to be placed correctly, but this drawback can be avoided by inserting it up to two hours before sexual intercourse is anticipated. Normally a diaphragm/cap won't be dislodged by urination, a bowel movement, or other normal activity, but the position of the cap or diaphragm should be checked prior to the time of intercourse.

Female Condoms

The female condom is a relatively new contraceptive device that also offers some protection against sexually transmitted diseases. These condoms are made of polyurethane—prelubricated plastic about twice the thickness of the latex condoms but still very thin. They are one size, soft, and have a flexible ring at each end. The condom is closed at one end, like a male condom. The flexible ring that inserts into the vagina is positioned over the cervix, much like a diaphragm. The condom acts as a barrier between the penis and the vaginal wall. The condom extends outside from the vaginal opening and is visible. At first it may seem disconcerting and cumbersome to the users who are not accustomed to seeing a vaginal/vulva contraceptive.

Interrupting the Journey of the Egg by Tubal Ligation

A surgical procedure altering the fallopian tubes so that a mature egg cannot travel through the tubes is an effective, permanent form of birth control. As with vasectomy, before choosing this method women should carefully consider whether a pregnancy could be desired in the future. *This method is not reversible.*

The procedure is commonly done through a laparoscope, which is a unique telescopic instrument inserted into the abdomen. As with any medical procedure, complications can occur. Research shows that about 2% of these procedures have some type of medical complication. Other than the need for a brief period of sexual abstinence immediately following surgery, this procedure does not impact sexual function.

Preventing Implantation of a Fertilized Egg

The "morning after" pill, a high-dose estrogen or a combination of estrogen and progestin, can be administered under medical supervision within 72 hours after intercourse; its effectiveness most potent within 12 to 24 hours. This hormonal intervention alters the lining of the uterus so that a fertilized egg does not implant, and it alters the corpus luteum so that fertilization cannot occur. It also changes the character of the cervical mucus, alters tubal motility, prevents ovulation, and may cause nausea and vomiting, depending on the hormonal composition of the pill used. It has a 75% rate of effectiveness—which means that one out of four women using this method get pregnant.

PREGNANCY

> "When the results of the pregnancy test were positive, my feelings came in a flood. I felt scared and happy and anxious all at the same time."

The significance of pregnancy for our discussion about female sexuality is that girls and women generally associate their sexuality with reproduction and often view their bodies in the context of having the capacity to bear children. This capacity is inextricably linked with being a woman, and each woman has to manage this complex awareness in her own way.

The ever-present issues surrounding conception—as much a part of being a woman as are breasts, ovaries, and a vagina—have tremendous significance in the course of a woman's life. Think of the challenges a 24-year-old single woman faces if she decides to have a tubal ligation because she does not want to be a parent. Think of the grief of a couple coping with invasive and expensive technology in the hopes of conceiving, or a 14-year-old girl who ignores obvious signs of pregnancy because she can't bear to consider the consequences. Consider the 38-year-old single woman who is considering donor insemination because her "biological clock" is ticking and she is not in a relationship. Reflect for a moment on the agonizing choices many women have to make between career and motherhood. Imagine the challenge confronting the lesbian couple who may face multiple layers of "coming out" to employers, coworkers, and family members because of their choice to become pregnant. There are as many personal and poignant stories about reproduction as there are individual women in the world.

Prenatal care cannot begin too early to help assure a healthy outcome for woman and child. Books on pregnancy focus on all possible aspects of pregnancy, labor, delivery, and the postpartum period and are an excellent and easily obtained resource. Your midwife or physician can guide you toward the resources most relevant to your needs.

Our goal here is to provide an overview of possible sexual activity during pregnancy and the postpartum period. In addition, we address the possible impact of infertility treatments on sexuality. We are not at all suggesting that the areas we have selected to discuss are the most important issues regarding pregnancy, only the most pertinent for our consideration of sexuality.

Sexual Activity during Pregnancy

Sexual activity during pregnancy refers to masturbation or activity with a partner resulting in high sexual arousal, including lubrication, blood engorgement of the genitals, and often orgasm. Pregnancy, of course, brings enormous physical, emotional, and hormonal changes, as well as the anticipated presence of the new baby. Each stage of pregnancy—and, in some cases, special circumstances related to pregnancy—tend to create different challenges and raise questions about sexual activity.

> "When I was pregnant, I got worried that sexual activity or my exercise class might hurt the baby."

A developing fetus is well protected against physical sensations from the outside. The cervix has a mucus plug that blocks any direct passage of foreign material into the uterus—the baby's growing place. The fetus is enclosed in a protective amniotic sac of fluid, so jarring movements are experienced by the developing baby as a rocking or bobbing. Sexual activity should definitely be suspended, however, if there is any bleeding, loss of amniotic fluid, contractions, or on the advice of your healthcare provider.

Pregnancy, Previous Miscarriage, and Sex

In her book *Men, Women and Infertility*, Aline Zoldbrod (1993) describes the distress of a woman who suffered a miscarriage: "[She] was frightened of having sex while she was pregnant and said that she pictured the 'fetus attached to my body by only the thinnest of threads.' This woman saw her husband's penis as a 'giant intruder that will destroy the baby' " (p. 55). Women in a similar circumstance may find that they entertain fearful scenarios about sexual activity during pregnancy. The dangers may not be in line with reality, but women who are apprehensive because of previous loss will not find simple reassurance adequate. We recommend talking—early and often—with your prenatal health practitioner if you find you identify with these concerns. The practitioner can talk with you about your specific fears and help you prevent those fears from escalating further. Any sexually stimulating activity, including masturbation, should be cleared with your healthcare provider as well.

Sex in the First Trimester of Pregnancy

Breast tenderness is common during early pregnancy. Most women experience some breast growth along with increased breast sensitivity. Touch that once was fun, playful, and arousing may become uncomfortable. The additional rush of blood to sore breast tissue during sexual arousal may make breasts exquisitely tender for a time. Couples can compensate for this by experimenting with controlled touch and nipple stimulation, being careful to avoid anything the woman finds uncomfortable, and maintaining a special awareness of the need for gentleness.

Early pregnancy often includes two other physical experiences that are incompatible with feelings of sexiness: nausea and extreme fatigue. It is helpful to remember that these early symptoms tend to diminish after the first three months, although feeling tired and needing more rest are normal for the duration of pregnancy.

One liberating factor for women who have just become pregnant and their partners is that they don't have to put energy into *not* getting pregnant. Some women who were constantly anxious about getting pregnant discover that, once pregnant, they can relax and enjoy sex.

Even in the first trimester of pregnancy the genitals and vagina swell and engorge with blood, contributing to a feeling of pelvic and genital "fullness." This, in turn, can lead to enhanced sensitivity and arousal during sexual stimulation. Vaginal secretions are also increased.

Sex in the Second Trimester of Pregnancy

Pregnancy is a time for you to learn about your body in ways you never have before. Typically, you will ask questions about your body, its changes, and the baby's development. You can take this opportunity to learn about, and practice control of, your pelvic floor muscles—muscles involved not only in labor and delivery but also in the pleasurable contractions of orgasm.

The second trimester is generally physically more comfortable than the first. Vaginal tissues have engorged with blood, making them similar in appearance to tissue engorged during sexual arousal. The extra blood supply often changes the color of the tissue to a more vivid or darker color. When these factors combine—increased blood engorgement making genitals more sensitive, alleviation of some of the uncomfortable symptoms of earliest pregnancy, more self-awareness about your body, and increased confidence in the pregnancy's viability—you may find yourself more sexually aroused, interested, and responsive than ever before. In fact, some women experience their first multiple orgasms during this phase of pregnancy. In some cases, pregnancy creates an increased blood supply to the pelvic area, which can also contribute to increased arousal and orgasmic response *after* pregnancy.

Even if you are highly sexually responsive and desire sex, however, your partner may not share your enthusiasm. The partner who is overly anxious because of fears of hurting the fetus should find the time to talk openly, ask questions, and explore these concerns with his or her health practitioner.

Sex in Late Pregnancy

Adjusting to body changes during later pregnancy becomes a unique part of a woman's sex life. If motivated to overcome the challenge of making love with a bulging, pregnant abdomen, couples can continue to have sexual contact throughout pregnancy, and you can continue to masturbate, unless medically advised not to.

Adapting sexual positions to accommodate pregnancy can give you an expanded sexual repertoire. Intercourse is far from the only sexual experience you can have, but if you desire penile penetration, you may find that rear-entry positions are both comfortable and erotic. Face-to-face sexual intercourse may work best in a side-by-side or sitting position. Sexual intercourse with you lying on your back and your partner on top will work best if he props himself up on his hands to avoid too much direct pressure on your abdomen. This isn't a precaution due to danger to the baby but because it might be uncomfortable due to pressure on your bladder and diaphragm.

Concerns about Sex Starting Labor

Orgasm causes uterine contractions, and nipple stimulation with hands or mouth frequently causes strong uterine contractions as well. However, it is important to note that uterine contractions are present throughout pregnancy. In fact, as pregnancy proceeds, a woman will be aware of "Braxton Hicks" contractions that aren't labor contractions but more of a rehearsal. Real labor is not going to start because of an orgasm, unless the body is ready to go into labor anyway.

There are hormones associated with both sexual activity and labor. Oxytocin is a hormone associated with the beginnings of labor and one of the hormones released during sexual arousal. The uterus becomes more sensitive to oxytocin as pregnancy comes to its last few weeks. The increasing sensitivity to oxytocin builds up and culminates in the spontaneous initiation of labor.

Prostaglandins may also be associated with the onset of labor. Because semen carries a higher concentration of prostaglandins than any other substance in the body, semen coming into contact with the cervix may sometimes help induce labor. In fact, engaging in sexual intercourse and allowing the deepest penetration possible, with the penis actually touching the cervix, is a method of using sex to start labor in a full-term pregnancy described by Sheila Kitzinger (1985) in her book *The Complete Book of Pregnancy and Childbirth* (p. 151). To ensure the effectiveness of this method, make sure your partner's penis remains inside of you for a few minutes after ejaculation, so that the cervix is in direct contact with the semen.

This natural method of inducing labor seems to work for some women, although discomfort due to the physical state of being at the end of pregnancy may be a barrier to trying. Also, it is very important to caution against trying this method if the mucus plug has loosened (there may be some bloody "show"), if there is any leaking of amniotic fluid, or any other medical contraindication. It is best to discuss this option with your healthcare provider before attempting it.

Sexual Activity after Pregnancy

A number of factors influence a woman's sexual feelings and responses shortly after a pregnancy ends. First, life is different. Even if the end of the pregnancy has been the uncomplicated birth of a much-wanted child, life is much more demanding and tiring for everyone in the household, particularly for you as a new mom. If the pregnancy has ended sadly, then grief and a pervasive sense of loss may affect your sexual feelings. If your baby is kept in a neonatal unit after birth and doesn't go home with you, you will be preoccupied and concerned about your baby's condition.

Hormonal and other physical changes postpregnancy can be profound. Some women experience postpartum depression and feel completely overwhelmed for a time. Mood changes, crying jags, and feeling overwhelmed are normal responses soon after childbirth but should be addressed with practitioners if you haven't rebounded by the time of your first postpartum visit. Estrogen and progesterone levels are low soon after childbirth, and this may cause vaginal dryness. Nursing mothers may also experience some thinning of vaginal tissue due to low estrogen.

You may be able to compensate for this condition by using supplemental lubrication or an estrogen cream, but first discuss the possibility with your healthcare provider.

Physical discomfort may be present to some degree after childbirth. Some women have to heal from an episiotomy (an incision in the perineum to prevent tearing of tissue during childbirth) or a Cesarean section. The episiotomy site may remain tender for weeks or months after childbirth, making the pressure and stretching of vaginal penetration uncomfortable for a time. For a few weeks after childbirth you may have heavy bleeding, like an extended menstrual period, and breasts may be sore from milk engorgement.

Body Changes

After childbirth, the vagina, cervix, and muscles in the pelvic floor may be changed. Although some changes are normal, you may experience them as *ab*normal for you. You may have to learn about your somewhat changed body by experimenting with new sexual positions and stimulation. The differences themselves may be very minor, but coupled with all the other recent life changes, they may lead to some distress that you did not anticipate.

For a number of weeks postpartum, you may want to take your time working back into a full range of sexual activity. This may mean holding off on penetration for some weeks or even months, perhaps rejoining your partner in tender and intimate activities like kissing, holding, and stroking. Some women heal very easily postepisiotomy, and other women take months before they are comfortable with penetration. It is important for a woman to attend to *her* feelings in this regard: it never works to grit one's teeth and endure uncomfortable penetration. This can easily set up a cycle of physical tension, hypervigilance, and anticipation of pain rather than experiencing comfortable sexual feelings or pleasure. Painful conditions should always be addressed medically if things aren't back to normal several months after childbirth.

Just after pregnancy you may wonder whose body it is, anyway! You seem to have more body secretions than you ever imagined would be possible. If nursing, your breasts may leak and sometimes even squirt breast milk when stimulated. Some women love and regret nursing, all at the same time; they cherish the bonding and closeness with their infant and, at the same time, sigh and wonder if they will *ever* have claim to their bodies.

Some couples like the wetness and earthiness of sex after pregnancy. They report that they feel freer than ever before because it is impossible to hold on to some high-gloss and/or pristine notion of sex. They enjoy the stickiness and fun of milky breasts that can squirt a stream of milk several feet, vaginal secretions that are more copious, and even the occasional leakage of urine during orgasm because of the temporary relaxation of pelvic floor muscles.

Those women who feel highly self-conscious because of the perceived "messiness" of sex during this time have yet to become accustomed to their body—which seems to change every day and doesn't feel like their own.

Partners are sometimes surprised to learn about the other's feelings as the postpregnancy adjustment continues. Occasionally couples have a misunderstanding about the territory of breasts during nursing. Some partners feel left out or even replaced if the new mother is uncomfortable with her partner fondling and stroking her breasts while she is still nursing—an activity the woman may have previously loved and enjoyed. Communicating openly, even about negative thoughts and responses, forestalls many potential problems.

What does all of this suggest about sex after pregnancy? First, some recovery time is normal, and adjusting to healing may involve a process rather than a set endpoint. Second, there will be environmental changes of a demanding nature. A sense of humor and patience will be helpful for both you and your partner as you integrate your new life state. You will do well to anticipate some of the demands of this particular time, and talk about it. You can remind yourselves that sex involves far more than intercourse. With this understanding, you can take advantage of even a few minutes of time to share physical and emotional closeness. (See also Chapter 2 for further discussion of this topic in *And Baby Makes Three.*)

Cesarean Section

If a woman has given birth by C-section, she is recovering from major abdominal surgery as well as childbirth. For a while, it may seem to her that it is all she can do to pull herself to a sitting position or get out of bed. Her healthcare team should give her information on C-section recovery, including care of her incision, abdominal exercises, and what she can expect in the healing process. In addition to the physical discomfort, there may also be feelings of not having had her baby the "right way." It can be very helpful for a woman to talk about these feelings with her nurse, midwife, physician, and other women who have had C-sections.

> "A few weeks after my C-section, Tashi and I tried to have intercourse. My vagina wasn't sore, and I wasn't bleeding much. But it hurt at my C-section incision. Thank goodness Tashi is very easy-going. He said we would take it easy—and we did. We kept asking each other how we were doing. In a way, it was like birth: Tashi coached me through my entire experience, and now I was coaching him through this one."

After a C-section, you will need to pace lovemaking and intercourse in concert with your returning strength and flexibility. Because you are recovering from major abdominal surgery, you may feel protective of the surgical incision and somewhat self-conscious about your shaven pubic hair. If the C-section was unexpected, you may also be recovering from the exhaustion of labor and the disappointment that things didn't go "naturally."

When a woman has a C-section, she becomes the teacher for herself and her partner. She will need to think about what feels good to her, where she would like to be touched. For some women, the incision scar remains extremely sensitive; for others it is a non-issue. If a woman has fear about the incision splitting open with the strain of lovemaking, she will need to talk with her healthcare provider to reassure herself. This may be true for her partner as well. (In reality, surgical incisions are closed in multiple layers and do not burst open.)

INFERTILITY

> "When the pregnancy test after our latest procedure turned out to be negative, after all we'd gone through, I was devastated and felt dead inside. We'd already long given up on some romantic notion of conceiving, and now I felt like giving up on the whole business."

Infertility is often a profound personal experience. Medically, infertility is defined as a year of being sexually active without using birth control during intercourse, and not getting pregnant. The term is also used for women who are able to get pregnant but have a pattern of repeated pregnancy loss. As many as one in seven women experience infertility, and about half of that number go on to successfully complete a pregnancy. Most infertility is traceable to a medically defined cause, but about 3% of the time, no cause can be determined—everything looks just fine but pregnancy doesn't occur. Even for those infertility cases where a cause is evident, treatment and intervention are not always successful.

Often treatment becomes a gamble with very high stakes. You may begin infertility treatment with very firm ideas about how far you will go, but the seemingly endless array of treatment options holds out the tantalizing possibility that the outcome will be a baby. For many couples, taking another chance seems worth yet another risk and investment of hope.

In the next sections, we're going to take a look at how infertility impacts a woman's sexuality and steps that can be taken to minimize this impact.

Sexual Difficulties Related to Infertility

Infertility and Postovulation Sex

If you are in active treatment for infertility, you probably have experienced sex as a means to an end: pregnancy. The timing of intercourse around ovulation is prescribed and planned and therefore may have little or nothing to do with pleasure or sexual desire. In addition, you may experience tremendous frustration because so little of your reproductive life or sexual life is in your control during the period of active treatment.

What we have observed is that a woman in this situation will often have perfunctory sex around the prescribed time for intercourse, will prop up her pelvis afterwards to get the ejaculate fluid moving in the right direction, and will thereafter do anything possible not to disturb any potentially fertilized egg. For many couples, the days following ovulation and active attempts to get pregnant are days of self-imposed abstinence. What they don't realize is that the uterine contractions caused by orgasm, the thrusting from sexual intercourse, and the fluid from semen will not keep a fertilized egg from implanting in the uterus or dislodge a newly implanted embryo.

Sexual Problems in Response to Infertility Treatment

It would be more common than uncommon for you to complain of temporary sexual difficulties at some point during infertility treatment. Having sexual intercourse not motivated by desire can be a daunting experience for anyone. Sometimes couples are successfully able to separate out their "functional" sex from what they consider to be the real essence of their sexuality together. This can be challenging, however, and it is common for one or both partners to find themselves avoiding sex at times. This is because sexual contact can be such a vivid reminder of what they are longing for (pregnancy); instead of being a source of relief and pleasure, sex in these circumstances is a reminder of pain and loss.

Sexual Problems Caused by Infertility Treatment

Sexual problems actually caused by infertility treatment are much less common. If this happens to you, you need to talk with your healthcare provider to determine whether the problem is occurring as a result of the infertility treatment or as part of a preexisting problem.

> Mavis was in her bed on her back with her knees flexed and her eyes tightly closed. She didn't want to disappoint Sherm, but she certainly wasn't into sex this time. Mavis hadn't noticed that Sherm reached for lubricant. His hands touched her body for several moments. When he inserted two lubricated fingers into her vagina, Mavis felt her stomach muscles go rigid. Her entire body became stiff with hyperawareness. Sherm's fingers felt like a speculum to her, and she flinched away from his hand. She began to cry with the intensity of her reaction.

Mavis was already tense due to a recent medical procedure related to her infertility evaluation. Afterwards, her reactions during sex with her partner were tense, anxious, and avoidant. In circumstances like the ones faced by Mavis and Sherm, it is likely such an emotional response would be disarming to both the woman and her partner. If this has happened to you, we would advise you to resume sexual activity gradually, paying particular attention to your responses and avoiding any circumstances, at least for a brief time, that can re-create the problem. This may mean that you will refrain from sexual intercourse temporarily. It may mean changing the time/place/initiation/position to see if that will alleviate the stress, or at least decrease it. Although couples who are in the midst of infertility treatment don't want to miss even one month of opportunity, we believe that ignoring sexual problems only compounds the stressful situation.

Body and Self-Image Problems

How can the hidden stresses of infertility impact your body image, self-esteem, and sense of sexuality? We can count the ways!

First, reproductive and sexual organs are pathologized or at least scrutinized for possible pathology; it's difficult to maintain a positive sense of self and body in the midst of infinitesimal medical assessments of what is going wrong. Second, you have connected your personal identity with being able to conceive a baby—a natural enough connection, given the circumstances. Third, sex becomes inadvertently paired with a sense of failure and loss; each menstrual cycle brings a reminder that the wished-for baby is yet out of your reach. Fourth, medical and hormonal treatments (if you are in such treatment) have their own impact on emotions and feelings. Fifth, infertility is socially isolating: you may be out of synch with your own goals to start a family, while your friends and family members may be proceeding quite nicely with the same goals. To make matters worse, friends and relatives can be everything from clueless to sympathetic regarding your plight, and often inadvertently cause you and your partner to feel even more isolated due to their lack of support and understanding.

What to Do about Sexual Problems Associated with Infertility

Just relax. What couple experiencing infertility doesn't cringe to hear those words? Still, there is something to be said for taking a break from infertility treatment for a few months if this is feasible. Some couples find it helpful to step away briefly from the stress of trying to conceive and to find comfort in being relaxed and enjoying lovemaking that isn't on demand.

Change the routine. As therapists, we are always stressing that sexual activity is much more than intercourse. Couples can experiment with non-demand (not focused on penetration or orgasm/ejaculation) sexual activities and be pleasantly gratified.

Don't focus on the success stories of others. We consider this a tar baby—the more you focus on the success of others, the more negative you feel about yourself. Along the same lines, be critical of much of the advice offered by others. For example, the exhortation, "Don't get discouraged, think about the positive things you already have" sounds good, but it's much easier said than felt. If you take such exhortations to heart, you may find yourself on a slippery slope to more social isolation. Your feelings of failure will only increase when you realize (probably quickly) that you can't live up to the well-intentioned but often naïve advice of others.

Our recommendation is to be sure that you have interests and activities that are compelling and important to you, preferably physical ones. One woman found something healing in tending her flower garden. If this seems peripherally related to sex and intimacy, consider it more carefully: if you identify and practice focusing on activities other than basal temperature and ovulatory cycle, you will have an experiential foundation for pleasure, sensuality, and other positive responses. You will be able to build on that success to explore enjoyable, not just functional, sex and intimacy.

THE SECOND PART OF ADULT LIFE: MENOPAUSE AND BEYOND

As life expectancy continues to increase, you can look forward to having as many adult years postmenopause as you have during adult reproductive years. Menopause indeed brings challenges—not since adolescence has your body gone through such developmental changes. But you are not an adolescent in your ability to cope with these changes. You are tested and tenacious. You have experience in problem solving, and wit and humor are on your side. See Chapter 2 for further discussion about sexuality and aging.

Menopause Terminology

Menopause has long been misunderstood, so it's not surprising that the terms used to describe phases around menopause are confusing. If a woman has hot flashes and irregular periods for a few months and consults her healthcare provider, she may be told she is menopausal, premenopausal, perimenopausal, in the climacteric, or in a "situation that will just bear watching for a few months."

Sorting out terminology might be a good place to start for understanding menopause. Although technically menopause refers to a woman's last period, commonly the term is used to refer to the entire span of time during which ovarian function declines and periods stop. This time period is normally years in duration, generally encompassing ages 45–55, but the onset of menopause occurs for some women in their 30s. The average age of last menstrual flow is about 51 years. It takes 12 consecutive months of no periods to determine when menopause happened, so the actual time when menopause occurs can only be established long after the fact. The *perimenopause* or *climacteric* phase occurs about 12 to 24 months (in some cases, longer) before the last menstrual period, and is characterized by symptoms such as irregular periods and hot flashes. *Postmenopause* refers to the period of life starting 12 months after the last menstrual period.

Physical Changes Associated with Menopause

There are a number of physical changes associated with menopause. We will briefly discuss them here and also refer you to the "Suggested Resources" list at the end of this book. In Chapter 4 we discuss the impact of menopause on sexual response.

Ovarian Estrogen Production

During the perimenopause, estrogen production by the ovaries declines to about 10% of the level of the estrogen produced prior to perimenopause. At menopause, the ovaries disregard the signals to produce estrogen. It's the body's way of indicating that the woman's reproductive time is coming to an end. Ovarian-produced estrogen is called *estradiol*; only this form of estrogen decreases dramatically at menopause. *Estrone* estrogen, manufactured by, and stored in, the body's fat cells and other tissue, continues to be present in the bloodstream because its production isn't controlled by ovarian function.

Changes in the Vulva and Vagina

The vulva and vagina are very responsive to estrogen levels. Elasticity, lubrication, and thickness of the vaginal walls are affected by declining estrogen, and the tissues of the labia majora and minora become less engorged during sexual arousal. The mucous membrane lining of the vagina is particularly susceptible to irritation, minor injury, and infection as the capacity to produce lubrication decreases. Normally thick and cushiony, the vaginal walls can thin during menopause and after. The actual size of the vagina shrinks, as does the uterus. The cervix may atrophy (shrivel) and flatten out to the wall of the vagina. The Venus mound, or mons (described in Chapter 3), loses plumpness and definition.

Changes in the lining of the urethra and bladder can cause irritation as well, leading to an annoying need to urinate frequently. Supporting muscles to the internal organs lose elasticity because of reduced blood flow to the pelvis. This is especially distressing if it leads to involuntary urine loss (urinary incontinence) when coughing, laughing, exercising, or having sex. Some women experience thinning of their hair, including pubic hair. This can be as distressing for a woman as it is for a man.

Hot Flashes

Hot flashes, or flushes, have sometimes been called "power surges." A hot flash may not seem so empowering to a woman overcome by a sudden flush of heat radiating to all parts of her body. She is more likely to feel claustrophobic than powerful. Hot flashes happen to most perimenopausal women as their bodies react to dramatic fluctuations in estrogen. Though not entirely understood, hot flashes often are triggered by a stimulus, such as sitting in an uncomfortably warm room or experiencing stress and pressure. Most women on hormone replacement therapy experience significant relief from hot flashes. Vitamin E and other herbal remedies are also reported to be effective, though you should check with your healthcare provider to make sure they are safe for you to take.

Secondary Health Concerns

Cardiovascular

Heart disease is the number one cause of death in postmenopausal women. Although men tend to have heart attacks during their 40s, women seldom do because of the protective effect of their estrogen prior to menopause. Estrogen and progesterone both influence a woman's cardiovascular system. As estrogen production declines, "bad cholesterol" (LDL) tends to increase because blood lipid patterns have changed. Once they lose the protection of estrogen, women are more prone to heart attacks and stroke. Hormone replacement therapy may help postmenopausal women regain some cardiovascular protection.

Osteoporosis

Osteoporosis means porous bones. As women age, their bones lose density. This is a gradual process of aging, but it's noticed most dramatically at menopause when estrogen levels drop. Bones can become significantly more brittle and, at the same time, take on a honeycomb quality, making them much more susceptible to breakage. Hormone replacement therapy and supplemental calcium can substantially help this serious health problem.

Mood Swings and Decreased Concentration

Menopause has been blamed for a number of emotional problems. If menopause caused such problems as depression, anxiety, and memory loss, it would stand to reason that estrogen therapy or homeopathic treatments would then undo these symptoms. In fact, estrogen and other therapies do not cure clinical depression. The bottom line is that menopause may bring some temporary emotional disequilibrium, but it is a normal, not debilitating, condition. If you find that you have lost interest in activities in which you have previously taken pleasure; if you have sleep disturbance that is not responsive to estrogen or homeopathic treatment; if you feel consistently sad or hopeless or unable to concentrate effectively; and/or if someone close to you expresses concern about your mood, get an evaluation for clinical depression. Don't delay or let a medical practitioner minimize or rationalize these concerns.

Hormone Therapy

Hormone replacement therapy, or HRT for short, most commonly involves estrogen, or estrogen combined with progestin, a synthetic form of progesterone. If you are one of the women who cannot take estrogen, there are now effective treatment alternatives that you can discuss with your healthcare provider.

HRT can greatly relieve the symptoms of menopause, but no decision about hormone therapy should be made without careful, individual evaluation and discussion with your healthcare provider. Fewer than half of women who are postmenopausal are on hormone therapy, despite the obvious, even life-prolonging benefits many women could receive from this treatment. However, hormone therapy is not for every woman. Women are complex individuals; personalities and preferences differ, and so do reactions to hormonal intervention. Tailoring the hormonal replacement to one's individual needs is most important.

We recommend that you discuss hormone therapy with your healthcare provider before you need it. If you're not satisfied with your healthcare provider's knowledge and interest in menopausal women, get another opinion. Pay attention to new information about hormone therapy as it becomes available, but be discriminating. Go with the "preponderance of evidence," not with the latest news flash. Some news-media stories about medications include incomplete information or initial findings that are later contradicted by further scientific investigation. Hormone therapy is no substitute for self-care. You've heard it before, but the essentials for managing your health are still good nutrition and exercise.

PART III

Making Peace with Your Body

If you're alienated from your own body, you're shut off from an important source of pleasure and deprived of a vital means of connecting with special people in your life. In our modern culture, the media incessantly remind women that their bodies are woefully imperfect and that the quest for happiness is a quest for youth and beauty. For many women, to engage in sex is to focus on their perceived inadequacies rather than on pleasure and intimacy. To feel sexual desire, women first have to feel desirable—no small challenge in a culture that pays homage to the beauty myth peddled by Madison Avenue.

Feelings of alienation from your body can be intensified even further if you have been sexually abused, have contracted a sexually transmitted disease, have been diagnosed with a serious illness, find sex physically painful, or live with a disability. In the face of any of these challenges, you may even feel betrayed by your body. As a defense, you may try to distance yourself from all physical feeling and sensation. You may try to retreat to a world of thoughts and words, devoid of any pleasure that can come from touch, caressing, or the mingling of bodies.

In Part III, we examine the challenges that can alienate women from their bodies and explore how they can take care of their sexual selves by making peace with their physical selves. In this section you can learn to have a positive sexual identity that includes your physical appearance. You can come to terms with your uniqueness as a female and learn to feel comfortable in your body. The following chapters provide specific self-help strategies to help you move from fear to knowledge and from victimhood to empowerment. Exercises for those who want to take this work further are in the Appendix.

Chapters 6–10 address the questions our clients frequently bring us:

- I haven't been able to rise above the media's portrayal of women and feel good about the way I look, so how can I teach my daughter to do it?
- I'd love to love my body the way my partner claims to love it, but how can I deny what I see in the mirror?
- Where can I get information about having a good sex life in spite of my cancer?
- Does disability have to mean asexuality for me?
- How do I deal with my developmentally disabled daughter's sexual maturation?
- Having sex hurts, and the more I try to "get over it," the tenser I get, and the tenser I get, the more it hurts—what can I do besides stop having sex?
- What kind of sex is safe for me if my partner has an STD?
- How do I tell someone I'm about to have sex with for the first time that I have an STD?
- I thought I had put that awful abusive experience behind me years ago—why is my sex life suffering now?
- When sex is supposed to be experienced with abandon, how can I keep enough control over it to feel comfortable when just kissing makes me freeze up?

CHAPTER SIX

Body Image

ARE OUR BODIES OURSELVES?

From the first flood of breath into our lungs to the last flutter of our final exhalation, we make our sexual journey in our bodies. For too many women, much of the journey is yearning to be elsewhere: anyplace but in this body. Our bodies are ourselves, to quote a well-known book title, but not as we intended! Our bodies aren't the selves we want. Our dominant culture cultivates girls to be dissatisfied with their bodies, and a high premium—the highest—is placed on changing the bodies they have. *Perpetually changing them*, we should add, because women attaining physical goals wouldn't be good for the marketplace. For women, body image, sexuality, and self-image are interwoven. Women frequently stake their happiness, their future, and/or their sexuality on some imagined weight loss or other such physical "improvement."

All women, not some women, are subjected to the impossible dilemma of not meeting a fictionalized standard. Some women may "make the cut" for a period of time, only to face its inevitable diminishment. Even those who are temporarily elevated for their beauty find it is a precarious perch.

> Rosa, 15, shivered in the chill of the stark room, curling her toes against the cold tile floor. She was nude except for a light cotton gown, and she waited nervously for what would happen next. She twisted a plait of her black silk hair nervously when two women, also wearing cotton gowns, entered the room. The

women smiled briefly at her, but with no real connection. Rosa needed connection.

"This is my, um, first time. My first shoot. Who decides, like about hair and stuff?"

One woman flicked momentary eye contact with Rosa and said, "We'll get to that."

The gown was slid to Rosa's waist. A huge brush, soft as down, dipped in an earthy colored powder was dappled on Rosa's shoulders and breasts. One of the women rouged her nipples, causing Rosa to blush vividly. No one but she had ever touched these youthful breasts before.

Weeks later Rosa stared at the glossy magazine picture of herself propped on the machine where she was working out. In the picture Rosa was wearing a creamy silk shift, and her rouged nipples were apparent under the soft material. The wind machine had pressed the material against her skin, creating an allure in the picture Rosa had never seen in herself. She took stock of the magnificent girl in the magazine ad who was supposed to be her. She had been buffed and tinted and curled and posed and lighted and dressed.

How is this me? Rosa wondered, as she climbed into her third hour on the Stairmaster, going nowhere.

There are women who rise above this socialization and deserve our admiration, but most women struggle with this issue for most of their lives. Most women are familiar with the statements we've just made about body image and probably agree with them, but this doesn't mean that their behavior or self-esteem is free of our society's oppressive influence on what is defined as desirable. Joan Jacobs Brumberg, a professor at Cornell University and author of *The Body Project: An Intimate History of American Girls* (1997), points out that *awareness* doesn't equal *behavioral changes*. The same college student who participates in a class discussion about how women are handled in the media could possibly be the one heard retching in her dorm bathroom later the same day, painfully caught in her own conflict about valuing two things at once. The student concurrently wants to be as physically close to perfection as possible *and* wishes to understand, and perhaps revolt against, the marketing and media misuse of women. Unfortunately, the only visible revolt that is going on is the student's revulsion inside herself, about herself. And sadly, she is not alone in facing this dilemma.

We all know—or are—women who vehemently denounce *The Beauty Myth* (Wolf, 1991) yet just as vehemently reject their own bodies' shortcomings. We have heard countless statements by women despairing over their inherited physical traits:

> "I feel like a frog. All of the women in my family seem to have inherited these skinny legs and barrel belly."

> "My hair is impossible: seaweed-on-a-rock."

"Is every girl in our family doomed to be five feet tall?"

"I hate my freckles" [or round, fat shoulders, or short knees—the list is endless].

Many women will exempt themselves from sexual activity, holding out for the perfect body, imagining that such a body will create a perfect sexuality.

The Journey: From Corsets to Ab Crunches

We've stepped over the threshold into a new millennium that will put its own particular stamp on the history of clothing and body image ideal for women. As girls stepped into the 20th century a hundred years ago, they did so by throwing off the corset and other cumbersome clothing and by the 1920s had adopted the chemise dress (Brumberg, 1997). This physical freedom was accompanied, however, by a new tyranny. When women were no longer laced from the outside through corsets, they began in earnest to establish internalized control of their bodies through diet.

The 1950s capitalized on the "sweater girl" ideals of the time to begin to sell, literally, the *foundation* of this image (Brumberg, 1997). "Junior figure control" became a marketing term—a term more revealing than it intended to be: If girls (and their mothers) could be convinced from an early age that girls' figures demanded molding and control, they would be consumers for a lifetime—never mind that much of it would be spent in personal dissatisfaction.

From the mid-20th century onward we appear to have thrown off the cultural construction of "genderized" clothing and its constraints. Girls and guys wear the same pants and shirts. Why hasn't this change brought freedom? Because Victoria's secret is that there is an alter-image to the woman who jumps into her casual khakis. The elastic that used to encase a woman's abdomen and bottom in a girdle now comes in a spandex form that passes for a dress, skirt, or top. The purpose isn't to modulate her form but to provide a new way to emphasize and focus on the rigidly developed and defined muscles and fat-free body that she has achieved by rigorous exercise. Blumberg (1997) observes that "the pressure to control the body has been ratcheted upward by an even more demanding cultural ideal: a lean, taut, female body with visible musculature" (p. 123).

Drastic Body Control Measures

The Surgical Solution

Liposuction—a procedure that professes to help go the extra mile toward body perfection—was unknown a handful of years ago and is now considered acceptable (Davis, 1995). Liposuction surgery is sought by women because it also contributes to the fantasy of physical perfection and desirability. It doesn't come without real physical risk, including death due to surgical complications. There was a time in history when women's feet were mutilated by means of a practice called "foot binding," which attempted to shape what was then considered to be the perfect foot: a tiny one. Nowadays, the mutilation of foot binding to achieve this goal would rightfully be considered abusive, and efforts to curb the trend undoubtedly would be swift. This is in sharp contrast to our benign acceptance of surgical intervention as a method of beauty enhancement.

Anorexia and Bulimia

No argument is persuasive enough to alter the perception of a woman who has been convinced by magazines, the mirror, the mall, or her peers (and sometimes even parents) that she is fat. How far can this distorted thinking go? It can go to starvation and death. Anorexia is a purposeful restriction of intake of food, and bulimia is a purposeful restriction of the body's retention of food. With bulimia, eating is not restricted but by induced vomiting or laxatives or both, the body disgorges the food it has taken in. Even if this is an occasional behavior, it is too much. We want to stress that marketing and media do not cause anorexic or bulimic behavior, but they do contribute to its prevalence as a disease.

Anorexia and bulimia are devastating to sexuality. The closer a woman comes to paring off all of her body fat, the lower her sex hormone production drops. In fact, her reproductive system shuts down: menses cease and getting pregnant becomes difficult or impossible without medical intervention. Sexual desire is dampened or nonexistent. Body hatred or extreme body self-consciousness tends to further quench the flickers of sexual interest that might remain.

Behavior close to starvation comes with hidden costs. The body and brain don't care if the behavior is intentional. Energy will be conserved toward survival, so creativity, production, involvement with others, normal alertness, and judgment are all impaired. The body systems compensate for the starvation as long as possible, but eventually life-sustaining processes will break down.

Women who deliberately starve themselves become obsessed with food, almost or entirely to the exclusion of other interests. This isn't voluntary. It is the brain's mechanism against life-threatening peril. Furthermore, it appears that engaging in anorexic/bulimic behaviors creates a cycle wherein the distorted thinking connected with these behaviors becomes reinforced, making it even more difficult to stop.

If you have binged and purged even once or twice, we advise you to have a consultation with a social worker, psychologist, clinical nurse, or physician who has expertise in eating disorders. If you are severely restricting your food intake and find that you are fearful about continuing (or stopping) this behavior, the same advice applies. If you are the parent, relative, or friend of a person whose eating behaviors worry you, you may not know where to turn or what to do. Many communities have support groups for concerned "others" at local medical centers. You can join an online support group such as *www.something-fishy.org* or find out more about eating disorders on websites such as www.healthlinkusa.com.

Fat: The World on My Plate

Fat: What Is It?

Fat isn't easily defined. One woman with the tiniest, normal, visible indent that her bra makes in her back under a tank top will declare herself "gross" and cover up with an oversize T-shirt; she feels ashamed if her body has any curve or contour. A woman of ample body size may comfortably wear a garment that doesn't seem suitable to the observer because it reveals too much fat. These women have distinctly different responses to their body size.

Is the opposite of fat *thin*, and if so, is thin ideal—some number on the scale that is always a bit out of reach? Do only thin women experience pleasure and freedom in sexual activity? In fact, no. Sexual response is not negatively affected by added weight but by body hatred.

When the Pounds Add Up: Overweight

Few personal stories have been as candid and inspiring and powerful as Oprah Winfrey's detailed account of her struggle with excess weight. Her diary account of winning an Emmy in 1992 is riveting in *Make the Connection: Ten Steps to a Better Body and a Better Life* (Greene & Winfrey, 1996). This gifted woman—perhaps the most influential entertainer of the century—allows us access to her most private thoughts and feelings:

> "And the winner is Oprah Winfrey." I was stunned. Stedman and my staff were cheering. I wanted to cry. Not because I won, but because I would have to stand before this audience of beautiful people and be judged. And not for being a winner.
>
> I felt so much like a loser, like I'd lost control of my life. And the weight was symbolic of how out-of-control I was. I was the fattest woman in the room. (p. 2)

Sometimes weight becomes a real problem physically, medically, emotionally, and/or psychologically. A woman who carries around many extra pounds has a bigger burden than the literal weight. She will be prone to measure herself first, before any personal accomplishment, by what she considers to be a primary personal failure. Weight is certainly no gauge of capability, talent, humor, skill, moral strength, intelligence, or success in relations with others, sexual or otherwise. But being overweight obscures these assets, as if it were a shield beyond which little else can be seen or appreciated.

How many times have we heard statements from women to the effect of, "When my weight is down, I feel sexy and interested, but the more I weigh, the less I desire"? Genitals, brains, hormones, and nerve endings do not go into dormancy as a result of additional weight. In many cases, however, the blunting of sexual feelings and response is so complete under the burden of weight, women experiencing this phenomenon would be certain there is a biological connection.

Desirable versus Desiring

A woman's sexual desire often emanates in large part—or too often, exclusively—from how desirable she sees herself, instead of what *she* finds desirable.

> "I have never stopped to think about what I like in sex. I've come to realize that I have always gauged my sexual response to what he wants, when he is ready, and whether I'm desirable to him. My role has been to have my sexual energy be an answer to my partner's sexual desire. So if I arouse him, sex is successful. Now I see this pattern leaves me out! I honestly never thought of it differently!"

In turn, how perfectly a woman presents herself to her partner becomes distorted in its prominence. She doesn't exuberantly enjoy her body in the experience of sex, but too often remains self-conscious to the point of distraction. If she is overweight, she may exempt herself from sexual desire (desirability) altogether.

Keepaway

If an unresolved, unaddressed conflict with a partner exists, the protection of additional weight can express what isn't being acknowledged or explored: *I don't want to make love while there is so much stress between us—so keep away.* Weight becomes a formidable stand-in for the real issues.

At times there are unaddressed psychological reasons why a woman wants to keep her distance from others, at least where physical intimacy is concerned. Weight may be a protection against the perceived dangers such intimacy presents.

If we eroticize women's bodies, it stands to reason that women's partners will have their own responses to bodies that deviate considerably from the standard *du jour.* Although most men would heartily say, we assume, that a "swizzle stick" body isn't necessary for them to feel appreciative and desiring of their partners' bodies, we're all subjected to the same institutions that fuel contemporary media and marketing. Both men and women may respond to their partner's overweight by withdrawing their own sexual desire and interest. One reason for this response is the lack of appropriate real-life models for sexuality. We don't see ordinary folks in their ordinary bodies depicted in passionate scenes on television.

Sometimes the withdrawal response is a stand-in for other more complicated relationship problems. At other times a woman's partner withdraws not because of the weight itself but because of her unresponsiveness. Here's how this looks:

Partner A [overweight]: I'm not desirable anymore because of this weight. If I was, my partner would still show interest in me.

Partner B: I can't understand why my partner is avoiding me sexually. I feel shut out. I am very uncomfortable making any sexual overtures at all.

Too Hot to Handle

"She's let herself go," we overheard one coworker say to another, chatting as they waited for the coffee to finish brewing. There are multiple levels of meaning in that statement. Where is she going, or where has she gone? One possible answer is that she is going her own way. If she is going on her own, what's the problem? If we listen to the voices of some of the feminist spokeswomen, we hear that added inches aren't the problem but the refusal to get in lockstep with the national preoccupation with the *body impossible*. What other explanation could there be for why a woman's body is not hers alone but is co-owned by the family, society, and culture she lives in? Do we want her sexually satisfied and comfortable with herself? Satisfaction doesn't sell anything, and comfort and self-assurance can be threatening to others who don't feel that way. As absurd as it is to have an entire faction of society willingly gripping the short leash of body obsession, such is the status quo with which we are all familiar.

Being overweight can also neutralize the notion of a woman's sexuality being dangerous. An overweight wife won't stray, won't tempt others. Perhaps both partners are afraid of this possibility, and it gets acted out by maintaining an unhealthy, overweight body. The overweight partner fears her own loss of control should she feel thin and attractive to others. The fact that attractiveness and sexual vitality are a part of an internal process is meaningless. The theory that sexual control and discrimination are also determinations that are made from the inside, not the outside, doesn't hold as much stock as the artificial boundary: excess weight. When this dynamic is present and unrecognized, it can be fatal to any weight management attempts. Neither partner will be able to maintain behaviors supportive of weight loss if the underlying fear is that fat is the only thing that stands in the way of the woman and her rampant sexuality.

CLAIMING OUR BODIES, OUR SEXUALITY

You knew before you opened this book that your perceptions of your body, and the perceptions of women you love of their bodies, have been negatively impacted by all kinds of social and marketing influences. But have you calculated what this might have cost you in sexual responsiveness and pleasure?

Imagine the sexual energy women could have available to them if they harnessed and directed the resources they expend in useless worry, envy, despair, rumination, negative comparison, and oftentimes financial expense to get somewhere that doesn't exist. Women don't just waste the valuable resource of their own energy in this quest. They squander the synergy of the relationship of themselves with others, women and men. If the selves women bring to all relationships (including to one's own self) are confined by the black hole of body despair, then all aspects of the relationships are limited and constrained.

In this section we outline specific suggestions for keeping a perspective about body image and challenging your negative thinking when it occurs. Exercise and its imperative role in sexual health are emphasized. We include talking to youth, because a natural outcome of self-awareness is outreach and mentoring. There are younger women and girls in your life who can benefit from your insights and experiences, even if they seem to be on another planet at times.

We've Come a Long Way: Women's Athletics

In 1972 Title IX became federal law, mandating that schools provide girls the same opportunities in sports as boys. Title IX was generated for economic reasons. Proponents contended that boys' sports, such as high school and college football, were lavished with money and attention, providing these boys with a later, unfair advantage in the workplace.

The American team winning the women's soccer World Cup finals in 1999 certainly showcased several outcomes of Title IX. During the years since its institution in 1972, schools have recruited and hired "real" coaches, rather than drafting any teacher, qualified or not. Scholarship opportunities now exist. Real attention has been paid to women as serious athletes, and this has resulted in a heightened interest in, and respect for, women's sports. In a subtle turn of phrase, many newspapers and cartoons profiling the soccer finals captioned: "She [Mia Hamm] played like a girl."

Women athletes have the strong, lean, taut bodies that come from years of dedicated training. Today's ideal female body is often presented in motion rather than posing prettily. Consequently, clothing is marketed not just to showcase these bodies but also to allow the freedom to move and to work out. We now have a generation of female athletes who have come on the scene, and many of them have felt the power and freedom that comes from being physically fit. They bring to their adulthood the knowledge of how great it feels to move.

Exercise

Not all women are or will be athletes, but exercise is the closest thing we have to a fountain of youth. It is life-sustaining. It impacts all areas of health and strength. It keeps us moving and flexible well into our latest years. It helps our bodies maintain nutritional and hormonal balance. It affects mood, and not just because we feel good that we're exercising when we do, but because it regulates important chemicals in the brain.

It is never too late to begin to exercise and reap its benefits. If you are 18 and "too busy to exercise because of school and work," prop your homework on a treadmill and get moving! If you are 80 and your doctor approves, get to the mall and start walking. Exercise should be consistent—three to five times a week for 30 minutes or more. An ideal exercise program includes aerobic exercise, strengthening and toning, and stretching. Your healthcare provider can offer guidelines. Many communities have a recreation center with personnel qualified to offer exercise advice and make recommendations for a balanced routine.

There are sexual benefits to regular exercise:

- Improved pelvic muscle tone enhances orgasm and sexual response. See Chapter 8 for a description of Kegel exercises, which can help maintain muscle control or improve it if the muscles have become lax.
- Physical flexibility contributes to the comfort and pleasure of sex with a partner. The more you can move, the more spontaneous and adventuresome you can be, the less you will concentrate on what you can't do. This can be particularly important for you as you age.
- Exercise is almost an "on" switch for hormones. It reduces fatigue, releases endorphins, and helps your body make the most effective and beneficial use of sex hormones, such as estrogen and androgens.
- Exercise helps your body become fit, toned, and energetic. When you see the physical benefits of exercise, it makes you feel proud of your efforts and you bring this pride (along with boosted confidence) into the bedroom. You will also bring the energy that comes from regular exercise and fitness into your love life!

Mentoring Positive Self-Awareness: Talking with Youth

Most of us snag the nearest teenager handy when we have a question about electronics. Teens seem to have mastered even the most complex equipment. We worry about the kind of information they are exposed to with the combination of their curiosity and skill. Despite the rating systems for television, movies, and music, and blocking devices for cable, satellite, or the Internet, young people move in a world that is impervious to those barriers. Even the most conscientious parents are going to have insurmountable technological challenges if their primary goal is to censor their children's access to information, even if it is terrible, destructive information. Blocking mechanisms become obsolete or there are easy ways around them. New information pours out continually. Like the self-inflating raft, once it's out of the box it is much more difficult, if not impossible, to confine it to its original space.

Because teens and young adults are exposed to so much information, we tend to attribute to them far more sophistication than they possess, particularly in the area of sexuality and body image. Their worlds are much larger now than we ever could have imagined just a few decades ago. We can throw out the television and pull the plug on the Internet, but even a walk through the mall or a glance at a popular magazine or even the Sunday paper becomes yet another source of confusing information and complicated messages.

A girl who feels chronically uncertain about her body, hence her appeal, carries this uncertainty into her decisions about sexual behavior. Mixed with this is the dynamic of the young woman being more tuned in to her desirability than her desire. If we now add to this mix continual overexposure to sex, from its most banal to bizarre forms featuring truly unbelievable bodies, we have a recipe for disaster. This is the challenging context in which we want today's young woman to be self-aware, assertive, and discriminating about sexual choices.

What do the youngest of the women among us need? These youngsters or young adults may be sisters, daughters, granddaughters, nieces, babysitters, or girls in some other life relationship to us, but they share something in common. They all need to hear the stories of women in their lives who have gone through body image crises and physical, emotional, and sexual development.

If a young woman we cared about was going to take a youth hostel biking trip far from home for a number of days, we wouldn't let her launch into the trip with unsafe equipment or uncertain preparation and plans. So it should stand to reason that she shouldn't launch into her sexual journey with less preparation and input from the adults who care about her. A significant aspect of her developing sexuality will be how she feels about her body. We wouldn't say to her, "Just say no if the road is slippery and your biking group is going ahead anyhow." Likewise it wouldn't be sufficient to say, "Just don't pay attention to all of that over-inflated perfect body stuff you see on MTV," or "Don't waste your money buying all that cosmetic junk."

All teens need exposure to the dilemmas and struggles of women who have gone before them. They will absorb the ways in which these women solved their own dilemmas and took their own stands regarding exaggerated focus on appearance and body "perfection." They will benefit from being exposed to women role models in their community or the nation or in history whose contributions—not necessarily their appearances—have been notable and strong.

Challenging Our Thinking: Moving from Punitive to Positive Awareness

Worth a Second Thought

As therapists who do a great deal of couples counseling, we know that if a relationship is going to even approach satisfaction or fulfillment, there is one variable that has to be present: the ratio of positive to negative statements between the partners must be heavily weighted toward positive comments. Probably something like five or six to one (Gottman, 1999). This means for every "I'm really tired of walking over your shoes every time I get near our closet," there need to be five comments that are positive, such as "I love it that you listen to my grandfather's stories of the Great Depression," or "Thanks for driving me to this appointment—I'm really nervous about it, and I know it wasn't easy for you to arrange to do this for me." The ratio of more positive to negative comments between partners is more predictive of their happiness and satisfaction with the relationship than their age or how long they have been together.

If this is true for couples, doesn't it make sense that the same equation applies to us as individuals? Unfortunately, when it comes to self-commentary on body image, the likelihood is high that the ratio is reversed—more negative observations than positive ones. We're talking about the tendency to take notice only of what we consider to be negative about our bodies, and emphasizing that to ourselves repeatedly. We install a jury in our heads and appoint ourselves presiding judge, often making harsh pronouncements about our perceived physical shortcomings.

If we apply the five-to-one ratio of positive to negative comments (whether this is statements or thoughts) about ourselves and our bodies, we would be unconsciously training ourselves to notice the positives more readily than we notice the negatives. It takes vigilance to see positives when we're accustomed to seeing negatives. We are not talking about blaming someone for what we don't like about ourselves or not taking responsibility for behaviors that would be healthier if we change.

Sometimes couples struggle when, as therapists, we ask them to describe the strengths in their relationship. Many times they have come to therapy expecting to focus on only weaknesses. The strengths, whatever they are, are minimized or overlooked completely. As individuals, we too often do this with our physical appearances. We chuckle as a teenager magnifies a zit on her forehead, declaring, "It looks like a beacon!" But we might look in the mirror, take note only of a bulging midriff, and ignore the lovely roundness of breasts or the silkiness of glossy hair. It took conditioning for us to see the negatives first. It will take practice—conscious practice—to change a pattern that is set in place.

Hold That Thought

> Alicia, occupying her usual chair in the sexuality class she was attending, listened intently as the instructor talked about "thought stopping." She was emphasizing, at the moment, how it is possible to change one's view of one's body, and how often women are prone to negative thinking where their bodies are concerned. Alicia's own thoughts were running rampant—*Now, how am I supposed to feel good about this body? It'll never happen. My stomach is paunchy and has stretch marks, and my thighs are dumpy and dimpled. I feel like two people—one pretty good-looking one from the waist up, and one pretty awful from the waist down.*

Gradually, however, through writing in her journal—a class assignment—sharing with the other class members, and listening to the teacher, Alicia's attitudes changed considerably. *I have a right to my feelings about my body, good or bad,* Alicia thought. *Maybe I'm holding on to something that isn't all that good for me.*

Most of us are probably holding on to attitudes that aren't all that good for us. Here are some steps that can help you let go of negative thoughts about your body that you have likely held on to far too long.

- ***Identify*** the negative thought when it occurs. Example: Alicia getting dressed in the morning catches a glimpse of herself in the mirror and is swamped by the thought, *I hate how my thighs look.*
- ***Stop*** the negative thought. Do it with words. Example: Alicia can think to herself, *I have a choice about what I think. I will not continue to describe my thighs as awful.*
- ***Refocus*** your observation. Example: Alicia can think, *I believe I will gain nothing with such self-destructive, negative thoughts. I need to remind myself that I have begun to exercise regularly, and I am proud of this accomplishment.*
- ***Substitute*** a positive thought for the negative one. Example: Alicia can think, *My legs are growing stronger as I exercise. I can feel the strength increasing every time I work out.*

We don't think of our thoughts as being conditioned into a certain pattern, but they are. Just as our routine of getting up in the morning or retiring in the evening has predictable patterns, so does our thinking. We talked about how negative body-imaging might come to be, but why does it continue even when we think we should know better?

Our charge to you is: One more time: *stop that negative thinking.* We know you have heard it before. We take time to reemphasize the point because, ironically, even those who teach positive thinking techniques can tend to hold on stubbornly to their own negative body image, as if this self-destructive thinking were really justified in their personal circumstance.

In Chapter 13 we explain how attitudes and thinking impact our experience of sex. Refer to this chapter for further insight into this issue. Libraries and the self-help shelves at bookstores are loaded with books describing how to modify behavior, beginning with attitudinal changes.

A Perfect Body/Perfect Life?

If we got the "perfect" body, what would happen *then*? Considering the obsession that is often connected with it, here's the way it seems: the traffic lights would forever be green, the bank statements would perpetually show a healthy balance, and love would come with little effort, all because we would be so ornamental. And: we could forget about having to work or study hard, ponder over difficult decisions and life challenges, and of course the medical diagnoses would always be in our favor.

No? Well, what *would* happen?

Consider answering these questions[1]:

- If I had the body I yearn for, men (or women) would . . .
- If I weighed what I want, I could . . .
- If I had the body I yearn for, my life would . . .

The answers to these questions can reveal a great deal if you are willing to explore your answers a little more deeply. For example, you might have answered, "If I had the body I yearn for, men would find me sexually attractive and would want to be with me." Now let's explore that further. Do men (or women) find you attractive now? If the honest answer is yes, then what is it they find attractive and what would happen if you felt you were even more attractive? If the honest answer to the question above is no, then ask yourself why. If your answer is "because I'm not thin/tall/pretty enough," then keep going. Ask yourself if you know other women who are as heavy/short/plain as you are and who have still attracted others. If you do know such a woman, what makes them attractive? If you don't, refer back to the discussion on negative thinking to help you see where your thinking has stalled.

The point is that physical appearance may be a factor in attractiveness, but it is not the sum. And physical appearance is not the road to personal fulfillment or lasting relationships. It does not insulate one against pain, disappointment, loss, grief, or illness. There are no shortcuts to intimacy in a relationship, and the work will be just as intense whether you're doing it in your size six or 16 jeans.

How Are You Feeling?

Information often tells our head what to think, but emotions often tell our feet what to do. If your car stalls on a railroad track, your brain takes in the information that you have stalled in a dangerous place. It is your emotions, however, mixed with the information, that will most likely get you to take the action and move out of the potentially dangerous situation.

When it comes to feelings, it is important to recognize and interpret the emotions correctly. This may seem obvious, but it often doesn't happen. Emotions are sometimes numbed, disguised, buried, or misinterpreted. This is a bit like having a compass when you need it, but not taking the cover off to get your bearings. You can hold the compass at any angle you want to, but with the face of it covered, it can of-

[1]Adapted from Meadow & Weiss (1992, p. 147).

fer you no assistance. You lose the keen advantage of feeling your feelings, understanding them, and using them to help determine behavioral choices.

If our emotions are routinely discounted, ignored, neglected, or subordinated, we lose the ability to trust ourselves. Once that has taken place, we are extremely vulnerable to outside influences. That is, we are more prone to believe or buy into the hype, the seductive promise that is held out to us if only we would believe in the products, the diets, hyper-exercise, liposuction, or cosmetics to improve our confidence.

Balance Is Beautiful

Obsession about one's body bleeds away personal power, and anxiety fuels the obsession that only becomes more disappointing. Obsession is doomed from the beginning: it will fail to deliver. Obsession can be masked as indifference or control. Paralysis—the inability to take important steps for the sake of health and well-being—is one way obsession manifests. If you are in the clutches of an obsession, you are seldom far from thinking about your problem (which could be overeating, overdrinking, or smoking, for example), but your obsession has a short tether. You can't muster feelings beyond powerlessness, so you are left impotent in the face of those problems. You cannot tap into your obsession to find the way to take the action you need to take.

"If there is a natural female shape," writes Naomi Wolf (1991), "it is the one in which women are sexual . . . and not always thinking about it" (p. 200). This is not about disregard for healthy standards. Self-pride and self-responsibility are imperative requirements, however, if you want to establish and maintain weight control, a healthy exercise regimen, or some other physical routine. This isn't the stuff of which obsessions are made.

Balance is beautiful. It implies an active, interactive, involved woman—you, absorbed in your life with all of its gifts and pains. It means that you maintain respect for your own boundaries and believe that you, like others who are significant in your life, need time and attention from yourself for yourself. The balance that you strive for encourages moderation and modification where it is needed. Perhaps this is about eating. Perhaps it is about challenging your self-focused negative and disempowering thinking. Perhaps it is about establishing a healthy exercise routine. Perhaps it is about monitoring and managing weight—but on your terms and for your own reasons.

CONTINUING THE JOURNEY IN YOUR BODY

Each woman's sexual journey is personal, though often shared. On this journey no one is immune to feelings of uncertainty and inadequacy. Even having an "ideal" body, however, doesn't provide exemption from these feelings and certainly doesn't assure happiness. We should care for and respect the bodies we have—they are our vehicles in our journeys. We are careful here to distinguish *care* from *punitive obsession*, which relegates us to a state of futile, powerless yearning. Focusing our thoughts toward what we appreciate about our bodies will provide us with the fuel (energy) to keep them in the best condition possible for their journeys.

CHAPTER SEVEN

Illness and Disability

Even though I was tired, I did pretty well during radiation treatment. I faced some hard days and came through them. When my energy returned, I wanted to make love, but my sexual desire was low and my vagina seemed so dry. I thought my doctor would have some ideas to help with these problems.

At my next appointment, I asked about increasing my sex drive. My doctor looked surprised and said, "I saved your life. What more do you want?"

The "more" I wanted was to be sexual.

If you are living with illness or disability, your sexuality may be challenged in several ways. For one, your healthcare provider may shut you down when you ask questions about sex, because he or she simply may not know how to answer. Sexual difficulties during illness and disability have multiple causes, and your doctor may not have the knowledge or time or desire to provide you with the customized solution you need. On top of this obstacle, when you have an illness or disability you have to cope with changes to your body, self-perception, self-esteem, and identity. Then there is the pervasive cultural bias that says if you're sick, you are no longer a sexual person; and if you were born with a disability, you're living in a world where sexuality is the domain of the able-bodied.

In this chapter, we discuss how you can take care of your sexual self in the face of illness and disability. First we consider important things for you to do if illness threatens your ability to enjoy sexuality. Then we look at disability and, if you are not able-bodied, ways to more fully experience your sexuality.

ILLNESS AND SEXUAL VULNERABILITY

When healthcare providers and the public in general consider the impact of illness, they often think in terms of life and death, physical discomfort, disfigurement, and return-to-work issues. What everyone, except for the person with the illness, often overlooks is the importance of sexuality and how it is affected by the medical condition. Sex is a quality-of-life issue. It gives pleasure to you and can connect you to others, even if your body is physically challenged. But how do you make this happen?

First Things First: Grieving and Moving Ahead

Whether you secretly suspected the diagnosis or were caught completely off guard, your first reaction to learning of your illness was probably disbelief and shock. You may have felt betrayed by your body, fearful of how the illness would progress, or pessimistic about your future. One thing is certain: coping with a serious or chronic illness can be an emotional roller coaster that can impact your self-image and sexual identity.

> "I manage my ostomy[1] well, but I still feel funny about it when I'm having sex. I'm not quite ready to have my partner see my stoma[2]."

> "I thought I was doing fine in chemotherapy until the day my hair started coming out in handfuls. I called my husband and sobbed. He came home from work with a buzz cut. I felt like his message was 'We're doing this together.' That night, he initiated lovemaking. It was so reassuring that I cried, this time because I loved him so much."

Even if a life marked by illness eventually turns out to be very good, it will be a different life from before, a "new normal." Grieving is a necessary part of adjusting to an illness. Grief requires that you admit there has been a loss in your life and that you allow yourself to experience all your feelings related to that loss. Grief demands that you get used to things being different in your life. Finally, in grief, you must learn to move ahead, despite the awareness that your loss and grief will always be a part of you (Worden, 1991).

> "Our bodies would twist and bend and become so entwined that it was sometimes hard to figure which leg or arm belonged to who. That was before my arthritis. Now just penetration is a major accomplishment. We're doing well; our sex is loving and tender. But I still miss my old body that could melt into Rory's embrace."

---

[1]A surgically created opening for discharge of body wastes.

[2]The end of the small or large bowel or ureter protruding through the abdominal wall.

Hemingway (1929) in *A Farewell to Arms* wrote that the world breaks everyone, and afterwards some are stronger in the broken places. This has been our experience of working with women, and those who love them, when illness or disability has disrupted their lives. It's a heartbreaking experience to develop a disability or to be diagnosed with an illness. But most women don't remain heartbroken; they pick up the pieces of their lives and put them together again. They go on, often stronger in the broken places.

This resiliency is especially true for their sexuality. Their bodies may become disfigured, their sexual response may be altered, their energy to make love may be diminished, but they choose to find pleasure in their bodies. They grieve their losses, including sexual losses, and move ahead. They find ways to become stronger in broken places. Sexuality, perhaps taken for granted in their "earlier life," becomes a priority in their "new life." Women who've decided to be sexual in their bodies can be very resilient indeed.

Getting Educated about Your Illness

How does your illness impact your sex life? Are certain medications notorious for destroying sexual desire? Do certain sexual positions minimize pain? It's essential that you get educated about your illness or disability. Books, healthcare professionals, support groups, and the Internet are valuable resources for learning ways to improve the quality of life, including your sexual life. The process of self-education also tends to push you into meeting other women who've been through similar circumstances. Whether it's in face-to-face support groups or chat rooms on a website, you'll connect with others for information and emotional support.

A good place to start is to ask for recommendations from the nurse or social worker where you receive your medical care. Some hospitals also have patient libraries with excellent resources. Many illnesses actually have entire support and research networks. For example, the American Cancer Society, American Lung Association, American Heart Association, Arthritis Foundation, Hemophilia Foundation, and American Kidney Foundation all provide information about adjustment to illness. Many of these organizations have excellent booklets about sexual concerns.

Internet websites provide information that specifically relates to your diagnosis or treatment. For example, if you have cancer, you can go to the website www.acor.org (Association of Cancer Online Resources, Inc.); from the menu of mailing lists, select Cancer-Sexuality where, after you register, you will find resource information, suggestions for overcoming sexual difficulties, and a "listserve"—a private mailing list for people who want to "talk" to each other through e-mail about their cancer-related sexuality concerns. Women are now "talking" to each other through listserves that have been established for most illnesses and disabilities. If you don't have a computer, you can use one at your local library. They'll explain to you how to obtain a free e-mail address, and you can pick up your e-mail at the library computer.

Reclaiming Your Sexuality: Self-Exploration and Masturbation

As a part of the process of being sexually active during the course of an illness, you need to touch and explore your body, determining what parts feel good when touched and what parts are uncomfortable. Surgical sites, areas around stomas or shunts, and scar tissue often feel uncomfortable, numb, or even painful. It's important to determine in advance what's off-limits during sexual activity with your partner.

Self-exploration should include looking as well as touching. If there's been a surgical or other body change, look carefully at the affected area. If it feels too threatening to do this alone the first time, ask your partner or your physician or nurse to be with you. If it's too hard now, go on to some other aspect of self-exploration and come back to this later. The goal is for you to see yourself as a whole person, not as a "stoma" or an "amputee."

Try to be curious about parts of your body that you might not have considered sexy before. Because skin is our largest sensory organ, you can slowly, deliberately touch all of your skin to find areas that feel good. You need to remember that your mind is your most powerful sex organ, rich with sensual memories, images, and fantasies. It may be helpful to review the material on sexual fantasies in Chapters 12 and 14.

Masturbation provides a means for you to explore your sexual response and how it may have been altered by your illness. It also can also be a valuable source of relaxation and pleasure. Try different positions for masturbating to see which give you the greatest sense of pleasure and comfort. Some women prefer lying on their back; some semi-recline with pillows behind them; and some lie on their stomach and increase pelvic pressure by holding a towel or small pillow between their legs. Some women touch just the head of the clitoris; other women like to stroke their inner labia and probe their vagina. Some women rock their whole body back and forth. Some women just move their hands. Some women use vibrators. Some women watch erotic movies. Some read romance novels and masturbate during the "good" parts. Some women heighten their arousal by imagining erotic fantasies. The point is, if masturbation is new to you, feel free to explore, experiment, and enjoy. If it is an "old friend," introduce it to your "new" body.

Overcoming Sexual Response Problems

A woman's sexual response can be affected by the illness itself, by the treatment, by fatigue caused by the illness, and by her self-image. You may find that it's hard to determine exactly what's affecting your sexual response, but you know that *something* is different. To determine what to do, begin by checking with your healthcare provider to make sure that sexual activity is not medically risky. If you get the "go ahead," think about what your sexual response was like before the diagnosis. We suggest reading through Part I, "Knowing Your Sexual Story," as a starting point for understanding your sexual response both now and in the past. Next, write down the areas you're concerned about now. Are these changes in desire, arousal, or orgasm? Are you experiencing increased pain? Do you feel that you have a poor body image? Ask your healthcare provider if other women have had these same concerns and, if so, what they have done about them.

Desire

Illness robs us of sexual desire, either by directly impacting hormonal levels necessary for normal sexual desire or by creating flu-like symptoms and fatigue. Sometimes medications and other treatments have side effects that dampen desire. Some illnesses, like congestive heart failure, compromise breathing and make every movement an effort. If these symptoms are familiar to you, or you simply recognize your loss of desire, the suggestions in Chapter 14 will be useful. In particular, be rested but alert for any sexual experience. If you're sleepy, woozy, or tired, your desire will be affected. Look for times of the day when you feel best, perhaps first going for a brief walk or taking a warm shower to enhance your sensory awareness. Make sure your room is comfortably warm. You can purchase small electric heaters to warm a particular space. Dress comfortably and use a semi-reclining position if lying down places too much stress on your heart or breathing.

Depression is a dampener of desire and is frequently linked with illness. Symptoms of depression can include loss of appetite, changes in sleep patterns (too much or not enough), loss of interest in activities and others, self-isolation, chronic irritability or dissatisfaction, and repetitive thinking of negative thoughts. If you're experiencing depression, counseling may help you overcome not only your depressed mood but also your low sexual desire. In some situations, antidepressant medication may also be helpful.

Arousal

Sexual arousal involves both your sense of excitement and your body's response to sexual stimulation. Normally during sexual arousal, your vagina becomes moist with lubrication, your genital region feels full because of increased blood flow to that area, and you have an all-over aroused feeling in your body. Neurological damage, spinal cord injury, vascular damage, chemotherapy, and various medications can interfere with genital blood flow by blocking blood vessels or preventing signals from traveling along the nerves that control vasocongestion (the swelling response in your genital region). Anticipating discomfort or coping with fatigue, depression, or worry can also affect your arousal. Chapter 15 may help with specific concerns. Some women also report that arousal improved for them once they had completed treatment or finished taking certain medications for their illness. For example, chemotherapy is an anticholinergic (drying) medication that can affect your lubrication and swelling response. If you're on chemotherapy, you may find that your sexual arousal will improve once you complete your course of chemotherapy. Be sure to read and ask questions about how your illness and treatment can affect sexual arousal.

Orgasm

Orgasm may be affected by treatment, medications, neurological or spinal cord damage, depression, distraction due to pain or restricted movement, and other factors. You may find it helpful to reread Part II, "Understanding Your Body," for a better understanding of how orgasm works. The suggestions in Chapter 16 may also be helpful.

Learning to Manage Pain

Nothing interferes with pleasure faster than pain. You may have chronic or occasional pain. It may be throughout your body or only in specific areas. In this section, we discuss general pain that results from your illness and ways to minimize its disruptive effect on sex. In Chapter 8 we focus on genital and pelvic pain, which may or may not be associated with an illness. In addition to reading the material in this book, we suggest that you talk to your healthcare provider, check the "Suggested Resources" section at the end of this book, and check websites dealing with your illness for other suggestions.

Pain is personal. People have different pain thresholds, and on different days pain can affect us differently. Fatigue and stress influence pain, and it's hard to remain emotionally steady when in pain. The longer we're in pain, the more depressed, frustrated, and hopeless we feel. Pain can rob *anyone* of sexual interest.

Being Believed

One of the most isolating parts of being in pain is the feeling that others don't believe you or that they're unable to appreciate how much pain you're experiencing. If you're in pain, you need support from your healthcare provider, your friends, and your partner. Being believed doesn't necessarily come from putting your suffering on full, open display. Instead, you can take care to educate others about what support or special assistance you'll need to make life easier.

> "Because my pain came and went, I'd forget that my partner couldn't know I was miserable. I'd get irritable about her advances to be sexual when I couldn't even lie down comfortably."

Taking Control

The management of your pain requires you to have confidence and believe in your ability to control and cope with it. This may include finding the right healthcare provider, undergoing physical therapy, getting a prosthesis, obtaining educational materials, attending a pain clinic, taking medications, or finding the right chairs, mattresses, and pillows that assist you in coping with pain. This may also include seeking therapy to learn to cope with pain and/or learning techniques of self-hypnosis to control pain.

Experimentation

The management of pain toward the goal of reclaiming your sexual life requires experimentation. Although there are general rules about what will help with certain kinds of pain, there's no substitute for trying different things and determining what works for you. You may find mornings better than nights for making love, and semi-reclining positions or being on top better than lying flat. Some women start with a warm bath or shower. Also helpful is scheduling sex according to a medication regimen if you have one, so that lovemaking takes place when pain management is optimal. Thinking about what soothes and gives pleasure and then incorporating that into sexual activity is an important part of managing pain positively.

Some couples develop alternate plans for times when the pain is too great to have sexual activity. They cuddle, read to each other, and find other ways to connect intimately. Sometimes this leads to masturbation for the partner who's not in pain. Ultimately the goal of sexual contact is pleasure and connectedness—feeling comfort and pleasure in each other's company and bodies. Sex is deeply personal and individual, as are the ways to connect.

When It Hurts Too Much to Touch

There'll be times that no matter how positive the attitude, no matter how creative the experimentation, pain still gets the best of you. If that happens, try to keep from making broad generalizations like "It's always going to be like this." Try to stay focused on the present moment. Focus on breathing evenly and try sitting or lying in a way that minimizes the pain. Continue to work with your healthcare provider to find solutions and to learn about new developments in pain management. Reread the section in Chapter 6 called "Hold That Thought," and see Chapter 13 for further suggestions in managing your thinking.

Sometimes pain is so great that it hurts even to be touched or held. If you have severe arthritis, migraine headaches, or fibromyalgia, you may find that being touched makes you feel acute pain or nausea. In these situations, trying to force sex is a bad idea. Instead, it's a time to focus on getting as comfortable as possible. Some women need to be absolutely still with no sensory input whatsoever. Other women listen to music, look at a movie, or light a scented candle and enjoy olfactory sensation. These are ways of taking in pleasure as sensory experience despite the presence of severe pain.

Overcoming Special Problems

Disfigurement

Sometimes coping with changes in physical appearance far exceeds any issue of a "wounded" self-identity due to illness. Gaining or losing weight, losing your hair, having a body port or shunt, or using prosthetic devices, whether they're wigs or crutches, is an all-out assault on your sense of being sexy. Some women refuse to get caught up in social definitions of beauty and sexiness. For other women, it's not that clear-cut. It's not just that they think others don't like their bodies. The bigger problem is that *they* don't like their bodies.

You may need time to reintegrate your sense of self when there's been an assault to your body. But don't wait too long. Challenge your isolation or negative thinking. Consider joining a support group or getting on the Internet and participating in a chat room for women with your particular concern. Sometimes speaking with a counselor or therapist can be very helpful. Make sure you don't try to ignore your concern.

Urinary Incontinence

Urine leakage can be caused by a number of illness-related problems. You will find a discussion of ways to cope with urinary incontinence in the Chapter 2 section "Accommodate, Don't Capitulate."

Heavy Menstrual Flow

You may experience sexual difficulties from illnesses that are bleeding-related. These can include bleeding disorders like von Willebrand's disease or gynecological problems like endometriosis. If your period is excessive in either duration or intensity and demands lifestyle changes, it can impact your sexuality.

> "I never worried about my period until I was in my 40s. Now I'm self-conscious about my heavy menstrual flow—correction, gush. I don't want to kiss because I'm afraid it'll lead to having sex, and I can't manage the heavy bleeding during sex."

If menstrual flow is not neatly assigned to a five-day period, is copious rather than discreet, and is turning you off sexually because of the mess, we have some suggestions.

If you have heavy or chronic menstrual flow, begin by thinking about how much risk versus nuisance you're willing to endure. If sexual activity is messy but enjoyable, try switching to dark-colored sheets or buying bath-size towels in navy and deep green and spreading them on the bed before making love. Talk with your partner in advance, share your concern, and suggest enjoying sex followed by taking a shower together.

If you don't want your partner to have contact with menstrual blood, you can wear pads and underwear and concentrate on nongenital stimulation, perhaps focusing on nipples, thighs, and buttocks. You can use a vibrator against the outside of your underwear as well as on other parts of your body. You can concentrate on touching your partner sexually. Because the vagina can expand, you might try inserting more than one tampon to absorb flow. This may allow you to engage in noncoital lovemaking without pads or underwear. Some women have been successful using a diaphragm during intercourse, not for contraception (which would require the addition of spermicidal jell) but as a means to catch menstrual flow. It's important to remember to remove tampons or diaphragm after sexual activity. A tampon inadvertently left in the vagina can cause toxic shock syndrome, which is potentially fatal. Remember to talk with your healthcare provider about your concerns too.

DISABILITY AND SEX

Living with disability requires adaptation, drawing from your resources and the support of others. Although you continue to be sexual, you have more than physical barriers to overcome—you must also deal with negative social stereotypes that portray you as asexual.

> "I have cerebral palsy and use a wheelchair. When I'm at a party, no one flirts with me. I'm everybody's 'best friend.' "

The following section offers a brief description of disabilities and associated sexual issues. As with illness, it's impossible to come up with one set of descriptors that will apply to all forms of disability and their accompanying challenges. Nevertheless, you should be able to find helpful information in this section that can be generalized to most disabilities.

> "I learned early to hold people with my voice and eyes. I was smart and witty, making people laugh. But when they saw I had no hands, I couldn't get them to laugh again. My left hand is missing entirely, but fortunately, my right hand has a functional finger and thumb and I can perform most tasks. The rest of me is 'normal,' and I don't have any sexual disability, but I've never gone out on a date."

If you have a disability, you've reckoned with the prejudices of others who may dismiss you without knowing you. You may have had unnecessary social limitations imposed on you by well-intended parents who didn't want you to be hurt, physically or emotionally. You may have been overprotected or ignored.

In our culture, people with disabilities are asexualized and marginalized by others. This is probably due in part to the overidealization of perfect bodies, which is so prominent in our dominant culture. In addition, the temporarily able-bodied (as some put it) may feel threatened with the disturbing awareness of their own vulnerability when they encounter a person in a wheelchair or someone physically disfigured, mentally challenged, or emotionally challenged. Because they don't want to dwell on how different their lives would be with such a condition, they try not to dwell on the presence of those who are challenged in these ways.

If you have a disability, you have developed resilience to cope with it. You know that you are sexual despite physical challenges. As you read through Part I, "Knowing Your Sexual Story," you'll note when you first "discovered" your disability and the impact it has on your sexual functioning. In Part II, "Understanding Your Body," you can assess which parts of your sexual functioning are affected by your disability. After reading these sections, make a list of any sexual questions you still have and take then to your healthcare provider. You can also check the Internet for websites that address your concerns. As with illness, getting educated and decreasing your isolation are both important.

Psychiatric Conditions

If you have a psychiatric condition, you may also feel that people treat your sexuality as if it were nonexistent. In fact, your sexuality is important and deserves your attention. Some psychiatric problems don't impair thinking and judgment, others impair thinking intermittently, and for some, judgment is impaired all the time. During times of impaired thinking you may make poor decisions regarding taking care of your sexual self or avoiding sexually dangerous people and situations. If you know there are intermittent periods when your judgment is impaired (for instance, with major depression, schizophrenia, or active psychosis), then these are times you will need others to help keep you safe.

We offer the following advice to help you maintain a healthy sexual life. First, maintain your physical health. Schedule regular physicals with a healthcare provider who understands your psychiatric diagnosis and will work with you to take good care of your body. See your psychiatrist regularly and especially when you feel your medication needs adjustment. If you experience an increase in psychiatric symptoms, don't wait for your next scheduled appointment; call your psychiatrist right away.

Don't isolate yourself from others who can be a positive part of your life. This may include family, friends, coworkers, and neighbors.. Many communities have local chapters of the National Alliance for the Mentally Ill (NAMI), a remarkable self-help group. NAMI also has an excellent website (www.nami.org) for education, support, and advocacy. Make sure your close friends understand your psychiatric diagnosis and the symptoms you'll have if your judgment becomes impaired. Ask them to remind you to see your psychiatrist if you're acting with impaired judgment. An example would be if you started frequenting bars and drinking a lot—often a convoluted attempt to keep your symptoms under control. At these times, you may not be taking your medication, making you vulnerable to sexual assault, exploitation, or consensual but unsafe sex. Having sex during the acute phase of your illness could result in pregnancy, STDs, or physical harm.

You may find that your medications have sexual side effects. Antipsychotic and antidepressant drugs can negatively impact all phases of a woman's sexual response. We want to stress, however, that even though sex is an important quality-of-life issue, mental stability has to take precedence. Little can be gained by alleviating the negative sexual side effects of medication if your well-being is placed in jeopardy due to unchecked psychiatric symptoms. Psychiatrists have respect for, and awareness of, the negative side effects of medication and will work with you to manage symptoms and minimize these side effects. When sexual side effects cannot be minimized, sexual counseling can help you find creative ways to maximize sexual satisfaction. You'll also find helpful suggestions in the "Illness" section of this chapter when addressing problems of desire, arousal, orgasm, or pain.

If you are taking medication for depression, bipolar disorder, anxiety, or obsessive-compulsive disorder and are experiencing an unwanted impact on your sexuality, you may find helpful suggestions in Chapters 14, 15, and 16.

Disability Due to Spinal Cord Injury and Neurological Disease

If you have a spinal cord injury or neurological disease, you know it can have a wide range of impacts on sexual function, depending on where the injury occurs in the spine and how severe—or "complete"—the damage is.

> "I think I've made a decent adjustment to living in a wheelchair. I do get frustrated with my body, especially during sex. I feel like parts of my body are floppy and unresponsive, and we've had to figure out sex all over again."

You may find that the most devastating sexual effect of spinal injury/disease is the impaired ability to physically feel sensations. Your spinal cord injury may also interfere with sexual activity by impairing movement, producing chronic pain, and/or triggering involuntary movements in the extremities. Neural pathways that help regulate arousal and orgasm can be disrupted, making lubrication, pleasurable body sensations, and orgasm more difficult to experience. As in our discussion of illness, you'll need to get educated about your disability's effect on sex. Look for specific resources on the Internet and in the library that pertain to your physical difficulty. Ask your physicians, nurses, and social workers for information about sexual adjustment. Your healthcare providers may also know of local support groups.

Self-exploration and masturbation are two important ways to enhance your sexual capacity. If you have use of your hands, explore how different parts of your body respond to touch. If you can't use your hands but you have a partner, guide your partner to do the exploring. In this way, one woman with quadriplegia discovered that the back of her neck, her ear lobes, and her eyebrows were extremely sensitive and sensual. Some women with paraplegia use vibrators, especially inside their vaginas, to experience pleasure.

If you can't use your hands and don't have a partner, you face difficult but not impossible challenges in masturbating. Creativity is important as you experiment with sensory stimulation from both the external environment and your inner world of imagery and fantasy. You'll need to be watchful to determine what's possible. Using environmental cues to heighten stimulation may include concentrating on the feel of water on your skin while bathing, of sheets against your body at night, of breezes as they blow against your face when outdoors. Visual erotica, music, and pleasant smells are additional environmental cues that can increase self-pleasure. Search the Internet for disability-specific resources.

Experimentation with different masturbation positions is important, too. It may work for you to lie on your stomach and press your pelvis into the sheets while gently rocking back and forth, or to press a pillow or towel between your legs to increase the sensation of pressure. Some women have found that lying on their sides gives them more control over their rocking motions. A care attendant may assist by placing a vibrator or positioning your body. The rule here is to experiment and persevere.

You may have experienced loss of bowel and/or bladder control that requires these body functions to be managed on a schedule. Sexual activity with your partner can and should be planned around this schedule. This hardly allows sexual spontaneity, and you may need to grieve that loss of spontaneity. In general, we feel that spontaneity is highly overrated and that a couple's sexuality can flourish in a context of planning, communication, and controlling your environment. As you learn to manage bowel and bladder continence, there may be mishaps during sex. Keep your sense of humor. Try spreading dark-colored comfortable towels on your bed before making love. Keep a supply of smaller towels for cleaning up accidents. Talk to your partner in advance about his or her feelings toward bowel or bladder incontinence. Make plans together ahead of time for what you'll do in the event an accident occurs.

There have been more scientific surveys and studies regarding sexual functioning on spinal cord injury than on any other disability. A woman's ability or inability to lubricate and orgasm after spinal cord injury have been the focus of many of these studies. Depending on the extent of the injury, a woman may retain the ability to lubricate if she becomes sexually excited. Even more interesting, about 50% of women continue to be orgasmic even with complete injury.

Beverly Whipple, PhD, and Barry Komisaruk, MD, have researched women with spinal cord injury and report:

> Women with complete spinal cord injury (SCI) have reported that they do indeed experience orgasm. However, these women have been told (on the basis of the literature) that they could not experience orgasm—or if they did, that it was "phantom orgasm." Nevertheless, we have documented that women with complete SCI can indeed experience orgasm from self-stimulation of the vagina, the cervix, and a hypersensitive area of their body. (Whipple & Komisaruk, 1998, p. 21)

Drs. Whipple and Komisaruk propose that the vagus nerve may provide a sensory pathway from the cervix and vagina to the brain that bypasses the spinal cord. Although sexual sensations associated with this pathway may differ from your experience prior to the spinal cord damage, the important message is that a complete spinal cord injury does not mean that you must surrender your ability to enjoy your sexuality. You can experiment by stimulating the area inside your vagina called your G spot. In Chapters 3 and 15 we discuss how to locate your G spot and stimulate it.

Other areas of your body may become more sensitive to stimulation. Try increasing sensation with stimulation of your nipples, neck, ear lobes, and lips. Use the exercise called Partner Work: "Sensate Focus" in Chapter 15 to increase your awareness of the erotic parts of your body. Read the descriptions of sexual fantasy in Chapters 12 and 14 and consider purchasing books about erotica and sexual fantasy.

If rehabilitation for spinal cord damage is a part of your life or the life of someone you care about, we encourage you to make sure that the rehabilitation includes sexual rehabilitation as well. We recommend that you do the following:

- Understand your disability as fully as possible.
- Insist on sexual rehabilitation (which would include a complete assessment of the physical sensations retained and lost; education about orgasm, lubrication, and spinal cord disease; and guidance in experimenting with positions for lovemaking).
- Include your partner, if you have one, in the sexual "reeducation" part of the rehabilitation.
- Seriously consider peer counseling where you can talk with others about their process of adapting to disability and reintegrating their sexual identity.
- Allow time—a crucial variable in sexual healing or rehabilitation.

Your sexual life doesn't have to end after a spinal cord injury. Not surprising to us as sex therapists, the best predictor of how you'll adjust to these challenges and to what degree you will be able to resume satisfactory sex after spinal cord injury is how things were *before* the injury. That and time—giving yourself and your partner, if you have one, adequate time to adjust to the injury and to make accommodations necessary to resume sexual activity—are more predictive of a woman's sexual experience than how severe the injury (Sipski & Alexander, 1997).

Developmental Disability: A New View for the Families

A developmental disability is a disorder that occurs during childhood or adolescent development and is expected to impair a person's ability to function independently in adulthood. Sometimes a developmental disorder is due to one condition, such as a child with Down syndrome. Sometimes it is a cluster of disorders. An example would be Debby, a woman born with cerebral palsy linked to brain damage at birth. Debby has a seizure disorder, can't walk, and is moderately mentally retarded. Debby's cluster of problems would be categorized as a developmental disability. Debby will need to have supportive care all of her life. Her education, mobility, cognitive ability, self-care ability, and potential to earn a living are permanently affected by her cerebral palsy and retardation. Her ability to make discriminating choices about sexual activity will also be affected, although Debby, like all women, will be a sexual person throughout her life. Debby will need the support and guidance of the people who love her throughout her life. She'll also need their respect for her sexuality as a woman and her need to be educated about sexual functioning and sexual choices that her disability will permit her to make.

Mental Retardation

Throughout this book we say that sexuality is a process of growth, development, and experience, and that the way a woman experiences her sexuality depends on biological and social factors as well. Mental retardation, one of the most common developmental disabilities, places an adult woman in double jeopardy: she has cognitive impairments making her dependent in ways other women aren't, and others view her sexuality primarily from the perspective of her perceived vulnerability. Her emerging sexuality, usually first apparent at puberty, is often met with vigilance and rigid control. Debby's parents' greatest fear is that she could become pregnant if someone takes advantage of the fact that she is easily influenced or manipulated.

There are two responses often seen when others equate a woman's sexuality with vulnerability. One is overprotectiveness, which actually has the effect of creating more vulnerability. The other is a denial that allows parents, family members, friends, teachers, and neighbors to see women with mental retardation as living in adult bodies but with a child's mind. Because it can be so disturbing and confusing to deal with the sexuality of an adult with a cognitive disability, it becomes easier for families to support the *perpetual child* than to deal with the *developing adult*. Society—collective social attitudes—follow suit.

Debby might be mentally retarded, but she isn't stupid. She knows that adults in her domain are uncomfortable with her curiosity about sex. Her interests and exploration of this fascinating subject become covert.

In Chapter 1 we talked about the fairy tale of Sleeping Beauty. This fair and vulnerable young girl is doomed from the beginning of the story. Her parents want to protect her from pricking her finger on a spindle and falling into a 100-year sleep. They make every possible effort to keep her from even knowing what a spindle is. Still, the parents fail in their total protection of Sleeping Beauty, even though they go to great lengths to ensure her safety. We wouldn't have much of a fairy tale if Sleeping Beauty's parents had given her a safe spindle education from the time she was small, so that when she finally did encounter a spindle, she would have some way of making a discriminating decision about touching it, or better yet, how to use it appropriately.

As sex therapists and educators we support more, not less, sex education and counseling for adults with developmental disabilities and mental retardation. Parents of adolescent and young adults with mental retardation have to face their fears and resist the urge to be overly protective. Because so much of childhood and youth is a rehearsal for adulthood, it is imperative that persons with developmental disabilities learn to make as many choices as possible as early as possible. This will help them make more discriminating decisions throughout their lives. We also encourage those who have a relationship with a child with mental retardation to envision that person's adulthood. Sometimes it takes courage to think beyond childhood and imagine an adult. There is no better way to begin those steps toward supporting adult life than by seeing a woman as a sexual human being throughout her life.

An adult woman with a developmental disability should have a complete physical, including a pelvic exam, to assure that she is in good health and to address any medical problems, including problems with menstruation. If the woman is not able to understand the purpose of a pelvic exam and expresses distress, ultrasound may be substituted. If a woman is not sexually active, her risk of cervical cancer is greatly reduced and she may not need annual pap and pelvic exams. Check with your healthcare provider about a gynecologist or "specialty" clinic that offers individualized health care for persons with developmental disabilities.

Sexuality education should be provided. Self-care in personal menstrual hygiene, a discussion of conception and contraceptives, and an understanding of sexual function (including desire, arousal, and orgasm) are important components of sex education for any woman with developmental disability who is capable of directed self-care. A discussion of masturbation and the meaning of self-pleasure is a further example of teaching a woman with developmental disability how to care for herself. This discussion can include an explanation of "public" and "private" with regard to sexual self-expression, and should be combined with an assessment of her living space to make sure she has privacy in which to masturbate. Women who are living independently or in group settings should also be taught about types of sexual interaction, from brief to committed partnerships. These conversations should be dialogues that are ongoing rather than one-time-only inservices. There are many websites and books discussing sexuality concerns for the developmentally disabled. A good place to start is The Arc of the United States (formerly the Association for Retarded Citizens), at www.thearc.org.[3] Sex education and training will also be important for group-home staff to ensure that they can respectfully handle sexual concerns as they arise.

[3]In addition to The Arc of the United States: American Association of Mental Retardation at www.aamr.org; National Down Syndrome Society at www.ndss.org; Autism Society of America at www.autism-society.org; and United Cerebral Palsy at www.ucp.org.

CHAPTER EIGHT

When Sex Causes Pain

There are few circumstances more daunting to a woman's sexuality than to have her experience of sex repeatedly associated with pain. If you are coping with such pain, you know what we mean when we say that this invisible condition affects your everyday life and many decisions you make. For example, if you have chronic burning pain in your vulva, something as simple as being invited to a concert becomes a challenge. Because of the pain, you have to factor in how long you can sit and what you can wear to make the discomfort manageable. If you are in a relationship, it is likely that you and your partner have found yourselves avoiding sex or even situations that could lead to sex. If you are not in a relationship, you may avoid the possibility of entering one—it becomes too painful to contemplate.

The bad news—as if you needed any more bad news—is that diagnosing the cause of chronic sexual pain is often difficult. If sometime in the past you sought medical treatment for sexual pain, chances are you were told that no physical abnormalities could be identified and that the problem may be psychological. And, unfortunately, without proper diagnosis and treatment, your chronic sexual pain probably didn't resolve itself.

The good news is that this trend is changing. Your healthcare provider is more likely today than in years past to take your experience seriously. We are now learning a great deal more about what causes sexual pain and how to treat it effectively. If you question whether you're getting appropriate care for your sexual pain, get a second opinion. You as a patient are in a better position than ever before to advocate for yourself. There is a wealth of information available on the Internet that can help you educate yourself about sexual pain, available treatments, and centers that specialize in this problem.

The majority of sexual pain for women falls into one of three categories. When pain during sexual activity occurs in the visible portion of the genitals, we refer to it as vulvar pain. Internal or vaginal pain occurs inside the body during vaginal penetration or thrusting. Pelvic floor muscle pain occurs in the muscles that wrap around the opening of the vagina and is triggered by vaginal penetration.

Many factors can cause or aggravate pain, so a thorough medical work-up is important. Sometimes the pelvic muscles become lax and internal organs begin to prolapse (slip down) into the vagina, or even up against the vulva. Infections, sexually transmitted diseases, masses on the uterine ligaments, tubes, or ovaries, or endometriosis can all be sources of pain. Sometimes medical conditions such as interstitial cystitis or irritable bowel syndrome cause pain during sexual intercourse or even attempts at penetration. Gynecologic cancer can be a cause of sexual pain, but usually only during the later stages of the disease. Sometimes pain can be associated with sensitivity to certain soaps, shampoos, fabrics, medications, douches, or topical ointments. Regardless of the cause, the first line of defense against painful sex is a thorough medical evaluation.

VULVAR PAIN

Chronic pain, burning, rawness, stinging, or itching in the vulva is called *vulvodynia*. If you have this condition, you might feel discomfort only when you attempt sexual activity, or the pain might be constant (or intermittent) and not restricted to sexual activity. For some women sexual arousal by itself, without penetration or even physical contact, can cause pain because of the vasocongestion that occurs in the genital region.

If you have experienced vulvar pain, you may be familiar with the term *vulvar vestibulitis*—a subset of vulvodynia that happens in a very specific part of the vulva. The vulvar vestibule starts at the hymenal ring and blends with the labia minora. Within this area, some women have distinct points of tenderness. The cause of vulvar vestibulitis is not known. It is not a sexually transmitted disease, so it's not something you can pass on to your partner.

Because vulvodynia can have many possible causes, it is important to have a gynecology specialist evaluate the problem. Seek medical help as soon as you can. Pain is a neurological process that follows neuronal pathways. It is a bit like a path in the woods: at first the path may be hardly noticeable, but if it is traveled enough, it becomes clearly worn. Pain is like that. The longer it is present, the more entrenched it becomes. This does not mean that your situation is hopeless if you have had pain of a longstanding nature. Check the "Suggested Resources" list for books and websites that provide a wealth of information on treatment options and symptomatic relief for vulvar and pelvic pain.

In addition to getting appropriate medical care, a cornerstone of recovery from chronic vulvar, internal, or pelvic pain is education and support. Join a chat room on the web and share ideas and concerns with other women. If you don't have a computer, go to the library and use one there. It will help you feel less isolated even as you find ways to advocate for quality care.

If you have vulvodynia, you may fear that sex will never again be pleasurable. Not so. Even in cases where pain is acute, a number of medical treatments are proving to be helpful. For example, vulvar pain can often be relieved by tricyclic antidepressant medication. The treatment seems to work by interfering with the nerve transmission of pain in the part of the brain where pain is perceived and processed. It is outside the scope of this chapter to offer prescriptive recommendations about medication and other medical treatments, but specialists who treat the problem will have many ideas. Instead, we will offer some self-help ideas to decrease the discomfort of vulvodynia and minimize sexual difficulties.

Relief for Pain and Itching

Measures that effectively relieve pain and itching differ from person to person, but some common recommendations include:

- *Clothing*: Use only white, 100% cotton underwear, not synthetic underwear with a cotton crotch. Avoid close-fitting clothing. Wash underwear in mild soap and put it through an extra rinse cycle.
- *Chemicals*: Be alert to chemical irritants that may be present in soaps, shampoos, panty liners, and so on. Use a gentle soap on the rest of your body, but avoid using soap on the vulva.
- *Hygiene*: Keep the vulva dry, but rinse often. Warm water cleanses the vulva adequately after urination. Cornstarch can also be used to absorb moisture.
- *Diet*: Watch your diet. There may be a correlation between "oxalates" in the diet and vulvar pain. Oxalates are a byproduct of oxalic acids, which are present in some plant foods (non-animal products) such as coffee. Many women find that cutting back on foods containing oxalates and taking calcium citrate (which decreases calcium oxalate formation in the urine) decreases vulvar pain and itching. You can learn about the low-oxalate diet on the Internet or from your healthcare provider. We recommend that you follow this diet under medical supervision. Over time you will be able to determine which foods, in particular, aggravate your vulvar condition and should be avoided.

Vulvar Pain and Sex

Couples coping with chronic sexual pain are naturally at a loss about what to do. The frustrating and intrusive association of pain with sex often means that nongenital sensual pleasure is lost as well. The default mode for many couples dealing with vulvar pain is to avoid all physical contact because of the fear that sexually stimulating activity is expected to follow.

If you have become touch avoidant because you have been coping with vulvar pain, openly discuss this with your partner. Reintroduce holding, hugging, kissing, and massage, making clear that these pleasurable activities are not to be associated with any additional expectations and are complete unto themselves. Touching and caressing should be valued for their own merits and not seen as an inevitable prelude to genital sex.

If you decide to have sexual activity with your partner while you have vulvar pain, there are a number of things you can try to decrease the discomfort. It's essential to realize, however, that you should never feel forced or pressured into having sex. A grit-my-teeth-and-get-through-it approach will almost always backfire in the long run; it can cause you to be fearful and avoidant of sex, and your partner, in turn, will feel confused, unfulfilled, and perhaps even guilty. If you decide to try the following suggestions, make sure it's because you *want to*, not because you feel you have to.

- Educate your partner about your condition.
- Learn about your own pain responses. Are there times of day when you have less pain? What parts of your vulva produce pain upon touch? Are there sexual positions that cause less pain?
- Figure out what still feels pleasurable. For example, do you enjoy having your breasts and upper thighs stroked as long as the vulva is off-limits? If your clitoris is a sore spot, is it pleasurable when you avoid the clitoris and stimulate inside the vagina?
- Check with your gynecologist about occasionally using a topical anesthetic (lidocaine, for example) to temporarily numb the skin.
- If you have pain with sexual arousal, try using an ice pack on your crotch (for no more than 20 minutes). You can also use the ice pack during or after sex.
- Urinate before and after having sex, rinsing yourself with warm water after urination.
- Make certain that you decide in advance which activities will and will not be included during sex, and remain in control of those activities.
- Use added lubrication such as Astroglide, K-Y Liquid, vitamin E oil, or vegetable oil. Some women find that the oils contain fewer irritants. Information about ordering lubricants online can be found in the section in Chapter 15, "Lubricants."
- If you decide to have intercourse, have your partner first put one finger into your vagina, then two fingers. Massage the pelvic muscle by gently rubbing the area at the vaginal opening. When it's time for penetration, guide the penis in and control the amount and intensity of movement. Your partner should

never push. Have penetration for just a minute. You don't have to thrust. Then have your partner withdraw his penis and go on to other sexual play. Build the intercourse time up slowly over many sessions of lovemaking.
- Never override your experience of pain. If you are in pain, *stop*.

After sexual contact with your partner, cuddle and communicate. Talk about at least one thing that went well, but avoid talking about disappointments or frustrations. You are trying to build a repertoire of success. Later, when you're dressed and in a neutral setting, you can analyze what went right and wrong, and what to do next time.

INTERNAL PAIN

Whereas vulvar pain is experienced in an area of the body (vulva) that we can see and touch, with internal or vaginal pain the sexual pain is experienced inside the body, in places we can't see but can certainly feel. It's pain that does not necessarily occur in the vagina but is triggered by a penis, finger, or a sex toy inside the vagina. Sometimes this type of pain is called pelvic pain or deep thrusting pain.

Causes and Treatments of Internal Pain

Lack of Arousal

A common cause of sexual pain is vaginal dryness. The excitement phase of the sexual response prepares the vagina for penetration by providing lubrication for the genitals (see Chapter 4 for more about sexual arousal). You can tell if you are aroused and lubricated by the vaginal opening, which becomes somewhat swollen and slippery. Lack of adequate lubrication can cause friction leading to pain, irritation, and rawness at the opening of the vagina. The walls of your vagina can also be irritated by penetration if lubrication is insufficient.

If you try to have vaginal penetration without enough stimulating activity to produce lubrication, penetration can be uncomfortable or painful. It's important that you gauge the timing of penetration not simply by your partner's urgency but by your own readiness and urgency.

Lubrication can be compromised by several physical factors such as medication side effects, low estrogen due to aging, or hormonal changes during nursing. If this is the case in your situation, you can compensate by using a supplemental lubricant such as Astroglide, K-Y Jelly or Liquid, or Replens. Different types and brands of lubrication last varying lengths of time and have different viscosities or textures. For example, Astroglide, Moist Again, K-Y Liquid, and Sylk, are thinner in viscosity, K-Y Jelly is thicker, and Replens lasts longer. Experiment to determine which lubricant is the most suitable for you. Your healthcare provider may have samples of various lubricants for you to try. You can order lubrications from several of the websites (like www.goodvibes.com or www.babeland.com) listed in "Suggested Resources."

If you are having problems with sexual arousal, see Chapter 15 for additional ideas on how to overcome low sexual arousal.

Pelvic Inflammatory Disease (PID)

Pelvic inflammatory disease (PID) is an infection in the uterus, fallopian tubes, or ovaries. As with any infection, PID can range from a very mild condition to a severe medical crisis requiring emergency treatment and hospitalization. Because sexually transmitted diseases can cause PID, you are at greater risk of developing this condition if you have been sexually active with several partners. Douching also can increase your risk of developing PID, because some of the douche fluid may enter the uterus.

Because there are many causes for PID, including sexually transmitted diseases, and because PID can lead to infertility, it is important to get medical treatment as soon as you suspect that you might have this condition. If you experience pain inside your lower abdomen when your cervix or uterus is jarred by sexual intercourse, and this happens over a period of time and not just as an isolated incident or two, get a medical evaluation. Other symptoms of PID include persistent abdominal pain, backache, fever, and a vaginal discharge that differs from your normal discharge.

Your medical care provider will order lab work such as blood tests and mucus smears. Sometimes a diagnostic laparoscopy is indicated (a common surgical procedure in which a tiny camera is inserted into the abdominal wall to see and treat what is going on inside the body). PID is often treated with a carefully monitored antibiotic regimen.

A Tough Hymen

A hymen that doesn't give way easily to finger or penis penetration can cause pain during penetrative sex. It isn't common, but sometimes the hymenal tissue is rigid and tough, and a simple surgical procedure may be necessary to correct the problem. The medical term is "imperforate hymen." If you suspect the opening to your vagina isn't as elastic as it should be, a pelvic exam will reveal whether there is an imperforate hymen. For more information about the hymen, see Chapter 3.

Uterus in the Wrong Position

Sometimes the internal organs or genital tract isn't in the correct position. A tipped uterus is an example of such a condition. If you consistently have a feeling of pressure or pain in your lower back and tenderness in the abdomen during intercourse, you may have a tipped uterus. You can experiment with sexual positions to see if a different one leads to more comfort during intercourse. Chapter 12 describes four common positions for intercourse.

We spoke earlier in this chapter about a prolapse, where the pelvic muscles become lax and internal organs can slip out of place; the cervix and uterus may even protrude into the vagina. If you have a prolapse, it will be very easy for your healthcare provider to make this diagnosis. There are both surgical and nonsurgical measures that can relieve this problem. If you continue to have pain after medical treatment for a prolapse, and experimenting with sexual positions does not help, consider seeing a sex therapist.

Muscle and Skeletal Problems

Muscle or skeletal problems can be a source of pain with sex. (Here we're talking about muscles other than the pelvic floor muscles, which we discuss in the next section of this chapter.) Scoliosis (curvature of the spine) is an example of a musculoskeletal problem that can cause discomfort during penetration. The discomfort may be due to spasms in the lower back muscles that have been working to compensate for the scoliosis. Another example would be a muscle strain in the abdominal wall that is aggravated during intercourse. The oversensitive muscles may go into painful spasms when there is vaginal penetration and thrusting.

Musculoskeletal problems can be difficult to diagnose. If you have chronic pain with sex and have had extensive diagnostic tests that fail to turn up any explanations for your pain, an evaluation by a physical therapist may be in order. In many cases physical therapy can help relieve symptoms arising from musculoskeletal problems. You may also benefit from biofeedback procedures discussed in the next section of this chapter. Also review the material on illness and disability in Chapter 7.

PELVIC FLOOR MUSCLE PAIN

Pelvic floor muscle pain (PMP) is also known as vaginismus. Pelvic floor muscle pain is a more accurate term than vaginismus, however, because the pain involves the musculature in the pelvic floor, not in the vagina. (See Chapter 3 for more information about the pelvic floor muscles.) These muscles can tighten near the vaginal opening and make penetration by a penis, finger, tampon, or any outside object painful or impossible. If these muscles involuntarily contract, there can be a painful spasm. In other cases, the pain does not come from muscular spasm but from the tightness around the vaginal opening caused by the muscular contraction. The penis or any other object trying to penetrate the constricted opening to the vagina can cause bruising of surrounding tissue, making it very tender or painful to touch.

Pelvic muscle pain can be primary, meaning a woman has always experienced muscle spasm when penetration has been attempted; or secondary, meaning the onset of PMP followed some event like an infection or trauma.

> "I had yeast infections one after another for a while. It made intercourse uncomfortable at first, and then downright painful. The thing is, even after the infections cleared up completely, I still had the pain. I had no idea what was wrong, and my doctor wasn't much help. She said I was clear of infection, and to just relax."

It is very common for pelvic muscles to involuntarily tighten or spasm following some form of vulvar or internal pain. It's the body and mind's way of protecting you—trying to avoid further pain by avoiding further penetration. Unfortunately, though well-intentioned, this attempt at self-protection inadvertently becomes the cause of further pain.

Pelvic muscle pain can *really* hurt. Women who chronically experience PMP report that the pain is excruciating. It is often described as a burning sensation. Anyone who has had a severe and sudden cramp in a leg muscle knows how painful a muscle spasm can be.

PMP sets up a cycle of pain and dread so that any attempts at penetration, or even circumstances in which penetration might be expected, create anticipatory anxiety. This anxiety can make it difficult or impossible for you to relax in sexual situations. The anxiety may also trigger, or contribute to, further muscular contractions—which lead to further pain—which leads to further anxiety. And so the cycle continues.

Most women with PMP experience muscular pain as soon as penetration is attempted, though some don't feel pain until penetration has been achieved. A rare few experience the spasm not at penetration but at withdrawal. Some women experience extreme muscle tightening without an accompanying painful spasm. Regardless of the pattern, PMP is tenacious. It doesn't usually go away spontaneously, but it *is* treatable.

What causes PMP? This is a little like trying to say what causes a fever. PMP is a symptom, not a disease. When pelvic muscle pain develops in response to another painful condition, such as after a vaginal infection, we can easily understand the connection. Pelvic muscle pain can also develop (though rarely) after experiencing a sexual assault or sexual abuse. We have seen pelvic muscle tightness develop after injury—even minor injury—to the pelvic area. An example would be a girl falling on the crossbar of a bicycle and perforating her hymen so that she bleeds. The injury is more frightening than serious, but because PMP is a protective reaction, it becomes a reflexive response when the vaginal area is "threatened" again at a later time, even if the "threat" is consensual intercourse.

When pelvic muscle pain is present and unaccounted for, the medical profession tends to assume that there must be a psychological cause. It is certain that pain with sex will always have psychological components. Feelings of alienation, isolation, and loss are common and normal psychological responses to chronic pain. The challenge in many cases is to determine whether the psychological distress develops because of the pain or whether the pain develops because of underlying psychological issues.

Treatment of Pelvic Muscle Pain

Physical Therapy and Biofeedback

Physical therapy (in combination with medical care and sex therapy) is the most effective way to treat PMP and is almost always helpful as an adjunctive therapy for vulvar and internal pain as well. The best person to provide this treatment is a physical therapist who has been trained specifically in the rehabilitation of the pelvic floor muscles. A physician referral is often required for this specialized treatment.

Why is this treatment so effective? If you have chronic pelvic pain, you may have learned to shut off the conscious sensations from these muscles, so you have difficulty identifying the muscles and exercising any voluntary control over them. In addition, the muscles may be chronically tense, chronically weak, or in a chronic state of spasm. The physical therapist can help you identify these muscles and gain better control over them. As you learn how to tense and relax these muscles, you can gradually relieve the chronic muscular tension and allow penetration without undue tightness or discomfort.

Physical therapy for PMP often includes biofeedback. Biofeedback is a treatment using a monitoring device that gives you feedback on how your actions are affecting a biological process like heart rate, blood pressure, or muscle tone. As you try different strategies to influence or control a body response, the biofeedback equipment provides information about your success. With this feedback, you can fine-tune your thoughts and actions until you develop good control.

For PMP, the biofeedback component of treatment uses a stimulation sensor that measures the degree of tension in the pelvic floor muscles. After you have been completely prepared and are comfortable, a tampon-like device called a periometer is inserted into your vagina. If you are uneasy about any penetration, the therapist works at your pace, never overriding your reluctance. The sensor stimulates the pelvic muscles to contract, and you and the therapist get immediate feedback on a computer screen about how the muscles are working. The therapist trains you to gain voluntary control over the pelvic muscles, then prescribes a home program for you to follow. This method works very well not only for patients who have overly tense pelvic floor muscles but also for patients with interstitial cystitis, vulvar pain, urinary incontinence, and some forms of vaginal or pelvic pain.

If you don't have medical insurance that would cover such treatment, don't give up. A consultation/evaluation session with a physical therapist can be invaluable and is worth saving up for a visit or two. The physical therapist can recommend inexpensive periometers that you can purchase and use at home. In one or two sessions, the therapist can teach you how to insert the periometer and how to program this biofeedback device to improve your muscular control. Additional information is located in the "Suggested Resources" section on pain.

Physical Therapy and Ultrasound

In some cases, a physical therapist may use ultrasound treatment to help with chronic pelvic muscle pain and tension. This treatment may precede biofeedback. Ultrasound is a painless, nonintrusive treatment that has been used extensively by physical therapists for patients with injuries, muscular pain, and muscular spasm. More recently, therapists have discovered that this treatment can rehabilitate pelvic floor muscles. Ultrasound introduces sound waves deep into tissues. It is sometimes referred to as "deep heat." It increases blood flow, promotes healing if there is trauma to the tissues, and helps to relax tightened muscles.

Kegel Exercises and Dilator Therapy

One of the problems women have with PMP is that they become unaware of how to exercise voluntary muscle control. Kegel exercises involve consciously squeezing and relaxing the pelvic floor muscles so that you gain voluntary control over these muscles. One way to identify how to control and relax these muscles is to experiment when you urinate. When you start to urinate, try to stop the stream of urine. When you can do this, you are contracting your pelvic floor muscles. When you stop trying and the urine stream resumes, you have relaxed the pelvic muscles. Once you've identified the muscles, practice contracting and relaxing them (Kegel exercises) when you're not urinating.

The goal of Kegel exercises is not to tense the muscles but to learn to relax them and exert voluntary control over them. When you contract the pelvic muscles, you are tensing them. To release the tension, stop contracting and push slightly, as if you were attempting to expel urine or a tampon. This is, in part, how you relax the pelvic muscles. Pay particular attention to what it feels like when you relax the muscles. These exercises should be practiced several times a day. Kegel exercises are best learned under the guidance of a physical therapist or healthcare practitioner during a pelvic examination, so that you can be certain that you are properly contracting and relaxing the correct muscles. Kegels can also be used to help strengthen muscles that have become too "relaxed," as with urinary incontinence.

Using your improved muscular control from the Kegel exercises, you can use vaginal dilators to train or retrain your body to allow penetration without involuntary muscular contractions. Vaginal dilators were originally designed for patients who had undergone surgery or radiation treatment for the vagina. They are cylinders with rounded tips that come in sets ranging in size from very small, about the size of a tampon, to large, approximating the size of an erect penis. Depending on the manufacturer, the dilators can be made of a material that is rigid or flexible and rubbery. We prefer the flexible dilators. Dilators can be ordered through your healthcare provider.

Dilator therapy is usually done alone in the privacy of your home. You begin by inserting the smallest dilator and keeping it in place for several minutes, commonly 10 to 20 minutes. This is repeated three to five times a week. Once you have comfortably mastered the smallest dilator, you move up one size and repeat the process until you can accommodate the largest dilator without difficulty or discomfort. You should clean the dilators with soap and water after each use.

Two important points: First, if you have pain when inserting a dilator, stop. Dilator therapy won't be effective if you are in pain, so proceed slowly and at your own pace. Second, the use of dilators can be a highly effective treatment for PMP, but we emphatically state that dilator therapy should be directed by a sex therapist, physical therapist, or healthcare practitioner. The practitioner or therapist can explain how to use the dilators, indicate when to graduate to the next size of dilator, and monitor your overall progress. Too many women have been given dilators and marginal instruction. Without ongoing guidance, the dilators often end up discarded in a dresser drawer, and the woman remains frustrated and confounded.

SEX THERAPY

Even when there are physical reasons for pain, psychological and relationship issues should not be overlooked. Research has continually demonstrated that pain management is best accomplished when there is a multidisciplinary treatment approach that addresses not only the physical cause of the pain but also the impact of the pain on the individual and the couple. In many cases of sexual pain, treatment with a sex therapist can be very helpful. See Chapter 17 for suggestions on how to find a qualified sex therapist. Just as physicians specialize in one aspect of medicine or another, sex therapists tend to specialize. Make sure your potential sex therapist has had experience working with chronic sexual pain.

A sex therapist can help you and your partner understand the symptom you are experiencing, where it is located in your body, the common relationship strains that may occur, and treatment strategies for overcoming the symptoms. Your sex therapist will be alert to whether the symptom of pain keeps some balance or serves some purpose in your relationship. For example, one couple coping with PMP disclosed that they were at odds with each other about when to try to get pregnant. The husband urgently wanted to begin a family, but the wife was not ready to take this major life step. In this case the symptom—chronic PMP—served a purpose; it kept the couple from dealing with their underlying conflict about pregnancy. Although the conflict didn't cause the symptom in the first place, there certainly was a covert reason why the wife may not have been completely eager to resolve the problem.

FINAL THOUGHTS ON PAIN MANAGEMENT

One of our patients said that having chronic sexual pain made her want to divorce her genitals. Compensating for pain can certainly make you want to live anyplace but in your body, and for this reason you may find yourself becoming further and further disconnected from the pleasures and benefits of movement and touch. We want to encourage you to live and move and relax in your body again. Massage therapy is a good place to start. It reminds you of sensations of connection, pleasure, and relaxation. Then select a form of exercise that you enjoy: biking, walking, swimming, dancing, yoga, martial arts, aerobics at your gym or YWCA. Experiment with ways to relax and enjoy pleasure in your body, even if it doesn't come directly from your genitals. Sexual pain can be a challenge, but it doesn't have to prevent you from taking care of your sexual self.

CHAPTER NINE

Sexually Transmitted Diseases

Sexually transmitted diseases, or STDs, are diagnosed in 15 million Americans every year, and as many as 65 million Americans are currently infected with an incurable STD (Cates, 1999). The rates of infection for some STDs in the United States are among the highest in the industrialized world (Eng & Butler, 1997). Although public health initiatives have had a significant impact on the incidence of syphilis and gonorrhea, other STDs like chlamydia, herpes, HPV (genital warts), and trichomoniasis (a parasitic infection) infect millions of Americans every year.

It is a sad irony that in this supposed age of sexual enlightenment, the incidence of STDs is rampant even though transmission is largely preventable. It is equally sad and ironic that STDs are not being addressed adequately in the classroom, in the media, or in the legislatures. In a recent Gallup survey (American Social Health Association, 1995), 26% of the adult and 42% of the teen respondents could not name a single STD other than HIV/AIDS. Television virtually ignores STDs and the consequences of unprotected sex, routinely portraying casual sex with multiple partners as normal, benign behavior but rarely depicting couples taking precautions. On TV, unprotected, casual sex may occasionally result in an unwanted pregnancy, but never an STD. STDs remain a taboo in our society, prompting many policy-makers to avoid dealing with the issue in a direct, proactive, and enlightened fashion. As a result, we face what a recent panel of experts referred to as a "hidden epidemic" (Eng

& Butler, 1997) that is exacting a tremendous toll in lives, productivity, and happiness.

STDs exact a particularly harsh toll from women. Because they are more susceptible biologically to some STDs, each year more women than men become infected. Women also experience a wider range of physical complications, including infertility, pelvic pain, ectopic pregnancies, and cervical cancer. One million women each year are treated for pelvic inflammatory disease (PID), a condition often caused by an untreated STD such as chlamydia or gonorrhea. Between 1973 and 1992, *150,000 American* women died from STDs and their complications (Eng & Butler, 1997).

Another toll often exacted by STDs is the loss of self-esteem a woman may experience when she becomes infected. Anyone can get an STD, the same way anyone can get strep throat. Nonetheless, the general reaction to STDs is a moralistic judgment that someone who had unprotected sex just got what he or she deserved. Let us be clear as we begin this chapter: a woman with a sexually transmitted disease is a woman with a medical problem who needs medical care, education, and support in order to care for herself. Spare her the moralizing; she doesn't need or deserve it.

STDs: FROM THE INCONVENIENT TO THE LETHAL

STDs refer to the more than 25 organisms (Eng & Butler, 1997) that can be sexually transmitted between partners, with results ranging from mild embarrassment and inconvenience to severe disability and death. Some STDs are bacterial and therefore they are curable when detected early and treated with appropriate antibiotics. Other STDs are caused by a virus, and a cure can be much more elusive if not impossible. Just as we have yet to come up with a cure for the common cold, we have yet to come up with cures for most viral STDs. When you take medicine for your cold, it's not to cure the cold: it can only decrease the severity of the symptoms and/or prevent further complications from developing. The same is true for the medical treatment of most viral STDs. Advances have been made, however, in the development of vaccines to help prevent infection by some viral STDs such as hepatitis B. Researchers hope one day to have vaccines to prevent the transmission of herpes and HIV. Other STDs are caused by neither bacteria nor virus, but by fungus, protozoa, lice, or mites.

Some STDs, like syphilis and gonorrhea, are almost always transmitted by sexual contact. Other STDs, like HIV or hepatitis B, can be transmitted in nonsexual ways such as sharing an infected hypodermic needle or receiving a tainted blood transfusion. And some STDs can result without any transmission whatsoever. For example, many women have yeast cells lying dormant in their genital area that can become active in response to pregnancy, birth control pills, antibiotics, diabetes, or spermicides containing nonoxynol-9. Their resulting yeast infection is not caused by sexual behavior, but it can indeed be transmitted to a partner. Many STDs can be transmitted from a pregnant mother to her unborn child.

Table 9.1 summarizes 11 of the most common STDs, listing symptoms, means of transmission, possible complications, and available treatments. For more detailed information about each STD, consult the "Suggested Resources" list at the end of this book.

ONE MORE TIME: SAFER SEX

STDs are spread by physical contact. Bacterial and viral organisms enter the body through a mucous membrane. The mucous membranes are warm, moist, and more permeable than other areas of skin. Mucous membranes include the mouth and parts of the vulva, urethra, vagina, and anus. Most sex education programs now stress using a barrier, such as a latex condom, for sexual activity like vaginal intercourse or anal sex.

STDs are transferred from person to person. Animals don't give humans STDs, and doorknobs, toilet seats, or other objects are rarely transmitters because bacteria and viruses are fragile and require fresh, warm fluid to survive. They die quickly when they remain outside the human body. Exceptions do exist, however, as noted in the table.

Although STDs can infect people of any age, younger people are infected more often. They're more likely to be exposed to different partners and may, because of the fearless sense of immortality in youth, see themselves as less vulnerable to "bad things happening." They may be less educated about transmission processes and take a new partner's word as reliable, even though their new partner may be less educated about STDs than they are.

There are many myths in our culture to which women naively fall prey. The myths about romance, spontaneity, and nice partners not having "dirty diseases" are some of the biggest problems. Some women refuse to be realistic about safer-sex practices. They think that if they pull out a condom or insist on testing for STDs, at best, they'll be seen as the "safe sex police" and, at worst, considered a cheap slut who sleeps around. Women don't insist on condoms because they're afraid of being judged. This is self-esteem that is so low it can literally kill you.

There are a number of strategies to help women become more comfortable taking precautions. Traditionally women have confided in each other. You can ask other women what they say when insisting on safer sex and learn from each other's experience. You can read everything you can find on the subject and become informed not only about HIV/AIDS but also about where to get condoms, spermicidal gels, and testing. This education should include ways to have fun with safer sex. Because condoms are absolute necessities for safer heterosexual sex, we recommend that you become more comfortable handling condoms by practicing sliding them onto bananas.

TABLE 9.1. Sexually Transmitted Diseases (STDs)

STD	Symptoms	Transmission	Complications	Treatment
		Bacterial STDs		
Gonorrhea	• Vaginal discharge, painful urination, or unusual vaginal bleeding • Often symptomless • Can be confused with yeast infections	• Genital sexual contact • Mother to newborn during vaginal delivery	• Can affect urethra, anus, vagina, cervix, and uterus • Spontaneous abortion or premature delivery • Untreated, can develop into pelvic inflammatory disease and broad systemic reactions like arthritis, skin disease, and heart damage	• Antibiotics
Chlamydia trachomatis	• Vaginal discharge, painful urination, or unusual vaginal bleeding • Often symptomless, up to 75% of infected women are unaware they have this STD	• Genital sexual contact • Mother to newborn during vaginal delivery	• Chronic inflammation of the cervix, rectal inflammation, pelvic inflammatory disease • Infertility • Ectopic pregnancy • Premature delivery	• Antibiotics
Syphilis	• Primary phase—ulcer at point of infection • Secondary phase—rash, low fever, aches and pains, sore throat, swollen glands • Following the above phases, the person can be symptomless for years, yet internal damage continues	• Genital sexual contact • Mother to fetus • Skin contact	• Paralysis • Blindness • Mental deterioration • Death	• Antibiotics
		Viral STDs		
Hepatitis B	• Jaundice (yellowing of skin and whites of the eyes) • Fever, headache, joint pain, skin rash, and dark urine	• Infected semen, vaginal secretions, blood, or saliva coming in contact with mucous membrane or breaks in skin • Mother to fetus • Breast-feeding	• Cirrhosis • Liver failure • Liver cancer • Death	• In some cases, an acute infection resolves and the virus clears • For a chronic infection, no cure. Supportive measures include antiviral medication and abstinence from alcohol • Inoculate partner with hepatitis B vaccine.
Herpes simplex virus type 2 (HSV-2)	• First outbreak (primary) is usually the most painful, often with flu-like symptoms—fever, swollen glands, general stiffness, aches and pains. Local symptoms include itching and burning, herpes sores (roundish, watery bumps) on genitals, cervix, buttocks, anus, or inner thighs • Recurrent episodes, symptoms usually milder and more local, marked by herpes sores	• Occurs when body is shedding the virus, which comes in contact with mucous membrane or breaks in the skin • Shedding can occur even when sores are not visible ("silent shedding") • Contact with towels, bedding, or clothing • Mother to fetus	• During primary outbreak, spontaneous abortion, premature birth, and low birth weight	• Zovirax for symptom relief, not cure

(continued on next page)

TABLE 9.1. *(continued)*

STD	Symptoms	Transmission	Complications	Treatment
Human papilloma virus (HPV; genital warts)	• Warts may be visible on genitals or anus, or microscopic and unseen inside the vagina or on the cervix	• Genital sexual contact • Contact with towels, bedding, or clothing (possible) • Mother to child during vaginal delivery	• Cervical cancer	• Many HPV infections are cured by body's own immune system • Removal by freezing, cauterizing, laser treatment, or surgery • Topical treatments with caustic chemicals • Alpha-interferon injections
Human immuno-deficiency virus (HIV)	• Initially symptomless or mild flu-like symptoms • After initial symptoms, often symptomless for a long period of time, yet still highly contagious • In later stages, weight loss, fever, diarrhea, and opportunistic infections	• Infected semen, vaginal secretions, blood, or saliva coming in contact with mucous membrane or breaks in skin • Mother to fetus • Breast-feeding	• Breakdown of body's immune system, allowing opportunistic infections • Tumors • Mental deterioration • Death	• Maximizing healthy lifestyle • Antiviral medications, such as AZT, that slow replication of HIV cells
		Other STDs		
Candida albicans (yeast infection)	• Genital itching • Inflammation of the vulva • Genital soreness, burning, swelling, pain during intercourse, painful urination • Vaginal discharge	• Genital sexual contact • Can occur without transmission from someone else	• Usually none, other than disruption caused by symptoms	• Monistat, Mycelex, Femstat, Nystatin, Nizoral • Wearing loose-fitting clothing, cotton-lined underwear
Tricho-moniasis (protozoan; a parasitic infection)	• Often symptomless • Itching, painful intercourse, burning or painful urination, frothy gray or yellow-green vaginal discharge • Fever • Symptoms may only occur during, or immediately following, menstruation	• Genital sexual contact • Damp towels or clothing recently used by an infected person • Mother to fetus	• Usually none, other than disruption caused by symptoms	• Metronidazole (Flagyl) or tinidazole
Pubic lice (crabs; different from head and body lice)	• Genital itching • Inflammation of the vulva • Small blue spots from louse bites • Pubic lice may also be found in armpits or eyelashes	• Genital sexual contact • Contact with objects (clothing, towels, and bed linen) infested with pubic lice or their eggs	• Usually none, other than disruption caused by symptoms or secondary skin infection due to scratching	• Over-the-counter preparations that kill lice and their eggs • Permethrin cream • Lindane shampoo (not recommended for small children or pregnant women) • Thorough cleaning of clothing, towels, and bed linens • Use of disinfectants for nonwashable items
Scabies (mites that burrow under the surface of the skin)	• Intense itching, red rash, welts, pustules • Most often infest the hands or wrists, but also genitals and other parts of the body below the neck	• Genital sexual contact • Any close body contact • Contact with objects (clothing, towels, and bed linen) infested with mites	• Usually none, other than disruption caused by symptoms or secondary skin infection due to scratching	• Lindane lotion or cream • For infants, young children, and pregnant women: sulfur ointment • Thorough laundering of clothing, towels, and bed linen

You should also seriously consider the relationship of drugs and alcohol to sex. A woman "under the influence" doesn't do her best thinking, and neither will her partner. "Getting high and getting laid" can lead to disaster. You can help yourself by thinking ahead, getting educated, planning for sex, and staying sober.

In their book *The New Our Bodies, Ourselves*, the Boston Women's Health Book Collective (1992) reflect on sex and power:

> For women, safer sex is about power. Power in terms of feeling valuable, feeling worthwhile, having a high enough self-esteem to want to protect ourselves. Power in our relationships: being able to hold our ground and persuade a sex partner to use protection. Power in our pocketbooks: being able to support ourselves and our children if we leave a partner who endangers us by not using protection. Power in our friendships to support us in protecting ourselves. The power of feeling proud of our sexuality. There is the power, too, of speaking openly about sex, even when it is hard to talk about. Finally, our power to protect ourselves is weakened by drugs and alcohol; if we are addicted, the power we need depends on access to affordable treatment. All women deserve the power to keep ourselves and our loved ones healthy. (p. 338)

This kind of power is inherent in getting educated about options for safer sex. Barriers that prevent or reduce the exchange of body fluids are the most common means of protection. Of these barrier methods, condoms are an excellent source of protection during penile-vaginal intercourse or anal intercourse. For vaginal intercourse, there is also a female condom, although many women consider it less practical than a male condom. Still, it is a good alternative if a male partner can't use a condom for some reason. For a barrier during oral sex, you can use nonlubricated condoms which you cut lengthwise on one side to form a rectangle, or you can purchase small sheets of latex called dental dams, available in some pharmacies. Nonmicrowavable plastic food wrap has also been suggested as a more economical and easier-to-use barrier for oral sex with a female "recipient," but its effectiveness has not been proven conclusively. The goal is always to minimize direct contact of the woman's genitals, anus, or mouth with the partner's body fluids and genitals.

Spermicides are gels that were originally developed for use with a diaphragm. They can be found near the pharmacy section of drugstores, where condoms and lubricants are sold. Spermicides that contain the ingredient nonoxynol-9 or octoxynol-9 are recommended. A woman can also apply an applicator of spermicide ("foam") inside the vagina before having sex. She'll also get some protection from STDs if she uses a diaphragm that contains spermicidal gel. But spermicidal gels and diaphragms *do not* offer the same level of protection as latex condoms.

It is important to remember that of all the sexual activities possible with a partner, mutual masturbation offers the least risk. We recommend that it not be overlooked as a great source of pleasure and intimacy.

Being thoughtful about precautions doesn't have to diminish the joy and pleasure of life. Like buckling up when driving your car, checking your downhill ski-boot bindings, or wearing a life vest while boating, the pleasure you take in something you enjoy is hardly affected by being safe—taking precautions can actually lead to more enjoyment over time by preventing mishaps or tragedies.

STDs: NO TIME TO DENY REALITY

Typically the first reactions to learning you have an STD will be fear and dread. You may even just try to ignore the whole thing. This is not, however, the time to deny reality, because you need treatment. If you don't currently have a physician or nurse practitioner, call your local hospital, public health department, or community mental health agency and ask for a list of local healthcare practitioners. If keeping costs down is important, ask if there are local agencies that care for women's medical needs at low or no cost, such as a women's resource center, a public health clinic, or Planned Parenthood agency. You can also ask the healthcare providers to whom you are referred about the possibility of a sliding fee scale.

Remember that early and consistent health care, including taking all medications prescribed and returning for follow-up appointments, is important to effective treatment. You will feel more inclined to pursue the treatment you need if you are confident that the healthcare provider will treat you with the respect you deserve. Simply put, don't consult any practitioner who treats you as if you're the problem. You should be treated with sensitivity and respect. Your examination and treatment for an STD should maintain your privacy; call ahead and ask about confidentiality. For some STDs, like HIV or syphilis, the law requires healthcare providers to get a more thorough medical history, including the names of your sexual partners so that they can be notified of possible exposure. In some situations, you won't be required to give the names of sexual partners if you agree to contact them yourself. If you decide to handle it yourself, be sure to follow through. Others' health, fertility, and well-being are at stake, and you're only doing what you would want to have done for you.

When you go to your appointment, consider taking someone with you for support (to reduce any feelings of loneliness or shame that you have—discussed later in this chapter) and as a second set of ears to listen to medical recommendations.

The laws in all states provide that minors can receive testing and treatment for STDs without their parents' permission, though in some states physicians aren't prevented from telling a young woman's parents that she was treated after the fact. So if you are underage, ask the clinic ahead of time about its policy regarding confidentiality and how billing or any follow-up occurs.

Questions and concerns about STDs aren't easy to bring up with a partner, but remember the old sex education caveat: when you go to bed with someone, you're going to bed with every partner with whom that person has had sex. Women who won't sit down on a public toilet seat for fear of "getting something" are often willing to have sex with a new partner without first talking about STDs, simply because they're too embarrassed to raise the issue. What's wrong with this picture? We believe that if a woman feels she can be naked with someone, she should be prepared to ask some pretty bold questions beforehand.

COMMON SEXUAL CONCERNS

Let's say you discover you have an STD. What happens next? After education and early treatment comes a period of adjustment in your sense of self. At first you may feel that you will never *ever* have sex again. You might feel angry or disgusted with your body and yourself. You may also feel angry or disgusted with the sexual partner who knowingly or unknowingly transmitted the STD. Acknowledging this diagnosis as a loss and allowing yourself to feel grief are a very real part of adjustment. Then comes the process of fitting this new reality into the rest of your life.

Whom to Tell and When

> Jill liked Scott so much. She'd been seeing him for several weeks. She loved how things were unfolding between them . . . especially the touching and kissing. Lately, Scott had made it pretty clear he wanted more. Jill did, too, except what was she going to do about her herpes? She'd have to tell him soon or he'd feel she'd been covering it up on purpose. That wasn't the case at all. She just didn't know what to say without turning him off. She was really scared of losing him.

Sorting out whom to tell about your STD and when is like those Russian nesting dolls—there are issues within the issue of getting the STD. If you are involved with only one person and got the STD from that person, immediately tell him or her. In some situations, the STD might have become symptomatic during the current relationship, but may actually have been acquired earlier. In any case, a healthcare practitioner will need to see your partner to determine whether the partner is carrying an undiagnosed or untreated STD.

We'd like to say that all partners will respond with kindness, but that's not the case. Sometimes partners get frightened and angry. At that point you are dealing with not only your own diagnosis but also the strain in your relationship. None of this is easy to get through, and you will need support and education as well as treatment. If support from a partner or friend isn't sufficient, seek out a support group meeting, an Internet support group, or professional counseling. Ask your healthcare provider for referrals to local groups. In some cases, couples break up because the strain of the STD is too great for their relationship to carry. Like the nesting dolls, there are losses within losses.

If you are single, you'll be faced with issues related to timing and honesty: thinking about what to say and when to say it to a new partner. It's dishonest not to tell a sexual partner about an STD. Moreover, in the case of HIV or AIDS, it's a felony in many states not to tell the partner. But do you tell your entire STD story to every person you date? It's such a dilemma that some women just retreat from any relationship involvement at all.

Here's what we suggest. First, think about what you'd like to get out of this relationship. Is this just for fun and friendship, with no anticipation of sexual involvement? In this case you don't need to tell your partner anything about yourself sexually, including whether or not you have a sexually transmitted disease. But what if you're not sure where the relationship might go? If you're not looking for sex but not opposed to it either, tell your partner about your STD once you know the relationship is getting physically intimate. When the relationship moves to intimate touching and kissing, when you or your partner says, "I don't want to rush this, but . . . " or "Why don't you stay?," it's time to be straightforward about the STD. The cues that a relationship is heating up might be different, but they're usually pretty unmistakable. The cue says "I want to get physical with you." That's when you need to tell your partner, "Look, I think this is terrific, but we need to talk about me physically. I've had genital warts [or whatever the STD is], and we need to make sure that we're careful so that you don't get it. I can tell you how we can best manage it. Let's talk."

Will this be easy? No, because nothing about STDs is easy. Will this cool some hot romances? You bet. Will this discussion look like an Oscar-winning scene on the silver screen? Probably not. People tend to stumble around when they're explaining things. They backtrack and repeat questions they've already asked. It's part of getting accustomed to the new reality. All we can say is, if it chills the relationship permanently, then the relationship wasn't meant to be. As in the rest of this book, we're promoting honesty as the best route to meaningful relationships, whether they're brief or long-lasting. The relationship you have with yourself is the most important one you'll ever have.

Rejecting Your Body

If you get an STD, you may very well withdraw from any sense of connection to your body. You may describe it as divorcing yourself from your genitals, being mad at your body for betraying you, or denying the importance of your natural sexual responses. When a person is frightened, it's normal to take a fight/flight stance, being either angry or withdrawing. But because you have only one body and need to live in it for a lifetime, it makes more sense to address the hurt, bewilderment, and grief through education, counseling, and support. Then you can figure out how to move on and feel whole again.

Guilt and Shame

If you were exposed to hepatitis at your workplace or to malaria on a vacation, no one would say to you, "You should be ashamed that you got hepatitis [or malaria]."

Instead, others would feel sorry for you and express their concern. It's one of the meaner aspects of human nature that we tend to blame people for anything that goes wrong with them sexually, whether it's an accidental pregnancy or a sexually transmitted disease. Although the Salem witch trials were conducted over 300 years ago, when it comes to sexual behavior, people are likely to put women on trial for their troubles, saying "She should have known better" or "It serves her right for doing what she did." To make matters worse, because her genitals contain more mucous membranes and can retain body fluids from another person for a longer time, a woman is more at risk than a man for contracting a sexually transmitted disease.

Someone once said that "guilt is the gift that keeps on giving," and shame seems even more generous. Even if others don't taunt us or shake their heads behind our backs, we chastise ourselves: "I should have known better." If you are diagnosed with any STD, talk to a healthcare provider, counselor, or other supportive person about the diagnosis. You can be sorry that it happened. You can be sad that it will cause adjustments in your sexual relationship with another person. You can be angry that life is not always fair. But remember that you're not a bad person because you have a sexually transmitted disease.

Continuing to Be Sexual

People often associate safer-sex techniques with casual sexual relationships, not long-term monogamous relationships. Many couples, however, face the prospect of having to use safer-sex techniques for the rest of their lives.

> "I used to love having a lover go down on me—but that was before I found out I was HIV positive. Dental dams are better than nothing, but there are times when I really feel cheated."
>
> "I'm finally in a relationship that works, but it feels like a layer of latex will always exist between us."

If you are in a committed relationship and have an incurable STD, you and your partner have an important decision to make. Do you nurse your bitterness, feel sorry for yourselves, and remain focused on what you can't do? Or do you decide to continue being sexual, focusing on what you can do and looking for creative ways to heighten eroticism in your relationship?

With an estimated 65 million Americans with incurable STDs, you and your partner are certainly not alone in facing this dilemma. Like countless other couples in the same situation, it will be important for you to put your challenges in perspective. Sex is wonderful, but no one ever said it was simple. Keep talking to each other about your sexual interests, your desire for physical closeness, and the affection you share for each other. Stay well-informed by reading articles and books about how other couples enrich their sex lives. Make informed decisions, be creative, and keep sex a vibrant part of your relationship.

> "Condoms and hygiene—a small price to pay for the hot sex we're having. The precautions have become automatic, but there's nothing automatic about our lovemaking."

> "When I met Jeff, I was upfront about my herpes. We used condoms religiously, and the sex was great. When we got married, Jeff said he didn't want to keep using condoms. At first, I really felt awkward—I'd feel horrible if he got the infection from me. But he said it wouldn't be the end of the world if he got it, and he was willing to take his chances. Since then, we've been careful whenever I have a flare-up, but otherwise, we just don't worry."

LIFE AFTER LOSS: THE STD ISN'T THE END OF THE WORLD

With loss comes grieving, and being diagnosed with a sexually transmitted disease usually triggers grief—a normal reaction. Adjustments to the disease come with time, education, and support. Reading widely, asking questions of healthcare providers, and seeking out others who've lived with a similar STD can help you make the adjustment from fear to empowerment. Resources to assist you in this adjustment are listed at the end of the book.

One final note about your health care: *it matters*. If you don't have medical insurance, then call the public health department or Planned Parenthood agency in your community for references to low-cost or free services. STDs may change your life, but they don't have to rule your life.

CHAPTER TEN

Trauma

Trauma leaves a scar that can disrupt every aspect of life, including sexuality, whether it comes in the form of being robbed, witnessing a murder, being the victim of sexual abuse, or becoming disfigured as a result of an illness, accident, or surgery. Although people vary widely in the severity of their response to trauma, it's not uncommon for women to feel alienated from their bodies following a traumatic experience. In this and other ways, trauma can most certainly affect a woman's sex life.

In this chapter we discuss how trauma can impact your sexuality and present ways to overcome these posttraumatic responses. Chapters 14, 15, and 16 provide additional suggestions for overcoming sexual difficulties. If you find any of these suggestions too difficult or if you need additional help, consider seeing a sex therapist. Chapter 17 provides useful information about sex therapy and finding a qualified therapist.

The suggestions we offer in this chapter should not be viewed as a substitute for obtaining professional help in the aftermath of a traumatic experience. Counseling can give you insight into why you continue to feel frightened, numb, or upset following a traumatic event. It can provide you with emotional support and psychological understanding that can help you feel better about your life.

In addition to counseling, you may find it valuable to read more about trauma. The websites www.traumacenter.org and www.trauma-pages.com provide excellent information and refer you to other informative websites, books, and articles. In addition, we list several books about trauma and sex in our "Suggested Resources" section at the end of the book. All of this material can help you better understand your trauma and ways to reclaim your life.

THE IMPACT OF TRAUMA ON YOUR SEXUALITY

By definition, trauma is a shock that follows a disastrous or terrifying experience. Your brain and nervous system interpret the traumatic event as a life-or-death crisis. Whether the trauma is physical or verbal, something that happens directly to you or something you witness, one event or a series of events, sexual abuse or something else entirely, your body immediately goes into a self-protective mode, preparing you to defend yourself or to flee from the danger. Unfortunately, even after the real danger has passed, the traumatized mind and nervous system continue to respond, sometimes for years, as if the threat still exists.

If you have experienced a traumatic event, you may have noticed that one of your self-protective mechanisms is to continually reorder the priorities in your life. In the face of terror, normal interests and pursuits lose importance. Only survival matters, so sex and pleasure quickly fall by the wayside. In this state of emergency, you are constantly on guard in anticipation of any further threat. This hypervigilance makes relaxation or an erotic focus during lovemaking very difficult. Instead, any unexpected sound or shift in your partner's emotions is carefully monitored for signs of imminent danger.

> "We lived with my grandparents, and my grandfather would have explosive rages when he was drinking. You didn't know when it would happen. Now I don't like things to ever get out of control. Whenever emotions run high, or even when my partner gets sexually excited, I withdraw because I can't tell what could happen next. I hate unpredictability."

Being constantly on guard means that your body is often in a state of hyperarousal: a racing heart, lack of regular sleep, anxiety, nervousness, tension, panic, and a strong startle response. Your body is responding as if it is about to encounter a lethal threat at any moment. Not surprisingly, this constant state of internal agitation can drown out any erotic stirring.

> "I can't tolerate being touched on my shoulders or back. That's where the mugger grabbed me. If my partner accidentally reaches for me from behind, I have a panic attack—my heart races, my knees buckle, and I can't breathe. I have to orchestrate every touch and movement in order to have sex."

A traumatic experience not only affects how you think about safety and predictability in the world but also can deprive you of self-confidence. You may no longer trust your emotions, and you may try to suppress any intense feeling, including passion and sexual arousal.

Sexual Trauma

When a traumatic event involves sexual abuse, factors directly related to the sexual abuse also interfere with normal sexual response. For example, if the sexual abuse was mixed with love and special attention, you could feel confused and have difficulty accepting the possibility that you may have "allowed" the abuse to occur because it brought you the attention that you craved. If you experienced arousal and even orgasmed during the abuse, you may feel ashamed that your body responded sexually. It's not surprising that this confusion or shame often spills over into future sexual situations.

Following a traumatic experience, certain cues or reminders often remain in memory and trigger unwanted flashbacks, emotional numbness, or panic. In the case of sexual trauma, a trigger could be a person who reminds you of the abuser, a place similar to where the trauma occurred, or any smell, touch, taste, sight, or sound that your memory associates with the trauma. The trigger may be quite specific, like having a certain part of your body touched, or general, like anything that has a sexual connotation. You usually know your triggers, but occasionally new triggers can catch you off guard. Your response to triggers will usually be worse when you are fatigued or upset.

> "While we were having sex, my hair got caught under my partner's elbow. The sensation of having my hair pulled triggered a flashback to being raped. I was terrified. The rapist had yanked me by my hair to keep me from moving."

To complicate a painful situation, women who are having sexual difficulties following a sexual or other trauma often condemn themselves for being weak or overreacting. Researchers are not entirely sure why the range of possible responses to a traumatic experience is so broad, but if you are having a troublesome response to a trauma, keep in mind that everyone has different amounts of fear and horror that they can endure before the body and mind begin to take desperate measures for self-protection. Suffering trauma does not make you weak or inadequate. And you can make efforts to reclaim your sexuality after a traumatic experience. We believe it is important that you do so, because it's a step toward reclaiming predictability and pleasure in all areas of your life.

Distorted Responses to Sexual Trauma

In dangerous situations human beings have an innate tendency to fight, flee, or freeze. In many cases of sexual trauma, women display patterns of sexual behavior that are distortions of these normal fight/flight responses (freezing is subsumed under *flight*). If you know that you have suffered trauma but are not sure of its effects on your sex life, the following descriptions may enhance your understanding.

Lack of Sexual Desire

Many women who have been sexually abused find that they have little or no interest in sex. Their lack of sexual desire is the mind's attempt to flee from, or avoid, something that has proven to be frightening and dangerous. Sometimes this lack of interest starts immediately following the sexual abuse, and sometimes it appears years later, after a long period of normal sexual activity. The delayed emergence of this defense mechanism (psychological way of coping) can be perplexing. It usually happens in cases where other defenses were first used to minimize the horror of the sexual abuse, only to eventually become ineffective. Chapter 14 provides a detailed discussion of low sexual desire, its causes, and ways to overcome it.

Sexual Aversion

Following sexual trauma, some women do not simply lose their interest in sex; they become disgusted and frightened by anything that is sexual. Sexual aversion is often a phobic reaction that can be traced back to earlier trauma. Because of the trauma, sexual cues trigger a strong emotional reaction. The aversion to sex serves as a way of avoiding, or fleeing from, sex. If you have a sexual aversion, you may react negatively to specific sexual cues like the sight of an erect penis, or you may find all aspects of sex, including nudity, hugging, and kissing, distasteful. An aversion can vary from a moderate dislike and anxiety about sex to the extremes of panic, disgust, and revulsion. Even the thought of these sexual behaviors may trigger a negative emotional reaction.

> "At first I thought I could cope with my disgust by avoiding certain sexual activities. As long as I didn't do the things that were done to me as a child, I felt I'd be okay. Unfortunately, my aversion got worse and I found myself wanting to hit and kick my partner anytime I was touched, as if I was being assaulted."

Although both low sexual desire and sexual aversion serve as a means of avoiding or fleeing sex, they represent two different types of self-protection provided by the mind. When a woman has low sexual desire due to past trauma, sexual cues produce no response. Her unconscious mind seeks protection by not responding to anything that could reactivate the buried pain. In cases of sexual aversion, the pain is often closer to the surface. Rather than experiencing no response to sexual cues, a woman with a sexual aversion experiences strong, negative emotions. Feelings of disgust prompt the woman to avoid sex, which is an unconscious means of trying to avoid a recurrence of the earlier trauma.

Similar to low sexual desire, sexual aversion may first occur right after the trauma, or may come about later in your life, even after a period of safe or pleasant sex. The late onset of a sexual aversion can be triggered by life events that the unconscious mind associates with the earlier trauma. Relationship problems, a life crisis, even hormonal changes due to aging can trigger sexual aversion in some women as a delayed reaction to an earlier trauma.

Sexual aversion has elements of anxiety and panic, which may respond well to medication. If you are in therapy, you can discuss with your therapist how medication might help you.

Dissociative Sex

Dissociative sex represents a third type of protection against sexual conflict or the impact of earlier trauma. Rather than losing sexual desire or pulling away from sex out of disgust, you may mentally distance yourself from your body during sexual activity. Sometimes this distancing, or dissociating, is achieved by using alcohol or drugs. Maybe you experience yourself going off into a trance-like state during sex. Or perhaps you feel disconnected from your body during sex, as if your partner is making love to someone else's body. In all these instances, mentally removing yourself from a sexual situation represents a desperate attempt to avoid reexperiencing the trauma of the past.

> "I go through the motions of having sex, but I'm not really present in my body. I know I'm touching and being touched, but I don't feel any sensation."

Dissociation can range from mild nonsexual daydreams during sex to totally blanking out so that you have no recall of what happened during sex. The latter response is rare, quite dangerous, and falls beyond the scope of this book. If your dissociation is so severe that you lose all recall, you should contact a therapist. If you don't blank out but do become emotionally distant or numb during sex, you may find the suggestions later in this chapter useful. You may also find it helpful to reread Part II, "Understanding Your Body," and Part V, "Overcoming Sexual Difficulties," for additional exercises that will teach you how to stay present in your body.

Sexual Compulsion

Some women who have been sexually traumatized will seek sex rather than avoid it. In a distorted way, they are fighting back against earlier sexual abuse by trying to conquer sex or prove that they no longer have something to fear. Sex becomes a compulsion over which they have little control.

> "I had sex with any guy anywhere. I was known as the campus slut and I didn't care. As long as I was having sex, I felt powerful and desired. Afterwards, I would get scared I wasn't loved and go looking for sex again."

If you have a sexual compulsion, sometimes called a sexual addiction, you probably find yourself in an endless cycle of seeking sex to overcome painful emotions, only to feel more miserable after each sexual encounter. Your attempt to gain control over sex ends up leaving you out of control. You expose yourself to countless dangers, including relationship conflicts and the risk of physical harm.

Sexual compulsion may be a way of reenacting the trauma—creating it over and over—in an attempt to master it. It may be that you masturbate 10 or 12 times a day but feel very little pleasure. Perhaps you pick up multiple partners at bars, but the sex is disconnected and you feel lousy afterwards. Your compulsive masturbating or lovemaking may be attempts to prove to yourself that you don't care about sex or that you can have sex with anybody without getting hurt. Or by making sex so meaningless, your unconscious mind might be trying to prove that what happened years ago was no big deal. Sex may temporarily make you feel wanted or powerful by seducing others and making them desire you. Afterward, however, you feel powerless and bad about yourself until you repeat the pattern of seduction. Compulsive sex can also be a way of devaluing yourself. Because others abused you in the past, you may feel that you don't deserve to be treated well. Regardless of the reason, compulsive behavior takes over your life.

Sexual compulsion is a complicated and dangerous reaction to trauma. If you suspect that you have a compulsive sexual disorder, we recommend that you find a therapist to help you disengage from this pattern.

Trophy Sex

Usually when we hear references to sex and trophies, we think of men in pursuit of sexual conquests. Trophy sex can also apply to women, however. It may be a response to sexual trauma, although just as commonly it is driven by different psychological needs. If you find that you get a rush from the hunt and capture of a guy, you may be engaging in trophy sex.

Consider the following scenario. Your search for a sexual conquest begins with an awareness—however vague—that you are dissatisfied and perhaps depressed. You set out to make something happen and feel your first rush of excitement when you identify your prey. Then you begin the game of teasing seduction to capture his or her attention. In the end, much to your delight, you have the person eating out of your hand. You've won—you have another trophy for your mantle. The only problem is, once you've won, you're no longer interested.

If this scenario is familiar or makes you laugh uncomfortably, you may be engaging in trophy sex. The sexual hunt may be an attempt to overcome feelings of powerlessness and exploitation you've had in earlier life experiences, often with men. Ultimately, trophy sex is without thrill; you're not enjoying it and you don't feel control over your need to seduce others. As in the case of compulsive sexual behavior, trophy sex may be an attempt to fight back in response to earlier experiences of abuse. By sexually conquering others, you may feel that you are conquering your perpetrators, past and future.

> "Men can be real bastards, but when you know how to handle them, they're harmless. I've had professional athletes, famous lawyers, an obscenely rich CEO, even an actor from one of the daytime soaps lusting after me. They were like putty in my hands—God, what a rush."

If you're aware of this pattern in your sexual activity, try using the suggestions later in this chapter to stay present in your sexuality. If you continue to find you can't control your trophy seeking, we recommend that you get counseling to help you gain greater control of your sexuality.

A Cautionary Note

Although low sexual desire, sexual aversion, dissociative sex, sexual compulsion, and trophy sex may be the by-product of sexual trauma, these problems can also have many other underlying causes. If you engage in any of these behaviors but have no recollection of previous sexual abuse, don't assume that you must have been abused. Work with a therapist to explore why you are resorting to self-defeating sexual behavior.

CREATING SEXUAL SATISFACTION

Overcoming trauma involves learning how to feel safe again and becoming empowered with sexual knowledge, self-assurance, and the skills needed to keep unwanted emotions in check. This is how you open yourself to experiencing sexual pleasure unencumbered by posttraumatic symptoms.

Be Present in Your Body

Sexual activity requires you to be fully present in your body, aware of your body's responses, so that you can enjoy the pleasure your body can produce. Dissociating, being distracted by intrusive thoughts, or experiencing agitation during sex prevents you from being present in your body. You can learn to be present in your body by *taking control* of your body, learning to *soothe yourself*, and *defusing triggers*.

Take Control

Taking control means making sure you feel safe and that your partner is supportive and respectful of your goals. Start by checking your environment to make sure it is safe, comfortable, and pleasing to your senses. Purchase items for your bedroom that create a comforting and pleasing ambience. Do this yourself—relying on your partner perpetuates the pattern of not being in control.

Make an honest assessment of your current sex life. Are you engaging in sexual behavior that puts you at risk or makes you feel uncomfortable? If so, tell yourself that you're "taking a break" from that behavior. If the activity involves a partner, tell your partner no and explain that you don't like what you've been doing and that you're taking steps to feel more comfortable with sex. If you feel awkward talking to your partner about sex, take a look at Chapter 12 for suggestions.

Soothe Yourself

In your attempt to create a better sex life, you may experience emotional numbing or hyperarousal, especially anxiety. There are excellent books on understanding anxiety and learning soothing responses to counteract anxiety and panic (see Wilson, 1996; Dupont, Dupont-Spencer, & Dupont, 1998). Soothing responses such as deep breathing, positive self-talk, calming imagery, muscle relaxation, and body movement can help you stay present in your body, decrease anxiety, clear your mind, and take control.

To learn how to soothe yourself, try the following four steps. First, start by practicing a breathing technique that you can use when you experience anxiety, panic, or numbing. Focus on your breathing. Take slow deep breaths from your diaphragm while counting backwards from 100. Another way to focus on breathing is to breathe in, hold for three counts, breathe out, and hold for three more counts. Repeat this sequence 10 times.

Second, once you've brought your breathing under control, you are ready to talk to yourself with a clear mind. Tell yourself that numbing and hyperarousal are normal responses to trauma triggers and that you can tolerate them. We call this positive self-talk, a useful technique for soothing. If you need suggestions for how to talk to yourself positively, see Chapter 13 for ways to challenge negative thoughts with positive ones.

Third, practice picturing soothing images in your mind. Examples of mental images that many women find soothing include a sun-swept seashore, billowy clouds, mountains, birds in flight, or a field of wildflowers. Some women use prayer or meditation as their soothing mental activity.

Fourth, as you picture your soothing image, notice where you feel muscle tension. Reduce the tension by first tensing the muscles further and then relaxing them.

Practice these four techniques for 10 to 20 minutes a day, until you feel you are able to do all four with some confidence.

Once your initial soothing responses are working, try additional soothing techniques involving movement and sensory awareness. Because trauma may have caused you to feel frozen with terror, it's important to learn to move your body and respond to sensory cues. In the presence of numbing or hyperarousal, you can find relief from these uncomfortable sensations by focusing on body movement and sensory experiences—things that keep you grounded in the here and now rather than snapping back to the terrifying past. Start by moving your body in ways that feel good to you. This may be standing, walking meditatively—or raucously—around the room, stretching your arms above your head, swaying, stomping, stooping, or moving from side to side. You can rock your body as if you're in a rocking chair, tilt your pelvis back and forth, or practice Kegels. *Any* form of movement that is comfortable and natural for you can be helpful. Becoming absorbed in how the joints in your little finger allow you to bend it can bring you back into your body.

Next, pay close attention to your sensory experience. Touch, taste, or smell something that pleases you; listen to music or the sounds of nature (if any) around you; gaze at the trees outside your window.

> "There are times when I'm suddenly overwhelmed by fear and dread. It feels like I'm suffocating. I've learned to calm myself by breathing slowly, reassuring myself, and moving around. When I can get a clear image in my mind or focus on something concrete around me, I feel grounded. It's like I get a grip on things, and the scary feelings seem to drift away."

Self-soothing requires practice, but it is worth it: self-soothing becomes the cornerstone for creating positive sexuality. It also serves as an effective tool to combat posttraumatic symptoms by freeing you to stay present in your body and to focus on pleasurable sensations of any kind.

Defuse Triggers

It's important to know your triggers in order to overcome them. Make a list of the different experiences that trigger dissociation, numbing, aversion, or hyperarousal during sex. Consider people, places, things, different forms of sensory stimulation, fantasies, and types of touch or physical activity in compiling your list. Write your list of triggers in the form of negative statements, such as "I don't like to be touched" or "I don't like kissing." Now write how each trigger makes you feel. For example, if being touched makes you feel anxious or angry, write those words next to your trigger statement.

I don't like to be touched.	Being touched makes me angry.

As you do this, you may find that just thinking about the triggers can lead to a trauma response like dissociation or hyperarousal. If this happens, *use your soothing techniques as you write.*

Next, read aloud your list of triggers and feelings. Now write a take-charge statement next to every trigger. "I don't like to be touched" can be paired with "I will decide who touches me and when." "I don't like kissing" can be paired with "There are a lot of activities I like that don't involve my lips!"

Developing this list of positive statements helps you lessen the power of triggers to elicit posttraumatic reactions by giving triggers more links, more possible responses, than reexperiencing the trauma. The positive statements can actually compete with traumatic recall when triggers are encountered.

Another way some women face triggers and minimize them is by using their imagination. They will write the negative trigger statement several times, each time making their handwriting smaller. They imagine shrinking the writing into a tiny pinpoint and sending it away from them. Or if they view themselves as scared and helpless, they conjure up another image of themselves as a stronger, more powerful person coming to the aid of the frightened self. They see this stronger person helping the scared person. They repeat to themselves, "I'm safer now; I'm stronger now; I'm in charge now."

As you continue using these strategies to defuse your triggers, you will become more adept at staying present in your body.

Predict and Modify Your Reactions to Sex

Once you've established how to remain present in your body, you're ready to predict your reactions to sex and plan strategies for change.

To begin, make a list of three sexual activities you'd be interested in trying. Your list might look like this:

Alone:	Masturbate for five minutes.
With my partner:	Try French kissing.
With my partner:	Try massaging each other's butts.

Next, think about possible negative reactions that could occur with these activities. Be as honest as you can and write the possible reactions next to each sexual activity. For instance:

Masturbate for five minutes.	Negative reaction: I start to dissociate.
Try French kissing.	Negative reaction: I jerk my head away and feel nervous.
Try massaging each other's butts.	Negative reaction: I hold my breath.

Think about how you could counter each negative reaction by using the soothing techniques you've learned. Write down the technique next to the reaction. If at any time while you're writing you experience a negative reaction, practice the techniques you've learned. For example:

Negative reaction:	I start to dissociate.
Soothing:	I breathe evenly. I begin self-talking, telling myself to stay present, and I concentrate on my fingers touching my skin. If necessary, I get up and walk around the room and then come back and try again.
Negative reaction:	I jerk my head away and feel nervous.
Soothing:	I breathe evenly. I look at my partner and tell [him or her] that I feel nervous but that I want to continue by first kissing [his or her] cheeks and closed lips. I stay in control of the movements.
Negative reaction:	I hold my breath.
Soothing:	I practice breathing evenly. I take my partner's hand and I guide my partner's hand across my butt. I continue my self-talk, telling myself this is something I want to do for me.

Predicting and modifying your responses will take time and planning. Reread the discussion about triggers and try to think about how each type of trigger might apply to your sexual activity. Think of soothing responses that include breathing, positive self-talk, soothing images, muscle relaxation, and movement.

Setting positive goals for sexual activity is another way of modifying negative reactions. If all you expect from sex are negative reactions, chances are that's exactly what you'll get. But if you set goals like pleasure, satisfaction, calmness, or closeness to your partner, you can counteract possible negative reactions by putting positive expectations in their place.

Revisit your list of three sexual activities that you are interested in trying. Next to each activity, write a positive goal. Try to be realistic when setting these goals. For example, an intense orgasm might be great at some point in the future, but for starters, perhaps feeling calm during lovemaking can be a positive improvement.

Activity	*Positive goal*
Alone: Masturbate for five minutes.	I can touch my body sexually and stay calm.
With my partner: Try French kissing.	I can initiate intimate contact face-to-face and stay present in my body using my soothing techniques.
With my partner: Try massaging each other's butts.	I can touch and be touched while breathing evenly and being aware of my ability to enjoy some physical contact.

Negative reactions to sex may never disappear entirely, but their impact will be minimized by your prediction and active control of them.

Practice, Practice, Practice

Being present and predicting/modifying reactions build islands of safety in your sex life, which gives you more control. Now it's time to build an island of pleasure also. Over time, practicing new goals for sexual activity and controlling your response to triggers will bring you both pleasure and a sense of empowerment.

To begin, test out your predictions and remedies by experimenting with various types of sexual activity, perhaps starting with the three activities you listed in the previous section. Later you can expand your list of the sexual activities you'd like to enjoy, arranging them from the easiest to the most difficult. Remember to tell your partner about the changes you're seeking.

We suggest you find a way to practice the first sexual activity on your list at least several times a week. You may find it helpful to start your practice with masturbation, getting comfortable first with your sexual response by yourself. If you feel unsure about masturbating, read more about it in Chapter 12. You will also find helpful suggestions for how to masturbate in Chapter 15. If you don't have a partner but would like to be in a relationship, then perhaps you'll want to start by making a list of ways to begin to meet people and gain confidence in forming relationships.

As you gain confidence through practice with masturbation, try increasing the intensity of what you're doing. Intentionally try to lose control: go faster, be noisier, let the intensity of the vibrator get stronger, and let your fantasies get a little wilder. Remember to keep being present. If you start to feel anxious, remember to soothe yourself. If necessary, return to the previous level of activity that was comfortable and continue practicing that until you're ready to move to something more challenging.

After you gain confidence by yourself, you can add sex with your partner. Decide what sexual activities you want to try and share in advance with your partner. It helps if your partner is also learning about his or her own sexuality while you're working on your own. Encourage your partner to masturbate and to be positive about sexuality as well.

The two greatest barriers to successful practice are negative self-talk and setting goals that are too ambitious. In Chapter 13 we describe ways to challenge negative thoughts. Reread your list of desired sexual behaviors and break down your goals into smaller, more manageable ones. For instance, if learning to kiss your partner on the mouth is a goal, but it proves to be too overwhelming right now, start with kissing the back of your hand or your forearm. Notice your response to moving your lips moistly over your own skin. When that's comfortable, explain to your partner that you'll begin cheek to cheek, by rubbing skin and enjoying the sensation. Build up slowly to kissing on the mouth. *The Sexual Healing Journey* (Maltz, 1991) and *The*

Survivor's Guide to Sex (Haines, 1999) give effective step-by-step suggestions for how to introduce new sexual activities at a slow and comfortable pace.

Practice takes commitment. You may find it helpful to ask a good friend to serve as your check-in to keep you practicing; decide on a way to report to your friend on a regular basis. Or, if you prefer privacy, keep a journal in which you note your progress toward your goals. If practicing is too difficult to do on your own, consider counseling to help you reach your goals.

Take a Break

What about taking a break from practicing if you feel too overwhelmed? Although time away from practice might be all right for a brief period, be careful that it doesn't become avoidance. Avoidance is usually driven by fear of experiencing negative reactions or shame over not being able to overcome them. Throughout this book, we've encouraged you to take responsibility for your sexuality, including your healing. If you find that you are taking a break not because you're turning your attention to other areas of growth but because you're avoiding your sexual discomfort, we encourage you to take responsibility by seeking counseling. Because fear and shame are both profoundly isolating and disconnecting, the sense of restored connection you'll feel through counseling will help you overcome your avoidance and feel more empowered about your sexuality.

Empower Yourself

Your sexuality can make you feel powerful or powerless. The goal of your work in creating a sexual life is to feel your own empowerment. Sexual activity should always be consensual, meaning that you agree to, and accept, the activity. If you're having sex with a partner, make sure that you know exactly what kind of sexual activity you want with this person. Make clear what you want and set limits for what you don't want sexually. Only have sex with partners who practice safer sex.

If you find you can't ask for what you want or can't set limits, you probably aren't ready for partnered sex. Continue the earlier exercises designed to help you be more present in your body and predict/modify your negative reactions. Practice out loud in front of a mirror or with a friend what you want to say to your partner when you feel ready for partnered sex.

Some women find a fantasy of forced sex to be arousing. Some women have sex play in which they have roles with their partners of dominance or submission. Many women have fantasies or engage in sexual role-playing in which they get turned on by being in control or out of control. In these forms of sex, women are experimenting with the "edges" of consensual activity, the line between pleasure and pain or pleasure and fear. If a woman is in charge of deciding what she does, what she fantasizes, and what she role-plays—and her partner is in agreement—then this is consensual sex. For these women, it's playful, not harmful. (See Chapter 12 for a discussion of fantasy and experimenting with erotic power play.) As a survivor of trauma, however, you may find that these activities carry extra meanings. If you want to engage in them, make sure that you are not dissociating or hyperaroused and that you're able to have flexibility in your sex life—that your sexual activity is not confined to "being on the edge." If your sex life doesn't seem consensual and under your control, we recommend that you see a therapist to help you regain control.

This chapter can be the beginning of change for you. Keep reading other books on sexuality and overcoming trauma. Continue to work on creating your sexual life. Many women also find it helpful to practice yoga, dance, do body work (see "Suggested Resources" for books about body work), or martial arts. Other women find sensory experiences healing, like massage, gardening, painting, or working with clay. These experiences support your efforts to take care of yourself and, because they are experienced in your body, contribute to a more positive sexuality.

Restoring safety, pleasure, and empowerment to your sexuality takes time. You may want to start a sexual acceptance journal in which you record your experiences with being present, predicting, and practicing. Give yourself permission to celebrate your successes by using "I" statements when you write your accomplishments. For example, your successes might read like this: "I like my sexual fantasies," "I like to masturbate," and "I like oral sex with my partner." Review your journal frequently.

Creating a sexual life after trauma takes courage, patience, and self-love. The more capable you become of having positive sexual experiences in which you are in control and remain grounded in your body, the better you will feel.

PART IV

Creating a Better Sexual Relationship

Many women enter sexual relationships with the expectation that sex, the most natural thing in the world, will come naturally to two people who love and desire each other. As one woman said, "I figured that my responsibility for good sex with my partner was to show up and not have a headache." Another put it this way: "I was naïve enough to think that just because I wanted to have a good sex life, it would fall out of the sky and into my bed." Unfortunately, sexual relationships don't work like that. Sustaining a satisfying sexual relationship, especially one that fosters mutual growth, requires honest communication, knowledge and exploration, experimentation and practice, generosity, understanding, and even a healthy sense of humor. When you have stars in your eyes, it's not easy to see the rigid gender scripts, cultural myths, and sexual ignorance that can stand in the way of your having the best possible sexual relationship with your partner. And when you've been together "forever," habit and entrenched expectations (or disappointments) can blind you to the possibilities for a fulfilling sexual future.

Part IV begins with a discussion of men and their sexuality. We certainly realize that not all sexual relationships are heterosexual, but the majority of our readers have been, are, or will be in a relationship with a man. They can benefit from understanding how their male partners function sexually. We then move on to explore the sexual challenges facing couples and ways to enhance a sexual relationship. Exercises to help couples improve their sexual communication and to open up new, exciting dimensions in their lovemaking can be found in the Appendix.

Chapters 11 and 12 are dedicated to helping you create a better sexual relationship, no matter what your ages or how long you've been together. By understanding your partner better, having accurate information about sexual behavior, developing effective communication skills, and avoiding the pitfalls that all too often challenge a sexual relationship, you will be able to experience more fully the pleasure that comes from making love. The first step toward achieving these goals is to uncloak the myths and misconceptions that blindside so many sexual relationships. Chapters 11 and 12 address some of the most common ones our clients bring to us:

- Is a man supposed to come that quickly?
- If men really do have a stronger sex drive than women, why do I want to make love so much more often than my husband?
- How do we get the fireworks back?
- Isn't fantasizing a form of cheating?
- Who should take responsibility for initiating sex?
- What's a normal size for a penis?
- If my partner is having trouble getting hard, is he losing interest in me?
- Does a man who's circumcised feel more pleasure?
- What if one of us wants sex a lot more often than the other?
- Shouldn't people who have a satisfying sexual relationship give up masturbation?

CHAPTER ELEVEN

Male Sexuality

Understanding your partner and his or her sexuality is an essential ingredient for achieving sexual satisfaction in a relationship. Whereas lesbian women are usually only as mystified by their partner's sexuality as they are by their own experience of sex, heterosexual women are often somewhat clueless about what makes their partner tick, especially in the bedroom. Sometimes their knowledge of male sexuality is limited to the popular myths floating around, or to biased, and often distorted, explanations provided by their partners. Misinformation is anathema to leading a healthy sexual life and enjoying a happy sexual relationship.

NEWS FLASH: MEN AND WOMEN ARE DIFFERENT

Although men and women have identical anatomical structures for the first six weeks after conception and are born, raised, and educated in the same environments, they nevertheless differ from each other dramatically. When women are frustrated, for example, they may find relief in tears; men tend to retreat into anger. When a little boy is hit by a pitched ball, the mother wants to nurture and console; the father insists that it will toughen him up. When women encounter conflict, they want to dialogue to find a solution; men will swagger, posture, and bump bellies with their opponent. Women can embrace; men settle for a handshake. When a special moment occurs between two lovers, women might say, "I love you"; men might think, or even say, "Let's screw." When lost, women will ask for directions. There are men, on the other hand, whose pictures appear on milk cartons because after ten years, they're still driving around searching for their destination.

Obviously these examples are stereotypic and admittedly unfair, but there's enough truth here to highlight something we all know: men truly are different, not superior or inferior, but different from women. Yet as different and mysterious as men might be, it is usually a man who becomes a woman's life-mate. It's often with a man that a woman faces the joys and challenges of life—leaving home, pursuing a career, raising a family, grieving losses, and growing old. Understanding men and their sexuality is therefore important, because it can help women to better love them, live with them, and be sexual with them.

Throughout the remainder of this chapter, we will attempt to remove some of the mystery about men and their sexuality. Because this is a book about sex, we're going to restrict our focus to men's sexual behavior. We'll look at how their bodies respond to sexual excitement and how their sexual ability is affected by worry, illness, and age. We encourage you to check the resource list at the end of the book for suggested reading on personality and behavioral differences between men and women and ways that men and women can relate to each other in more effective, respectful, and loving ways.

MALE SEXUAL ANATOMY

An understanding of male sexual anatomy is a prerequisite to understanding male sexuality. Once we understand the parts, we can make better sense of how they respond and work together in sexual situations.

Penis

The penis is often the epicenter of a man's sense of manhood, potency, and sexuality. The penis is made up of muscular and spongy tissue wrapped by an elastic sheathing. This organ performs two very basic and important functions. By means of the urethra, a tube that runs from the bladder to the tip of the penis, the penis allows the man both to void his bladder and to deliver semen to a woman's womb. Because of this latter function, for thousands of years the penis has had a mythical significance in many cultures around the world. Phallic symbols have often served as sacred icons in early religions that revered fertility, that mysterious process that participates in the power of creation.

The shaft of the penis consists of three tubes or cylinders, two of them resting on top of the third (see Figure 11.1). The top two cigar-shaped tubes are called the *corpora cavernosa*, and the bottom tube, the *corpus spongiosum*. The urethra runs through the bottom tube, from end to end. These tubes consist of spongy tissue, small smooth muscles, nerve fibers, and blood vessels. They're wrapped in a tough, elastic sheathing called the *tunica albuginea*. When the penis is aroused, the corporal bodies become engorged with blood, which expands the tunica the way air inflates a rubber tire. Just as the rubber stretches to its natural limit and the tire becomes solid, the tunica stretches until the shaft of the penis becomes rigid.

The tunica albuginea surrounding the bottom tube is thinner than the sheathing surrounding the upper corporal bodies. When erect, the bottom tube is not as rigid as the upper tubes, which is why it's called the corpus spongiosum, or the spongy body. During an erection, the corpus spongiosum looks like a ridge protruding along the underside of the penile shaft.

The end of the corpus spongiosum extends past the two upper tubes and forms the head of the penis, called the *glans*. During an erection, the glans becomes engorged with blood and grows larger in size, but unlike the rest of the penile shaft, it has no sheathing and will remain soft and spongy. This quality makes the glans a natural cushion for when the penis thrusts back and forth inside the vagina during intercourse. At the tip of the glans is the urinary opening of the urethra, called the *meatus*.

The place where penile skin meets the glans is called the *coronal ridge*. In newborn and uncircumcised males, skin extends from the coronal ridge forward to cover the glans (inner foreskin), folds over and double backs over the glans (outer foreskin), and continues back along the penile shaft to the abdomen. The foreskin is connected to the underside of the penis, just behind the glans, by a ridge of skin called the *frenulum*. This ridge or fold of skin is similar to the ridge of skin stretching between the underside of your tongue and the floor of your mouth. The frenulum pulls the foreskin over the glans when the penis is flaccid. The glans, coronal ridge, and frenulum have many more nerve endings than the shaft of the penis and are very

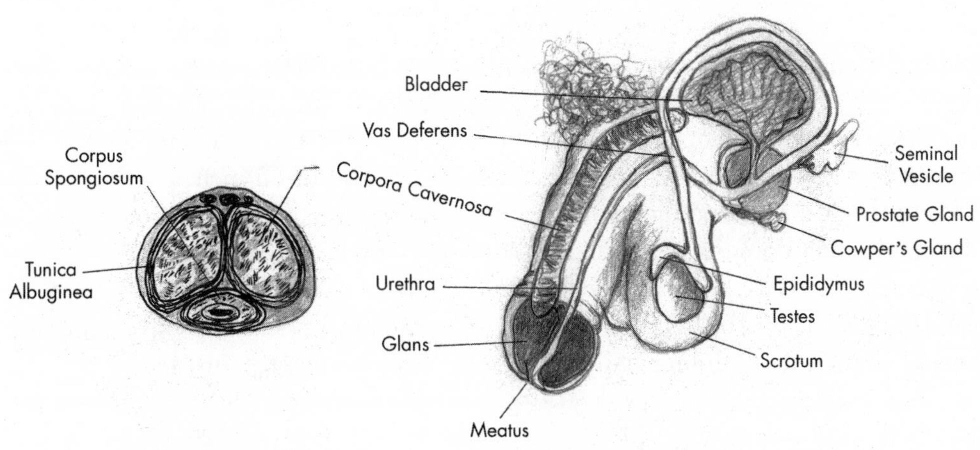

FIGURE 11.1. Male sexual organs.

sensitive to stimulation. During an erection the foreskin tends to retract, especially during intercourse, making these sensitive areas (glans, frenulum, and coronal ridge) more accessible to direct stimulation.

In a circumcision, the folded-over foreskin is cut away just beyond the coronal ridge, leaving the glans of the penis permanently exposed. Circumcisions are performed for cultural, religious, cosmetic, and health reasons. Today in the United States, there is a robust debate about the advantages and disadvantages of circumcision. Proponents argue that circumcision decreases the risk of developing infections and contracting sexually transmitted diseases. Opponents object to infants being subjected to the traumatic pain of a surgical procedure without the benefit of anesthesia. They point out that good hygiene and safer-sex practices reduce the reported risks of infection, some of which appear to be based on questionable scientific data.

Men have also wondered whether there are sexual advantages or disadvantages to being circumcised. It's a classic case of "The grass is always greener on the other side of the fence." Uncircumcised men have wondered whether absence of the foreskin makes intercourse more pleasurable for men who are circumcised. Circumcised men have wondered whether the foreskin makes it easier for uncircumcised men to maintain ejaculatory control. In truth, no evidence supports differences in the sexual experience of circumcised and uncircumcised men. In actuality, when an uncircumcised penis is erect and inserted in the vagina, the foreskin is pulled back so that the glans is stimulated in the same way as the glans of a circumcised penis.

What about Size?

While discussing the penis, we may as well address the age-old question about size. Rarely will you meet a man who, in his heart of hearts, does not wish that his penis were a little, or in some cases a lot, bigger. Men are hounded by the belief that to measure their manhood, you must measure their penis. They worry that anything less than a gargantuan appendage will disappoint and fail to satisfy their partner.

The average length of a flaccid penis is between three and a half and four inches. The average length of an erect penis is between five and seven inches. Size of a flaccid penis can vary depending on external temperature, mood, and even body weight. The penile shaft does not stop where it connects with the torso but actually continues internally and anchors to the pubic bone. When a man gains weight, more of his penis ends up inside of his body. Also, a shorter flaccid penis will expand proportionately, much more dramatically, when erect than a longer penis does.

Does Size Make a Difference?

Yes and no. These days the politically correct answer is: size makes no difference. But this is not totally accurate. Even though men often wish they had a larger penis, an extremely large penis can be problematic. On occasion we see couples who are distressed over not being able to have pain-free intercourse because of the excessive girth of the man's penis. For them, size definitely *does* make a difference, but unfortunately, a negative one.

Size also makes a positive difference for some women. They enjoy the feeling of surrounding and containing a penis that stretches the vaginal opening. They report that it's pleasurable when they feel like the penis "fills them up." Although this pleasurable feeling depends partially on adequate muscle tone around the opening of the vagina, the girth of the penis will also contribute to the "filled-up" sensation. In addition to girth, the length of the penis makes a difference for some women who enjoy the sensation during intercourse that occurs when a penis is long enough to stimulate the cervix directly.

So if size can make a difference, does this mean that a woman has been shortchanged if her partner is not well-endowed? Or that a man with a small or average-sized penis cannot be a good lover? Absolutely not. Sexual pleasure is the result of multiple factors. The presence or absence of any one particular sensation will not make or break the sexual experience. Although direct stimulation of the cervix or feeling stretched by penile girth can be pleasurable for some women, the major source of genital response is stimulation of the clitoris and nerve endings within the first two to three inches of the vagina. These highly erogenous areas, including the G spot, are well within the reach of even an unusually small penis. This is why it's not surprising that national surveys show that the majority of women downplay the significance of size. Research also shows that sexual arousal and satisfaction for women are dependent on much more than direct stimulation of the genitals. Affection, emotional intimacy, and communication are equally critical ingredients for a woman's sexual pleasure.

The Scrotum: What's in the Sac?

The scrotum is a pouch of loose, wrinkled skin that is lined by a thin layer of muscle called the *tunica dartos*. Hanging below the penis, the scrotum has two compartments, one for each of the testicles. The testicles are oval glands measuring about an inch wide and an inch and a half long. The testicles produce testosterone and sperm. Testosterone is an important hormone for sexual desire, sperm production, and the development of secondary male characteristics. If a man loses his testicles before puberty, he will be sterile as an adult; he will likely have little interest in sex; his voice will not deepen; and he will not develop the pattern of body and facial hair characteristic of adult men. Damage to the testicles after puberty can lead to sexual and reproductive problems.

Starting with puberty, sperm production is continuous throughout the remainder of a man's life. Fifty-thousand sperm are produced every minute in the testicles, but it takes more than 70 days for the sperm to mature fully. On the back, upper surface of each testicle, five to seven yards of tiny tubing are tightly coiled back and forth into an oval structure called the *epididymis*. After sperm are manufactured in the testicles, they move to the epididymis for storage and maturation. When a man becomes sexually aroused, as many as 500 million mature sperm are moved through the *vas deferens*, a tube connecting each testicle to the urethra. When a man has a vasectomy, the vas deferens from each testicle is severed, which prevents sperm from passing from the testicles to the penis.

Sperm need to be manufactured and stored at about two degrees lower than normal body temperature. This is why the testicles, unlike ovaries, are positioned away from the torso. It's probably advantageous that sperm can't survive very long at the normal body temperature. Otherwise, once they were deposited in the vagina, they would be free to set up housekeeping and wander around until they could impregnate an ovum. Pregnancy rates would be incredibly high, arguably at a rate that would be maladaptive for the species.

As the thin muscle lining of the scrotum expands and contracts, the testicles are positioned farther away from, or closer to, the torso, thereby regulating temperature. When a man comes out of the shower or a hot tub, his scrotal sac looks distended—the body is trying to cool the testes by removing them from heat generated by the torso. On the other hand, during exercise, sexual arousal, or when a man feels anxious or threatened, the testicles are drawn up closer to the torso, protecting them from being fully exposed to possible harm.

It's normal for one testicle to hang lower than the other. This uneven positioning provides protection for both testicles by preventing them from being squeezed together between a man's legs.

Seminal Vesicles

Males have two seminal vesicles, which are small glands located behind the bladder. The opening of this gland joins with the vas deferens and connects to the ejaculatory duct in the prostate. When a man orgasms, the seminal vesicles contract, secreting a fluid rich with fructose that helps nourish the sperm. Fluid from the seminal vesicles makes up about two-thirds of *ejaculate*, which is another name for semen emitted, or about to be emitted, during ejaculation.

Prostate

The prostate is a muscular gland that surrounds a man's urethra at the base of the bladder. Inside the prostate, the urethra forms a bulb where the semen collects just before ejaculation. On either side of this bulb are circular bands of muscle. At the top of the prostate, where it joins to the opening of the bladder, the urethra can squeeze shut during orgasm to prevent ejaculate from going up into the bladder. This section of the urethra is called the *internal urethral sphincter.* At the other end of the prostate, the *external urethral sphincter* tightens as the urethral bulb fills with ejaculate. This action keeps the semen in the bulb until it's time for ejaculation.

Secretions from the prostate gland make up about a third of ejaculate which combines with sperm from the vas deferens and fluid from the seminal vesicles. Even though there may be as many as 500 million sperm in an average ejaculation, sperm make up only a minuscule part of the ejaculate. For that reason, men do not experience any noticeable change in their ejaculation after a vasectomy.

When a man ejaculates, the prostrate gland squeezes shut the opening of the bladder, and the urethra and pelvic musculature go through a series of contractions to expel the semen from the urethral bulb. Because the bladder is shut off and the external urethral sphincter is relaxed, the semen can go in only one direction—down the length of the shaft and out through the tip of the penis.

Some men develop ejaculation problems when the prostate is damaged. A common treatment for an enlarged prostate that is blocking the urethra is called a transurethral resection of the prostate (TURP). During this procedure, an instrument is threaded through the urethra, and excess tissue inside the prostate is clipped. If, in the process, damage is done to the opening of the bladder, it may not close properly during orgasm. If this happens, during ejaculation semen will seek the path of least resistance. Rather than going down the length of the penis, the semen will go into the bladder. The man will experience the pleasurable sensations of orgasm, but he will have a dry ejaculation, called *retrograde ejaculation*. With this condition, he may notice white fluid in his urine when he voids after sexual activity. This is perfectly normal; the retrograde ejaculate is voided from the bladder during urination. Diabetes can cause similar problems by interfering with the nerve fibers that control the opening and closing of the bladder during sexual excitement.

If the prostate is surgically removed, a man will still be capable of experiencing an orgasm, but he will not ejaculate. With the removal of the prostate gland, the vas deferens and seminal vesicles no longer connect to the urethra. Prostatic fluid, seminal fluid, and sperm are no longer available to create ejaculate.

Cowper's Glands

The Cowper's glands are two small glands that connect to the urethra below the prostate. During sexual arousal, these glands secrete a mucous substance into the urethra that protects the sperm cells by neutralizing any acidity that may remain in the urethra from earlier urination. The discharge from the Cowper's glands also serves as a lubricant for the glans of the penis.

SEXUAL RESPONSE

As for women, it's easiest to understand the male sexual response by dividing it into the phases of desire, arousal, and orgasm.

Desire

The desire phase of the male sexual response precedes erection and orgasm. Put simply: to have sex, normally the man needs to want sex. To have sexual desire is to respond to sexual cues—"being horny" is the slang equivalent. It's looking for, welcoming, and being receptive to sexual invitations and opportunities. Men, like women, can become aroused and orgasm without sexual desire, but the presence or absence of desire will greatly influence sexual frequency and satisfaction.

As is the case for women, hormones play an important role for men in generating sexual appetite. Research has shown that the frequency of sexual thoughts and fantasies increases and decreases in tandem with rises and drops in testosterone levels. Testosterone is one of a number of steroid hormones that can alter a "sensory threshold," which refers to the lowest level at which a stimulus can trigger a response. If a woman's coy smile is normally a sexual cue for a man, he will be more likely to pick up on it and respond to it if his testosterone level is in the normal range. If his hormone level is below normal, he may miss or ignore the cue. Research also suggests that testosterone levels increase genital sensitivity to stimulation. Testosterone therefore affects sexual desire not only by increasing the chances of a man picking up on a sexual cue but also by increasing the probability that he will respond physically.

Is there a gender difference in sexual desire? Are men biologically driven by a stronger sex drive than women? If you gave any credence to all the corny jokes about men who think with their penises and women who have perpetual headaches, you might believe that men are innately more highly sexed than women are. It's not true. Both women and men are capable of having strong sex drives. If there is a gender difference when it comes to sexual interest, it's not that biology makes men want sex more than women do but rather how our culture conditions women and men differently.

Throughout this book we have touched on how culture can inhibit the development of a woman's comfort with her sexuality. Our dominant culture tends to evaluate the significance of sexual behavior differently for women and men. Most men, for example, have been programmed to interpret having sex as the ultimate evidence of their desirability and masculinity. Early in life, having sex is equated with conquest; only losers can't "get any." Men learn that having sex increases not only their worth but also the worth or value of any occasion during which it occurs. A date, a special evening, or a vacation is always best if there's sex; without sex, the event is less than perfect.

That's not necessarily the case for women—at least, not as often. Sex can be great, but for many women it's not as critical an ingredient for making an event or occasion special as it is for most men. Being sexually desired by a man can be nice, but it isn't necessarily a compliment. Women are well aware that men have been enculturated to seek sex for sex's sake, and they certainly know that sexual attention may not always be a sign of affection. For many women, being held, respected, and listened to—not sex—signal that they're special, cherished, and desired. None of this is intended to imply that men enjoy sex more than women or that men have an innately stronger sex drive than women. But men and women tend to assign different roles to sex, and that difference can give the impression of a general difference in desire. Even though social stereotypes suggest that men are always ready for sex, in truth, men, just like women, have sexual appetites that fluctuate not only according to hormonal levels but also emotional state, health factors, energy level, and external circumstances.

Arousal

As is the case with most natural body functions, the erection process appears simple and straightforward, but in reality, it is quite complex and susceptible to a wide variety of things that can go wrong.

There is a network of small, smooth muscles in the corporal bodies that, when the penis is soft, are in a natural state of contraction. Blood enters the corporal bodies through arteries running down the center of the tubes. The blood nourishes the penile tissue and flows back to the torso through a series of veins located just beneath the penile sheathing, the tunica albuginea.

When a man becomes sexually aroused, impulses are sent along parasympathetic nerve fibers in the penis that trigger the release of cyclic GMP, a chemical that relaxes the smooth muscles. As these muscles relax, pockets form and blood quickly pours in. The spongy tissue expands as these new spaces are filled with blood, and the tunica begins to stretch. When the corporal bodies push out against the tunica, they pinch the outgoing veins. Pressure builds in the penis as blood pours in but can only trickle back out because the veins are pinched. As a result, the man has a rigid erection.

In order for this process to work, the blood vessels and nerve endings must perform flawlessly. If the arteries are blocked, blood will not flow in quickly enough to create the pressure necessary for an erection. If the veins have leaks in them, the penis will inflate initially but, like inflating a tire with a pinhole, will keep deflating. If injury, surgery, or illness damages the nerve fibers, the signal for the smooth muscles to relax will never arrive, and the penis will remain limp regardless of what kind of sexual activity is taking place. The signal to the smooth muscles can also be overridden by the effects of certain medications and by stress and distraction.

While the penis is becoming erect, a number of additional changes take place throughout the body. Breathing, heart rate, and blood pressure all increase. Blood flow to the skin may cause a rash-like appearance, called a sex flush, over various parts of the body. This blood flow also makes parts of the body, including the earlobes, lips, and nipples, more sensitive to stimulation. The testicles become engorged with blood and increase in size. The *tunica dartos*, the muscle lining the scrotal sack, thickens and contracts, drawing the testicles closer to the torso. A drop or two of a clear, slippery fluid from the Cowper's glands appears at the opening of the urethra.

Orgasm

Emission Phase

Male orgasm occurs in two phases: emission followed by expulsion. The emission phase begins when sexual arousal reaches the necessary level of intensity. A series of contractions in the *vasa deferentia* (plural for vas deferens), the seminal vesicles, and the prostrate gland force sperm and ejaculatory fluid into the urethral bulb, which is located inside the prostate. At the same time, the urethra at the base of the prostate (external urethral sphincter) and at the opening of the bladder (internal urethral sphincter) contracts, keeping the ejaculate inside the prostate. Once this emission phase occurs, ejaculation will occur, regardless of any distraction.

Expulsion Phase

During the next phase of orgasm, the external urethral sphincter relaxes, opening up the passageway for ejaculation. At the same time, the urethra and muscles at the base of the penis go into involuntary, rhythmic contractions spaced about 0.8 second apart. The timing of these contractions is identical to the timing of a woman's muscular contractions during orgasm. The external urethral sphincter relaxes, and the ejaculate is expelled down the length of the penis and out the urethral opening.

Numerous factors can affect *ejaculatory latency*, which is the length of time between the start of stimulation and ejaculation. A man may take longer to ejaculate if he is fatigued, distracted, or lacks desire. Alcohol and some medications and other drugs can also delay or even prevent ejaculation. Anxiety, heightened sexual excitement, or a lack of recent sexual activity, on the other hand, can cause a man to ejaculate more rapidly than he is accustomed to.

Postorgasm Changes

As noted, when a man becomes erect, impulses travel along nerve fibers (part of the parasympathetic nervous system) to relax the smooth muscles inside the penis. Shortly after orgasm, impulses are sent along a different set of nerve fibers (part of the sympathetic nervous system) to the same smooth muscles inside the penis. During a process called *detumescence*, the nerve impulses signal these muscles to contract. Enzymes are released to break down the cyclic GMP, the chemical that relaxed the smooth muscles in the first place. As a result, the muscles return to their normal state, and the pressure-squeeze on the outgoing veins is released. As the little muscles begin to contract, blood is literally wrung out of the pockets, into the veins, and back out into the body cavity. The penis becomes flaccid again.

As the blood-flow pattern is reversed following orgasm, a man enters into a refractory period, which is a period of time when the body is not capable of re-arousal and orgasm. This refractory period can be very brief for young men—so brief that they may be ready to orgasm again before losing their original erection. The refractory period varies dramatically from man to man and often increases with age. As men approach their senior years, the refractory period can increase the downtime between orgasms to hours or even days.

AGING

A number of years ago, a man in his late 40s made an appointment with one of us because of an erection problem. He explained that he could get erect during only about half of his attempts at intercourse. This was particularly upsetting because he was in a new relationship, and he felt frustrated and embarrassed over having difficulty responding to his new partner. His partner was beginning to question whether she was doing something to turn him off, or worse yet, that perhaps he didn't find her attractive. He was desperate.

We agreed that a 50% failure rate certainly suggested a problem, so we pressed for more details. The man explained that he had just ended a very bad 20-year marriage, the final years of which had been sexless. Now he was madly in love with his new partner. On the nights he and his partner got together, they would make love, and it would be wonderful—so wonderful that minutes later they would want to do it again. They were in the "honeymoon phase" of their relationship, and the novelty and excitement of a new relationship triggered a sexual appetite that the man had not experienced since he was in his 20s. But always during the second attempt, things wouldn't work—he couldn't get an erection. That's how he figured that he had an erection problem 50% of the time: the first attempt of each evening would be successful; the second attempt would not.

It never occurred to this man that the difficulty he was experiencing was perfectly normal for his age. When he was in his 20s, he could make love two, three, four, or even more times during the course of the evening. It had been years since he'd had any interest in making love multiple times, so he was unaware of normal body changes that slowly occurred over time. He had no idea that his refractory period had increased so that now it might take an hour or two after an orgasm before he would be able to become erect again. Had he known about this normal, age-related change in his sexual functioning, he and his partner could have been spared a great deal of worry and grief.

This example highlights the importance of awareness of the normal sexual changes that occur as men grow older. Many of these age-related changes in male sexuality can become evident in a man as early as his 30s. These changes will continue slowly through each succeeding decade of life. In no way do these changes prevent men and their partners from enjoying sexual intimacy. Age alone will not eliminate sexual desire; it will not prevent a man from getting or staying erect; and it will not take away a man's ability to orgasm. Aging may slow down and modify how the body responds sexually, but it will not prevent a man from enjoying sexual activity. Men in their 80s can continue to have highly satisfying sexual experiences even though their bodies may no longer respond like the body of an 18-year-old. Knowledge of these changes prevents needless performance concerns that can easily distract and dismay both the man and his partner.

In this section, we look at common changes that most men experience as part of the course of normal aging. When changes in sexual function are more dramatic or extreme than the changes described below, they may be due to more than aging: they may be the result of injury, disease, or psychological inhibition. Sexual dysfunctions, which are abnormal changes in sexual response, are discussed later in this chapter.

Decreased Sexual Drive

During their teens and early 20s, men may feel like they're walking erections. It can seem like sex is always on their mind. If they're in a relationship, they'll tend to emphasize sexual frequency and initiate lovemaking every chance they get. As they move into their 30s, men still have strong sex drives, but the novelty of sex has begun to wear off, and job and family responsibilities compete for their energy and attention. By their late 40s and early 50s, many men find that their sex drives are beginning to decrease. A large part of this change is due to slowly decreasing levels of testosterone, the hormone essential for sexual appetite. Sexual desire, along with testosterone levels, continues to decline slowly as a man approaches his senior years. In later life, the man will respond with interest when presented with a sexual opportunity, but spontaneous thoughts about sex and an unrelenting drive to initiate sex will be much less common than during his younger years.

Psychological factors can inhibit sexual desire for men as they age. Men are not immune to vanity. As they grow older, many become distressed by graying hair, receding hairlines, protruding bellies, disappearing chins, drooping eyelids, and reading glasses. Gym memberships, hair coloring, and hair restoration products are part of a multimillion-dollar-a-year industry that caters to men trying to retain a youthful appearance. But changes in appearance don't seem to have a big impact on men's sexual desire. Whereas women often need to feel desirable to feel sexual desire, men apparently do not. Instead, men are highly concerned about sexual prowess. Some men, when they note subtle changes in their sexual response, feel threatened and pull back from sexual activity. Better not to be tested, they reason, than to be tested and fail. By avoiding sex, they avoid the potential humiliation of erectile failure. Unfortunately, in the process, they also miss out on opportunities to share physical and emotional intimacy with their partner.

Takes Longer to Get Hard

Whereas teens often fight to keep their erections down (outside the bedroom, of course), as men get older, it can feel like a fight to get and keep their erections. Accustomed to having instant erections in response to any sexual situation, middle-aged men may be threatened by finding that it takes longer to get an erection. This change is normal and should in no way interfere with lovemaking. Unfortunately, if the man begins to panic because he doesn't have an instant erection, he can worry himself out of responding.

Need for Fiction and Friction

Sex therapists like to say that an erection requires fiction and friction. The *fiction* refers to mental activity: think sexy thoughts and nature takes its course. *Friction* refers to the direct stimulation of the penis. When he's a teen or in his early 20s, a man only needs one of these two ingredients. Either wearing jeans that are too tight or seeing a girl in a sweater that's too tight is often all that is needed to produce an erection. As he gets older, however, sexy thoughts or direct stimulation by themselves will usually not be enough. For a middle-aged man to become and stay erect, his mind will have to be focused on erotic thoughts, and his penis will require ongoing stimulation.

A common occurrence for a man as he gets older is to panic when his erection decreases during foreplay. When he was younger and became erect, it would seem that nothing short of an orgasm or an act of Congress would make the penis go down. Later in life, however, a disturbing change occurs. One night he goes to bed with his partner, and during the initial groping and caressing, an erection develops. Nothing out of the ordinary so far. Having learned to be a "good lover," the man focuses on pleasuring his partner further before attempting intercourse. He dutifully does all the things the sex manuals instructed him to do. He gently plays with her nipples, strokes her thighs, caresses her clitoris, maybe even tries to find and stimulate her G spot. Finally her quiet moans and pelvic rocking signal that she's ready for him. But, lo and behold, when he looks down, he finds that his erection has abandoned him. He panics and desperately struggles to regain the erection. Unfortunately, desperation is the slayer of erections, and he ends up having nothing to show for his efforts other than a cold sweat.

What is important for this man to realize is that as he gets older, his erections will require continued physical stimulation. Stop direct stimulation, and erections will likely go down. It's normal for an erection to go temporarily soft during love play. If the man doesn't panic, the erection will typically come back when the penis is directly stimulated again. It should take limited effort because he's not starting from scratch: the penile tissue is already stretched and additional blood has already collected in the pelvic area. The important thing is for the man not to fret.

Stress, fatigue, or distraction can occasionally cause difficulty in regaining or maintaining an erection. It's important for the couple to remain flexible. Contrary to the myth that good sex equals intercourse, partners can be highly sensual with each other without the presence of an erection.

Greater Variability in Erections

Most young men have two kinds of erections—rock-hard and rigid. As men get older, however, erections become much more variable. A man in his late 30s or early 40s may find that on one day he has an erection reminiscent of his early youth, and on the next day, an erection that's usable but pliable. Over time, rock-hard, rigid erections will appear less often, but the penis will still be able to become sufficiently erect for vaginal entry and thrusting. Sexual activity will continue to be highly pleasurable.

Another quite normal change in erections, but one that worries men, is the angle of their erection. Typically when standing, a young man will have an erection that points toward the ceiling, sometimes at a 50-degree angle away from the body. Young men often delight in the strength of their erections, taking pride in silly things like being able to hang a bath towel on an erect penis. Because of changes in penile blood flow and the elasticity of pelvic musculature as men grow older, the erect penis will eventually stop pointing to the ceiling, but instead to the wall, and in time, perhaps, even to the floor.

Takes Longer to Ejaculate

One often positive age-related change in a man's sexual response is the lengthening of the time it takes before ejaculation occurs. Age can be a surefire cure for rapid ejaculation. Young men tend to ejaculate very rapidly. With age and increased sexual experience, they are able to last longer. As they enter their later years, however, some men find that it takes so long to ejaculate that, on occasion, they will end lovemaking before having an orgasm.

Although most women are quite accepting of the possibility that not every sexual encounter may lead to orgasm, men have been conditioned to think differently. The lovemaking might be the most beautiful and exciting experience imaginable, but if they don't climax, men tend to write off the experience as a failure. Some men in later life even avoid lovemaking altogether rather than going through the frustration of not ejaculating.

It's important for men—and the women who love them—to realize that, as they get older, not only will it take longer to orgasm, but on occasion they might not be able to ejaculate. More important, older men need to discover what many women already know from experience—that lovemaking can be very satisfying even if there isn't an orgasm.

Ejaculation Changes

Even in his 30s, a man will begin to notice changes in his ejaculation. It is very normal for the amount of ejaculate, the force of expulsion, and the number of muscular contractions to decrease with age. Young men can shoot a tablespoon of ejaculate a foot or more into the air. Older men may note that when they orgasm, perhaps less than a teaspoon of ejaculate will dribble, rather than spurt, from the urethral opening. These changes are normal and should not interfere with sexual satisfaction.

Detumescence Is Quicker

It takes a young man much longer for his erection to go down after ejaculation than it does for an older man. After an orgasm during intercourse, a young man may remain in his partner's vagina for minutes enjoying the few additional moments of physical closeness in his postorgasmic glow. An older man may find his soft penis slipping out of the vagina almost immediately after ejaculation. All, however, is not lost. The older man also can enjoy physical closeness with his partner during his postcoital glow by holding and caressing her. Like all the changes described above, quick detumescence is a change that should have no impact on sexual satisfaction, unless the man or woman is misguided by misinformation or unrealistic expectations.

Thoughts on Sex and Aging

When looking at age-related changes in a man's sexual response, we might be tempted to conclude that aging has only negative effects: less desire, slower and less rigid erections, and delays in ejaculation. As we've already said, however, these are normal changes and need not affect a couple's sexual pleasure and satisfaction.

It's important to realize that there are definite positives that emerge as men grow older. The sexual drive of an older man is often more closely attuned to his partner's drive than when he and his partner were younger. Many men in long-term relationships become more comfortable with physical and emotional intimacy. They have learned to feel more secure about their manhood and sexuality, and as a result, become far more sensitive lovers. We have often seen older men who have become much more responsive to touch. When we work with older couples, we're impressed hearing them talk about how much they enjoy massaging, cuddling, holding, and caressing each other. Women will marvel at how much their physical relationship has changed from the early years when sex involved "copping a feel, having a quickie, and falling asleep." They describe how genital sex has become only one portion of an extended, loving, physical connectedness between the two partners.

SEXUAL DYSFUNCTIONS

Slight alterations in the phases of sexual response are perfectly normal with aging. Sometimes, however, the phases of sexual response can be totally disrupted or shut down by psychological or medical factors. These sexual dysfunctions can be very alarming, both to the men who experience them and to the women who are their sexual partners. Understanding why they occur can ease the minds of couples and steer them in the right direction for help.

Loss of Desire

According to social stereotypes, real men want sex, and lots of it. It's women, not men, who get headaches and try to avoid sex. But it's just not true. Loss of sexual desire is a common problem for both men and women. In a 1994 study of over 1,300 men aged 18 to 59, almost 16% acknowledged lacking interest in sex (Laumann et al., 1994). Causes for this problem can include medical illness, testosterone deficiencies, adverse reactions to medication, depression, relationship problems, sexual conflict, reaction to erection problems, and stress.

It's very difficult for men to admit to others, or even to themselves, that they have lost their interest in sex. They will deny it, bury themselves in their work, and when pressed, make excuses to avoid sexual intimacy. If they're directly confronted about their avoidance of sex, they may try blaming their partner, suggesting that their weight gain, past history of sexual indifference, or unwillingness to experiment has finally beaten down the man's interest in sex.

If a man loses his sexual desire, a physical examination should be the first step in trying to understand and resolve the problem. A healthcare provider can make sure that there are no medical problems affecting the man's sex drive. If a medical problem is discovered, the healthcare provider can prescribe appropriate treatment. For example, when hormone levels are abnormally low, testosterone supplements can help to restore sexual desire in many cases. Despite claims often made in the popular press, however, testosterone is not a miracle drug and offers no advantage when hormone levels are already normal.

If the man gets a clean bill of health, consulting a sex therapist may be a helpful next step. For more information on sex therapy, see Chapter 17.

Erection Problems

The sexual problem that strikes the greatest fear in the hearts of men is not being able to "get it up." Potency and manhood are immutably connected in the male psyche. Many men cannot escape the belief that to be impotent is to be less of a man. As a result, erection difficulty can lead to significant personal and relationship problems.

Unless there is an injury or a psychological trauma, erection problems usually don't happen suddenly. More often, over a period of months the man notices that it is more and more difficult to get and stay erect. Noticing the dramatic decline, the man will often say nothing to his partner. Instead, he begins to pull back sexually, often as a form of denial or self-protection. The man may rationalize that avoiding sex spares his partner the frustration of "being left high and dry." All this goes on, often without a single word being spoken between the partners.

Meanwhile, the partner notices his withdrawal. How can she miss it? A man who for years has had a robust interest in sex is suddenly asexual. In time, it's not uncommon for the woman to start worrying. *Is it something about me,* she wonders, or *is he seeing someone else?* Frightened, hurt, and concerned, she may withdraw, become irritable, or turn to a Victoria's Secret catalog in hopes of reigniting his interest. And still, often all this goes on without a single word spoken between the partners.

Erection problems are common. In a study of men between the ages of 18 and 59, 10% were unable to achieve or maintain an erection (Laumann et al., 1994). Difficulty increases with age, so that in a study of a cross-sectional sample of men between the ages of 40 and 70, 52% reported some form of erection difficulty (Feldman, Goldstein, Hatzichristou, Krane, & McKinlay, 1994).

Not all that many years ago, practitioners assumed that the majority of erection problems were due to psychological factors. Performance anxiety was seen as the main culprit. We assumed that most men with this problem were so worried about performing well that the pressure and anxiety actually overrode the body's signals to respond sexually. Thanks to new diagnostic technology and increased understanding of how erections occur, we've come to realize that the majority of erection problems are due to medical problems. Medication can interfere with erections. The penis may have damaged blood vessels due to poor diet, smoking, or high blood pressure. Injuries, surgery, or diseases that impact the nerve fibers controlling erection can also lead to erectile dysfunction. There are still many bona fide cases of erectile failure caused by psychological issues, but a medical evaluation should always be the first step when addressing an erection problem.

How can doctors determine whether the erection problem is medical or psychological? Tests can measure blood flow in the penis, check for leaking veins, and determine whether the nervous system is working properly. One particularly helpful and easy diagnostic procedure is monitoring to see if a man gets an erection when he's sleeping. Most every man is familiar with what is called, in the vernacular, a "piss hard-on." Every few mornings, a man will wake with an erection. He gets up, urinates, and the erection goes away. He assumes that the erection was the result of a full bladder, thus the term, "piss hard-on." The penis, however, is not a water balloon, and the erection has nothing to do with the condition of the bladder. Normal sleep consists of 90-minute cycles, and one of the stages of these cycles is called the

REM, or rapid-eye-movement, stage. During the REM stage, the body goes through a number of physiological changes including the pooling of blood in the pelvis. As a result, every 90 minutes during sleep, men generally get an erection lasting 10 to 15 minutes. Likewise, women lubricate every 90 minutes during their sleep. Morning erections occur only on those mornings when the man happens to wake up during the REM stage of sleep. On other mornings, when he awakes during other stages of the sleep cycle, he won't have an erection—but he'll probably still have a full bladder.

We have been able to capitalize on this phenomenon to help assess the cause of erection problems. By simply asking the man about his morning erections, we can get a good idea about whether his penis is still capable of functioning normally. If the man is in doubt, we can send him home with a special monitoring device. If the man's erection difficulty is due to psychological problems, he should still get erections when he's asleep. The reasoning is that when he's sleeping, performance concerns and sexual inhibitions shouldn't come into play. Without the negative influence of the mind, the body is free to respond normally to physical cues. If, on the other hand, he can't get erections when he's awake or asleep, chances are there's a medical reason.

In recent years there have been a number of exciting advances in the treatment of erection problems. Let's take a look at some of these treatment options.

Hormones

Although testosterone primarily affects sexual desire, it also appears to influence genital sensitivity. When a man has an erection problem and his testosterone level is abnormally low, testosterone injections or a testosterone patch may improve erectile functioning. This is particularly likely if the erection problem is caused or complicated by low sexual desire.

Corrective Surgery

Sometimes surgery can change an underlying condition that is preventing a normal erection. For example, some men develop small leaks in the veins leading away from the penis. Every time there's an erection, the penis can't maintain the internal pressure necessary to sustain it because blood keeps leaking back into the torso. Surgery to tie off the damaged veins can restore potency in some of these cases.

Vascular surgery is sometimes performed to repair or bypass damaged arteries supplying blood to the corporal bodies in the penis. This is a specialized procedure that is not often used in the treatment of erectile dysfunctions. In carefully screened cases, however, this surgery has improved erectile functioning for some men.

Sometimes the erection problem is due to a condition called Peyronie's disease. In this condition, the sheathing surrounding the corpora cavernosa develops a fibrous plaque or scar. As a result, when the penis starts to expand, the sheathing can't stretch uniformly, which causes the shaft to curve. It's similar to pinching a balloon when inflating it: the balloon will curve around the point where it can't expand. In cases of Peyronie's disease, the curvature can be so severe that the penis is unable to become sufficiently erect for intercourse. Oral medication or steroid injections may be used initially in efforts to dissolve the plaque. In extreme cases, surgery to patch the affected sheathing has been successful. As a last resort, penile implants are sometimes used.

Vasoactive Medications

Certain medications can improve erections by increasing blood flow to the penis. Yohimbine, a natural vasodilator available by prescription, is a popular treatment that has been used for many years. Yohimbine does not act specifically on the penis but dilates blood vessels in general, causing flushing and elevated blood pressure in some men. Men with very mild blood-flow problems or with erection problems caused by psychological inhibition have been the best candidates for this treatment. Yohimbine also appears to help counteract sexual side effects caused by some medications.

Medications delivered directly to the corporal bodies can be very effective. Up until recently, the best way to concentrate a medication effect on penile blood vessels was to inject the medication into the corpora cavernosa. This self-injection method was particularly effective for diabetic men with nerve damage in the penis. Undaunted by needles because of years of injecting insulin, many diabetic men found that they could produce good erections by injecting drugs such as alprostadil (Caverject, Edex). More recently, a gel-like suppository containing alprostadil (MUSE) has been developed for insertion into the tip of the penis, bypassing the hassle and anxiety associated with needles and shots.

The use of vasoactive medication has really taken off, however, with the development of oral medication that specifically targets penile blood flow. In 1998, sildenafil (Viagra) became big news. For the first time in medical history, by simply taking a pill an hour before sex, many men with long histories of erectile failure are able to gain usable erections. As you read earlier in this chapter, erections occur when cyclic GMP is available to relax smooth muscles in the penis. Many erection problems are due to impaired blood flow or damaged nerve fibers. Because of these problems, the penis requires more cyclic GMP than is available for producing an erection. Viagra inhibits an enzyme that breaks down cyclic GMP, allowing even a limited amount of the chemical to have a maximum effect. As a result, a simple little blue pill is having a dramatic impact on millions of couples worldwide.

Side effects from Viagra are rare and usually mild and reversible when they occur. They can include headaches, facial flushing, nasal congestion, stomach irritation, muscle cramping, rashes, difficulty differentiating the colors blue and green, urinary tract infections, and shortness of breath. A number of highly publicized deaths attributed to Viagra, however, have alarmed the public. Most of these deaths have been due to a lethal drug interaction. Men taking nitrates should not use Viagra. Because nitrates dilate blood vessels, they are often prescribed for angina, which is chest pain caused by constricted blood vessels. Because Viagra also dilates blood vessels, the double impact of Viagra and nitrates can relax the blood vessels so much that blood pressure drops too low, triggering a fatal heart attack.

For the sake of safety, Viagra should be taken only under a physician's supervision. Ordering this medication off the Internet or buying it on the black market can be dangerous. Working with a physician not only ensures safe and effective use of the medication but can also uncover medical causes for the erection problem. Many men now taking Viagra were unaware of cardiovascular problems until they were screened for their erectile dysfunction. In some instances, this discovery was lifesaving.

Other oral drugs that use slightly different mechanisms from those of Viagra for producing erections are in development. Because of the significant number of men with erection problems—perhaps 20 million in the United States, and with the "baby boomers" quickly approaching their senior years—we anticipate a continued flurry of research and development to produce new and better treatments.

Penile Implants

When damage to the blood vessels, nerve fibers, or the structure of the penis is irreparable, penile implants may be a treatment option. A surgeon will implant cylinders into the corpora cavernosa, the top two spongy tubes in the penis. The cylinders may be either bendable rods encased in silicone or inflatable tubes. With the bendable rods, the penis is permanently enlarged. During nonsexual situations, the man bends the penis downwards to remain inconspicuous. When the man wants to make love, he bends the penis upward to position it for intercourse. This style of implant is particularly popular with older men who prefer something simple and who are less likely to spend time in gym locker rooms. Walking around in a locker room or shower area with an erection doesn't help to make new friends.

Men not wanting to contend with a permanently enlarged penis often prefer inflatable implants, because the penis appears flaccid during nonsexual situations. During sexual situations, the man squeezes a small pump in the tip of the implant or in the scrotal sac, which transfers saline solution from the back of the implant or from a reservoir placed in the abdominal cavity. As the fluid fills the tubes, the penis becomes rigid. When the man releases a seal on the pump, the fluid recedes back to its reservoir, and the penis becomes flaccid.

After surgery, the size of the erect penis is decreased slightly, but this change should have no effect on either the man or woman's sexual pleasure and satisfaction. Because the corpus spongiosum, the corporal body surrounding the urethra, is not affected by this surgery, a man's ability to urinate and ejaculate remains intact. The man usually retains normal sensations in his penis, unless sensation had already been lost due to injury or disease. The erect penis should feel normal to the woman; it will not feel like a foreign object poking at her.

Inserting the implants will damage delicate tissue in the corpora cavernosa and destroy any remaining ability the penis might have to become erect naturally. Implant surgery, therefore, should be considered a last-resort treatment. In cases where there were no other viable options, penile implants have allowed men to resume a full, active, and satisfying sex life.

Vacuum Constriction Device (VCD)

This treatment option involves the use of a large plastic tube with a pump on the end of it (this device resembles a breast pump). When the man places the tube over his penis and flush against his torso, he creates a vacuum by pumping air out of the tube. The vacuum draws blood into the penis, causing it to expand and become erect. The vacuum is usually powerful enough to overcome even severe blood-flow problems. Once the penis is erect, the man slips a specially designed rubber band off the tube and onto the base of the penis. The band traps the blood in the penis, which keeps it erect after the vacuum tube is removed. The band can remain on the penis for up to 30 minutes without risk of the restricted blood flow causing tissue damage.

The VCD is a safe alternative for men who do not want to deal with medication or surgery. Many men with erectile problems prefer this surefire mechanical approach to making the penis erect. The resulting erection can be a source of pleasure for both the man and his partner. This device does not interfere with orgasm, although ejaculation may be difficult. Because the band exerts pressure around the base of the penis, semen can be blocked. This is not a birth control device, however. If ejaculation is forceful enough, the semen can still be discharged.

The VCD does have some potential drawbacks. Some couples complain that the process of using the equipment to inflate the penis takes away the romantic ambience. Many couples have worked around this complaint by having the man generate the erection before he joins the partner to begin their love play. Some men don't like the VCD because of the subtle differences between normal erections and erections created with it. VCD-assisted erections tend to "hinge" or bend at the point where the band is located. (Remember that the penis continues past the abdominal wall and is anchored to the pubic bone.) With a VCD, the corporal bodies are engorged only from the constriction band forward. Behind the band, the penis is flaccid. As a result, it can be more difficult to align the penis with the vagina for entry and thrusting. Some men are distracted by subtle changes in skin coloration and temperature when the penis is erect. Because normal blood flow is greatly restricted, the penis may have a slightly blue or grayish hue and may be cool to the touch. None of these changes—hinging, color, or temperature—should prevent a couple from enjoying intercourse. Some men or their partners, however, are turned off by these changes and opt for another solution.

Despite the drawbacks, tens of thousands of men and their partners have been happy with this inexpensive, safe, and effective device. Men who take blood thinners or who are at risk for internal bleeding may not be good candidates for this treatment option, however.

Sex Therapy

For erection problems largely attributable to psychological causes, sex therapy (see Chapter 17) can be very helpful. Even when the erection problem has a physical cause and responds to medical treatment, counseling can help the man adjust to changes in his erectile functioning and their effects on his self-esteem. Counseling can also help the couple overcome the aftermath of the blame, embarrassment, or self-doubt that they may have experienced before the erection problem was diagnosed and treated.

Rapid Ejaculation

As common as this problem is—28% of our sample of 18- to 59-year-old men complained that they climax too quickly (Laumann et al., 1994)—rapid ejaculation is very difficult to define. How quick is too quick? Experts have disagreed for years. In the past, many doctors and therapists would use length of time prior to ejaculation or the number of thrusts as the criterion. For example, if a man ejaculated within two minutes of entering the vagina or before completing a hundred thrusts during intercourse, he would be diagnosed as a rapid ejaculator. But something was missing with this approach. Not only did it encourage people to bring a stopwatch into the bedroom, it also failed to take into account other important factors such as the duration and quality of the overall lovemaking experience. According to this definition, a man could last three minutes but skip any foreplay or afterplay, and feel reassured that everything was normal. We don't think so.

Some experts have suggested that a man is a rapid ejaculator if his partner fails to orgasm at least 50% of the time. The problem with this definition is that we have learned that more than half of all women have difficulty experiencing orgasm from intercourse alone, regardless of how long it lasts. Other experts have defined rapid ejaculation as occurring when a man does not have control over his ejaculatory response. But as most men will attest, a man at best may have partial control over when he is going to ejaculate, but certainly not total control.

Again, how quick is too quick? Certainly when a man ejaculates before getting out of his clothes, or before he enters his partner's vagina, or within seconds of entry—that's a problem that should be addressed. But beyond these extreme cases, a more general factor should be taken into account. How satisfying is the lovemaking experience for both partners? If lovemaking is reduced merely to the time the penis is in the vagina, satisfaction may be unlikely. Some writers make the distinction between *intercourse* and *outercourse*. Lovemaking should typically involve talking, holding, caressing, and stroking both before and after intercourse. When this is the case, the length of time that intercourse takes place becomes far less significant; satisfaction will come from the whole experience, not just part of it.

Rapid ejaculation rarely has a medical cause. Some have actually argued that rapid ejaculation was bred into the human species during the early millennia of evolution. The theory goes that the individual who could quickly impregnate his mate before having to fight off competing males was more likely to contribute to the species' gene pool. Consistent with this line of thinking, copulation for virtually every animal species is very brief. Others, however, argue that unlike for other living species, rapid ejaculation is not very adaptive for humans. Because humans are social and capable of emotional bonding, making babies is not the only function of sex. For humans alone, mutually satisfying and enjoyable sex facilitates an emotional bond between the two partners.

As for why some men tend to ejaculate much more rapidly than others, there is no agreed-on answer. Some people suggest that rapid ejaculation is a learned response going back to adolescence, when a male would masturbate quickly to lessen chances of being caught. It's clear that experience and frequency also influence ejaculatory control. Most young men ejaculate very quickly, but with experience their ejaculatory latency—the time it takes to ejaculate—increases. Likewise, the frequency of sex influences ejaculatory latency. If a man goes without sex for an extended period of time, he will ejaculate much more rapidly than if he has sex two, three, or four times a week.

Anxiety may be another possible factor contributing to rapid ejaculation. We know that the ejaculatory response is partially controlled by the sympathetic nervous system. Men who are very sensitive to the physical effects of anxiety, which are mediated by the sympathetic nervous system, appear to be susceptible to rapid ejaculation. In our clinical practice, we have noted an increased incidence of rapid ejaculation in patients with anxiety disorders, phobias, and obsessive–compulsive disorders.

Rapid ejaculation can affect not only the man but also his partner and their relationship. Unless he is so self-centered that his partner's satisfaction is of no consequence, a man who ejaculates too rapidly will often feel embarrassed and humiliated. The partner, too, may struggle with a variety of possible reactions. Some women blame themselves, assuming that they must have done something wrong to make the man ejaculate so rapidly. Many women feel cheated when the pleasure of being physically connected is cut so short. Some of these women resent repeatedly having to hide their disappointment and feeling obligated to comfort and reassure their partner. Others can't accept normal feelings of disappointment but instead feel guilty over what they inaccurately label in themselves as insensitivity. Any of these responses—embarrassment, humiliation, guilt, disappointment, or resentment—can lead to stress and strain in even the best of relationships.

Sex therapists have found a number of behavior-therapy techniques to be helpful in extending ejaculatory latency for the majority of men experiencing rapid ejaculation. The success rate for treating this problem has been encouraging. For the really difficult cases, we have found that small doses of select antidepressants can also increase ejaculatory latency. Perhaps most important of all, however, is for the couple to expand their understanding of what it means to make love. As we described earlier, lovemaking should be much, much more than merely intercourse.

One final word about length of time. As you've read above, we've tried to discount the significance of actual seconds or minutes that intercourse lasts. We also want to dismiss a fallacy that is perpetuated by porno films and locker-room bravado. When we ask men how long they think most other men can go during intercourse, it's not uncommon to get answers like 20 minutes, 30 minutes, or more. Believing that to be true, even when sex is good, many men still feel inferior, thinking that they have far less ejaculatory control than normal men do. In reality, however, based on survey data, it appears that the average length of time between entry and ejaculation is somewhere between four and seven minutes.

CHAPTER TWELVE

Taking Care of Your Sexual Relationship

"Some nights, I want passion and excitement—I want fireworks. I settle for Letterman."

Most people want sex to be exciting and full of passion, and even though we might not be able to tolerate fireworks every night, once in a while would be nice. But if we put any credence in what we see on MTV or on the big screen, other people are having great sex all the time and we're somehow missing out. Many of us feel that our sexual relationship has become routine, or a source of conflict, or a low priority, or a constant reminder that we're somehow sexually inadequate.

Can this state of affairs be turned around? Is it possible to supercharge your sex life? We think so. In this chapter we present a number of ideas for how you and your partner can bring variety, playfulness, novelty, and passion into your sexual relationship. If enough people follow these suggestions, Letterman's ratings are sure to go down!

GET REAL

There's a host of sexual gurus out there today who proclaim on talk shows and in books that they can tell you how to have stupendous sex. Even if you have a good, loving sexual relationship, if you listen to these "sexperts" long enough, you'll start to wonder whether you're missing out on something. The truth is, sex can be wonderful, but not every time. Sex can be beautiful, but it will never become the center of the universe. Sex brings us moments of pleasure, but it doesn't ensure happiness. This may sound strange coming from a trio writing a book about sex, but we feel that it's important for people to have realistic expectations. On some occasions, everything—mood, energy level, events earlier in the day, the ambience—will line up perfectly, and as a result, lovemaking *clicks.* And on those occasions every nerve ending explodes upon touch and the resulting orgasm rivals those described in the sexiest paperbacks. Those experiences, if and when they occur, should be enjoyed and cherished. But these magic moments are the exception, not the rule.

Sex between lovers varies dramatically from one occasion to the next. Sometimes you'll climax, sometimes you won't. When you do orgasm, one time it might feel like a tidal wave crashing over you, and the next like a quiet ripple washing gently across your body. On one occasion you'll feel incredibly connected with your partner, and perhaps on the next you'll feel that he or she merely came along for the ride.

Disappointed that there are no secrets to nonstop, earth-shattering sex? Or perhaps relieved? Well, it's reality. If we approach sexuality with realistic expectations, we spare ourselves the pressure of trying to perform like Olympic athletes. Instead, with each sexual encounter we can try to approach our partner with an attitude that says: *Well, here we are. The next few moments may be great, or they may be just okay, but because we're sharing them together, they'll feel good. Let's speak to each other with our bodies rather than with our words. And whether we climax or not, whether the earth moves or not, we'll try to hear each other's message—I love you.*

GET ATTITUDE

Probably the most important ingredient for experiencing satisfying sex is not technique but attitude. With the right attitude—the sense that you are comfortable with your body, interested in eroticism, and ready to pleasure and be pleasured—you create a sexual aura around yourself. You bring to lovemaking a sensuality and energy that can excite and fulfill both you and your partner. Admittedly, for many women, being comfortable with their body and their sexuality is easier said than done. You may have brief periods when you either feel you measure up or you don't care about measuring up. But then, thanks to years of conditioning by cultural myths and values, once again you're flooded with old feelings of inadequacy and insecurity.

It would be nice if all we had to do to escape self-defeating attitudes about sexuality was to tell ourselves, *Don't think that way!* Unfortunately, it's not that easy. As we discussed earlier, changing sexual attitudes takes self-examination, ongoing awareness, and hard work. The good news is that it can be done, and the fact that you're reading this book shows that you've begun the process. Chapter 6 on body image is one good place to start, and making a commitment to work on your sexuality by doing some of the exercises in the Appendix is a good way to continue.

DISCUSS, DISCUSS

Many couples have been together for years or decades, yet in all that time have never openly discussed sex with each other. Talking about sexuality can make people feel vulnerable as no other topic can. When sharing what turns them on and what turns them off, they might feel that they're exposing too much about their identity, quirks, hang-ups, and insecurities, standing psychologically naked in the presence of their partner. "So why get naked?" you might ask. Because getting emotionally naked is like getting physically naked—it may not be absolutely essential, but it can make sex much more rewarding and enjoyable. More important, it helps to prevent misunderstanding and fosters greater intimacy in the relationship.

It is important for couples to communicate about sexual issues such as their wishes, fears, and insecurities. We're aware that this type of dialogue is challenging, but discussing sex openly with your partner is a critical ingredient for a satisfying sexual relationship.

LIGHTEN UP

Now hear this: **Sex is not serious business!**

It's amazing how our society has made sex—this simple, beautiful gift in life—so terribly complicated. Sex can certainly be profound—it can be a powerful means of communication; it can be a sign of commitment; it can even generate life. But it doesn't have to be serious. Sex can occur during serious moments, such as when partners seek comfort from each other during times of personal or family crisis. But, for the most part, sex can be joyful, playful, and perhaps on occasion, even slapstick.

Hopefully, there is always a place for humor in a healthy sexual relationship. When we can laugh at ourselves, enjoying our own quirks and foibles in the bedroom, we reduce the destructive impact of self-criticism, performance anxiety, and resentment. A couple might mentally catalogue their own sexual bloopers and, as the years pass, recount them with delight. They can revel in retelling the time that the husband woke up his in-laws by falling off the bed during lovemaking; the time that the five-year-old thought Mommy was praying because she kept saying, "Oh God"; the time that the six-year-old took Daddy's "balloons" to school for a classroom party; and the time that, in the midst of beautiful lovemaking, complete with body oil, lit candles, and soft music, the husband unexpectedly made the wind rather than the earth move. Sex can be a source of great humor and joy—it doesn't have to be serious business!

GET OVER IT

Sex can be a two-edged sword in a relationship. It can serve as a profound act of love between two people, but it can also serve as the flash point for conflict. Sex is a common trigger for conflict because of our increased vulnerability when dealing with sexual issues. Our partners can disagree with us about the weather, the economy, politics, or religion, and unless the disagreement is particularly vicious and personal, it's unlikely that we'll feel deeply wounded. We may become irritated and conclude that our partner can be a real jerk at times, but these areas of dispute seldom touch close to home. But when our partners challenge our sexual beliefs, criticize our performance, or make light of our desirability, look out—they're venturing into a minefield. Because we live in a culture that equates appearance and sexuality with personal worth, any ridicule of our bodies or criticism of our lovemaking strikes at the very core of our self-esteem.

Conflict over sexual issues can be highly toxic to a relationship. Rather than confronting sexual disagreements directly, couples often harbor their resentment or resort to sarcasm, name-calling, or game-playing. The result, all too often, is misunderstanding, hurt, anger, and disillusionment. To minimize the harm that can result from sexual conflict, couples need to understand the issue, talk about it with open minds and mutual respect, avoid games and power plays, and work toward a win-win solution.

Let's look at two of the most common sexual conflicts that arise in sexual relationships.

Frequency

Two people can have perfectly normal sex drives yet differ dramatically on how frequently they want sex. There is no ideal or correct frequency that applies for all people. Among normal, healthy, well-adjusted adults, there can be a wide range in sexual desire, with some people desiring sex on a daily basis, and others desiring sex on a weekly basis or less. The desire for sex can also vary dramatically over time in response to factors such as stage of life, quality of the relationship, level of fatigue, and the presence or absence of stress or illness. As we discussed in the last chapter, however, it is not due to inherent gender differences. Because of this variability in sexual desire, it's inevitable that most couples will, at times, face a discrepancy in their preferences for sexual frequency.

The reasons why the frequency of sex can become a major issue for couples are varied and complex. At the most basic level, people tend to get upset if they're deprived of something they want. If another person repeatedly tells us, "No, you can't have it," chances are we'll become resentful over time.

For some people, being denied sex goes beyond the simple disappointment of being deprived a moment of pleasure. For many people, sex has a lot of symbolic significance. Some people, for example, equate having sex with being desirable. As a result, if they're told, "No sex!" they hear, "You're not desirable." Other people may believe that the true sign of love and a strong relationship is the presence of a torrid sex life. It's not surprising if, after being turned down by their partner enough times, these folks begin to question the merits of their relationship.

At a deeper level, a couple's struggle over the frequency of sex may really be a reflection of a struggle over more basic issues. For example, consider Jim and Char, a couple who have been feuding for months. Rarely home, Jim has been immersed in a project at work. Char complains that he's so wrapped up in his own world that he ends up showing little or no interest in her. Jim dismisses her complaints and accuses her of being hypercritical. Against this backdrop, each time Jim turns away from sex, the anger Char ends up feeling does not simply come from "not getting any" but from feelings of being ignored, minimized, unimportant.

Or consider Michael and Tanya. Michael has strong emotional needs and looks to Tanya as a substitute mother—he wants her to constantly hold his hand as he encounters life. Tanya, however, feels as if a noose is tightening around her neck. She loves Michael, but his dependency is suffocating her. For survival, she pulls back at times to create distance. Saying no to his frequent requests for sex permits her to keep that distance; otherwise, lovemaking would become one more way for him to cling to her emotionally.

What steps can a couple take if one partner consistently wants sex more often than the other? Because the causes can be varied and complex, the solution is usually not a simple one. Having sex with your partner out of a sense of obligation is not the answer—resentment will surely be the long-term result. Likewise, shaming and trying to make the partner with the less-intense sex drive (or vice versa) feel guilty will inevitably create tension in the relationship.

The challenge of addressing desire discrepancy will often be part of the larger challenge in any relationship: two people trying to meet their individual needs while respecting the needs, values, and sensitivity of the partner.

Dressed only in his boxers, Riad leaned over the sink and vigorously brushed his teeth. *I think I'm ready for tomorrow,* he thought. The slides are done and the handouts are in my briefcase; the boss should be impressed by the presentation.

Hands came from nowhere and began to play with the thick, black hair on his chest. Startled, he looked up and, in the mirror, saw Rana peering over his shoulder with an impish grin.

"What's a girl gotta do to get laid around here?" she asked playfully.

Riad rinsed out his mouth and turned. Taking her hands, he said gently, "Normally that would sound great, but tonight's a bad night."

"Seems like there's been a lot of bad nights lately," Rana said, the smile now replaced by a look of disappointment.

"I know," he sighed. "I guess I've been in a slump lately. But I do love you."

"I was starting to wonder," she said, her smile returning.

"Don't ever question that," Riad said, squeezing her hands for emphasis. "I'm not up for sex tonight, but it would be nice to hold you."

Riad didn't want to have sex. While making clear his own preference, he acknowledged the validity of Rana's request. Instead of becoming defensive or resorting to sarcasm, he reaffirmed his love and desire for his wife. He attempted to come up with an alternative—holding each other—that would at least partially meet both of their needs. This vignette shows how any disagreement, whether it involves sex, money, in-laws, or parenting, can be better handled when the communication is marked by honesty, sensitivity, and mutual respect.

Who Initiates

Closely related to the issue of sexual frequency is the issue of who initiates sexual contact in a relationship. Surveys show that most people believe that ideally both partners should initiate sex with equal frequency. Surveys also show, however, that in the vast majority of relationships, this equality doesn't occur—usually one person initiates sex much more frequently than the other.

Even when the non-initiating partner readily accepts the invitation to make love and participates enthusiastically, his or her failure to initiate can still create tension in the relationship. The offended party (the usual initiator) tends to read significance into his or her mate's failure to reciprocate. The initiator may reason that if two people are attracted to each other and enjoy being sexual, both should be equally inclined to initiate sex; because the partner doesn't initiate, deep down he or she must not really enjoy their lovemaking.

Although the preceding reasoning appears to be logical, when it comes to sex, the rules of logic don't necessarily apply. Yes, normally when people want something, they take steps to get it. But because sex is such a loaded issue in our society, many people find it awkward to initiate lovemaking, even when they desire it and thoroughly enjoy it. Many women and men who have been raised with the belief that sex is dirty, for example, may shy away from suggesting erotic behavior. They may enjoy lovemaking, but the burden of feeling awkward or ashamed of wanting it too much inhibits them. If a woman or man feels sexually insecure, initiating sex can be intimidating. The ever-present possibility of being turned down or ridiculed makes the overture too scary. In both cases the non-initiator may gladly accept when his or her partner takes the initiative.

Surveys show that men are initiators more often than women. We suspect that this trend (and it is only a trend, because in many relationships women are the primary initiators) may be due to upbringing and differing arousal patterns. Many women were raised hearing the message that good girls don't ask for sex or that sex should be reserved for special moments of intense emotional intimacy. On the other hand, cultural myths give men permission to initiate sex without shame or remorse. Unlike women, they have not been conditioned to associate sex with special moments of emotional intimacy but instead have been taught that "real men" will try to have sex whenever possible.

In addition to upbringing, differences between women and men's patterns of sexual arousal may account for men being more inclined than women to initiate sex. First of all, in an erotic situation, a man may become more quickly aware of his arousal than a woman will. A man's major physical sign of arousal, the erection, is more apparent than the more subtle signs for a woman, such as genital swelling, warmth in the pelvic area, and vaginal lubrication. The more readily a person becomes aware of arousal, the more readily he or she will tend to act on that arousal.

Another difference may come from what causes a man to become sexually aroused, in contrast with what arouses his partner. It appears that, in general, men are more responsive than women to visual cues. A man watching his partner undress is more likely to feel arousal than the reverse. Some professionals believe that this is due to differences in culture and upbringing. They point out that women's bodies are more often glamorized, and exploited, in our culture. Peepshows, "girlie" magazines, topless bars, and stag films are ever-present messages to young boys and men that seeing a woman's naked body is something to be desired. It is a valued response, even something to brag about. Other professionals have suggested that the different way many women and men respond to visual cues may be due to minor differences in the structure of women and men's brains. They suspect that cues from a man's visual cortex (the part of the brain that mediates vision) may be more directly connected to the sex-center of the brain. Whether it's due to nurture or nature, men are often trained or conditioned to respond to visual cues more quickly than women.

Regardless of the reasons, it's dangerous to overinterpret the meaning of a partner shying away from initiating sex. It isn't proof positive that the partner doesn't enjoy sex. Instead, it's usually a reflection that the partner's arousal pattern is different from the initiator's. The partner is just more comfortable being the pursued than being the pursuer. As long as a couple can enjoy physical intimacy, our response to the initiator who complains that his or her partner doesn't initiate is "So what?"

MAKE TIME

We're living in an era of fast-paced, action-packed lifestyles. More and more families now have two breadwinners; indeed, for many it's become an economic necessity. In addition, parents are often called on to become much more active in their children's lives than was the case in previous generations. Parents are expected to attend school meetings and recitals; chaperone field-trips; supervise the lunchroom; carpool for dance lessons, soccer practice, and scouting; coach Little League; and serve as committee members at the local church, mosque, or synagogue. In addition, parents typically provide an on-call taxi service for their children, whose busy social schedules often go beyond the bounds of their immediate neighborhood. With all these activities, couples often feel burdened and overwhelmed. They feel little sense of control in their life. Rather, it seems as if they're swept through the days, weeks, and months by a tidal wave of responsibilities and obligations.

And then there's sex. Is there ever time for lovemaking? Is there sex after kids? Many couples in the throes of modern living seriously wonder.

Just as creativity and ingenuity are required to juggle finances, shuttle the children about, and maintain the household, they are likewise required for sustaining a satisfying sex life. If we wait for sex to occur spontaneously, the wait could be endless. Couples have to plan, schedule, adjust, be flexible, and support each other if they hope to find the time to make love. They also have to let go of myths like "Only spontaneous sex is good sex" and that "For sex to be good, it has to be frequent."

Preplanned sex may not always have the passion-driven, rip-off-your-clothes excitement of spontaneous sex, but it still can be wonderful. In a fast-paced lifestyle, sex often has to be planned far in advance, sometimes with the same logistical genius that couples display when scheduling their car-pools. And even with good planning, sex may not happen as frequently as both partners would prefer. But whether spur of the moment or planned weeks in advance, whether the fifth time this week or the first time this month, each act of making love remains a powerful and important connection for two very busy people. We easily lose sight of the fact that each time two lovers touch, hold, and make love with each other, they have the opportunity to abandon themselves for a few precious moments in the joy that comes from the intimate sharing of their bodies.

STIMULATE THE MIND, NOT JUST THE BODY

Lying on her side, Laura hugged her pillow. As she drifted off into that twilight state between consciousness and sleep, she was startled by a body pressing up against her. Clearly Barry was aroused—his firm penis poking her buttocks left no doubt about that. Not an unpleasant way to end the day, she thought.

"Are you trying to tell me something?" she asked playfully.

Barry answered by reaching under her nightshirt and cupping her breast. As he gently pinched her nipple, Laura felt a warm rush radiating from her pelvis. Very definitely a nice way to end the day, she decided. Despite her fatigue a few moments ago, she rolled on her back and began kissing and stroking Barry's body.

Barry shifted so his penis could penetrate her; she was amazingly moist, given the brevity of the foreplay. Within seconds of him entering her, Laura picked up the tempo of his thrusting and began moving in concert with his body. She was immersed in pleasurable sensations until she suddenly heard the telltale moan forming deep in Barry's diaphragm. *No, not yet*, she thought. Barry began to shudder, then his body went limp and lay heavy on top of her. Laura couldn't move; breathing became an effort. Fortunately, within seconds of his climax, Barry rolled off her.

"Thanks, hon," he whispered.

"You're welcome," Laura answered, trying to mask her disappointment.

"That was really nice," he sighed before drifting off into blissful sleep.

Yeah, I guess it was, Laura thought without conviction. *But am I wrong to want more than nice?* she wondered. *Sex has become so ordinary, so predictable. We never try anything new or different. God, when we first made love years ago, it was always an adventure. When he touched me, every nerve ending exploded. There were times when we'd be in public and just looking at each other would drive us crazy—we wanted to rip off our clothes and do it right there. But after fifteen years and doing it at least a thousand times together, I'm probably being silly wishing for more. I guess we're lucky that we're still doing it at all.*

Today, unlike 50 years ago, the media bombards us with suggestions that sex should be breathtaking and exciting. Against this standard we look at our actual experience, and especially if we have been with the same person for many years, odds are the sex just doesn't match up in comparison.

"What do you expect?" many people will argue. Like Laura, people often assume that once the novelty of a new relationship wears off, sex between the same two partners is destined to become routine and boring.

But is this necessarily so? Is a new partner a prerequisite for sparks to fly in a sexual relationship? Do partners in long-term relationships inevitably lose the ability to have great sex together? We don't think so. As one colleague confided, "Each time my husband and I can get away for a weekend—without pagers, telephones, car pools, and deadlines—we rediscover that there's actually nothing wrong with our sex life." Many couples have made the same discovery. If your routine sexual encounters lack excitement, it doesn't necessarily mean that you and your partner have lost the potential or capacity for exciting, satisfying sex with each other.

So why does sex become boring in a relationship? The answer is that exciting sex is the result of more than just physical stimulation—it requires stimulation of both the body and the mind. That's why sexual encounters with a new partner can be so exciting. It's not the novelty itself but the intellectual and emotional stimulation that the novelty creates. With a new partner, there is the excitement of discovery and the satisfaction and validation that come from feeling desired. With a new partner, there is intrigue and the possibility of previously unknown pleasures. There is also a sense of intimacy created when two people allow each other to move beyond private boundaries, such as seeing each other naked for the first time.

For many couples, sex over time ends up on autopilot. To their credit, they find time for sex in their busy schedules, but they rely too much on stroking the vital spots for arousal. Sex becomes an exercise in stimulating the body with little attention given to stimulating the mind. That's the problem with many "how-to" sex manuals; they teach three ways to stroke the clitoris and six variations of oral sex, but they often overlook the importance of bringing one's mind and emotions into the sexual experience.

Before going into specific suggestions for bringing more excitement into your sexual relationship, we want to make two points. First, while we are saying that a long-term sexual relationship does not have to be boring, it doesn't mean that every sexual encounter has to have nail-digging intensity. Sexual encounters, like orgasm, vary from the dramatic explosion to the quiet shiver. Not every sexual encounter has to be dramatic or explosive for a sexual relationship to be exciting and satisfying.

Second, we urge you to give yourself permission to take the initiative in your sexual relationship. As we've noted, this can be a challenge for many of us, especially for women. But society's rule that men should take the lead in sexual relationships is archaic and needs to be revised. There is no reason women shouldn't feel free to initiate sex, voice their wants and needs, and suggest variations. Old roles are hard to break out of, however, so the first time a woman says, "Let's try something a little crazy," she'll probably feel awkward. Risking a new recipe or attempting to repair the plumbing for the first time will seem easier for many women than risking new sexual behavior, even with a partner of many years.

It's important to be able to trust the relationship enough to take chances, to try new behavior, to stretch oneself in pursuit of growth. A woman may feel self-conscious the first time she suggests making love in the shower or the back seat of the mini-van, but it can be worth the initial uneasiness if the resulting novelty sparks a moment of excitement and passion.

Now let's look at ways to stimulate the mind and create sexual excitement.

Fantasy

Sexual fantasies are perfectly normal and, indeed, a part of the sexual experience of people everywhere. It is important to note that some people find the idea of sexual fantasies awkward; during sex they rely solely on the physical and emotional sensations of the moment. Still others may be intrigued by the idea but feel too conflicted about sexual fantasies to experiment with using them. Perhaps they were raised with the belief that sexual thoughts—which are fantasies—were sinful and to be avoided. This type of upbringing can create confusion, conflict, and even shame about having sexual fantasies. For vast numbers of people, however, fantasies freely accompany sexual arousal without reservation or guilt.

What goes through your head during lovemaking will impact how pleasurable and satisfying the experience will be. Research has shown that the most common cause of loss of physical arousal in healthy people is the loss of erotic focus. *Erotic focus* means having your attention focused on sexy, arousing thoughts and sensations during lovemaking. Assuming physical health, if during lovemaking you focus on the pleasant tingling radiating from your vulva, the feel of your partner's skin, or mental images that are sexual, nature will take its course. If, on the other hand, during the midst of your partner's passionate foreplay you're trying to remember whose turn it is to pick up the kids from soccer practice, you can say good-bye to arousal. Sexual fantasies—those thoughts, ideas, and images that you find exciting—provide a valuable way to sustain erotic focus.

Why does sexual fantasy "work"? Remember that your mind has an extremely powerful influence over your body. When you see a movie where the hero is dangling over a cliff, your heart races, your breathing speeds up, and your body tenses. You know it's make-believe, but for a few moments you suspend your critical judgment and allow this two-dimensional picture to become your reality. Your body reacts accordingly. The same thing happens with sexual fantasy. This is why sexual fantasy is one of the most powerful (and free) aphrodisiacs available to us.

Fantasies Unlimited

Because people are unique, there will be a great deal of variability in what each person finds to be arousing in a sexual fantasy. Fantasy is an adaptive resource that can serve as a rehearsal for how you want to change something in your life, or it can be a fleeting, fictitious time-out from reality. Some people enjoy having the same sexual fantasy every time they make love. They say it is a sure way to arousal. Some have a smorgasbord of fantasies. Some draw upon passionate scenes from a book or movie, some recall past experiences with their partner, and others create imaginary scenes involving strangers or people they know only in passing.

Imagining sex with someone other than one's partner is a concern for some people. It's important to remember that fantasies are not necessarily wishes. As a matter of fact, research has shown that people often fantasize about things they would never act on in real life, even if the opportunity presented itself. Heterosexual women and men may, on occasion, fantasize about a homosexual encounter. In real life they may have no interest in making love to someone of the same sex, but within the safety and anonymity of fantasy, the unthinkable can lead to novel excitement. Women and men may fantasize rape (sexual force is a common fantasy theme), but this does not mean they would want to sexually exploit or be exploited in real life. Within the safety of make-believe, however, sex without consent may be an exciting image for some people.

Fantasy Detractors

When you fantasize, you're taking advantage of the novelty that imagination can create to heighten your sexual excitement. Fantasy allows you to flirt with outrageous and totally out-of-character sexual behavior without any risk of harm, whether alone in masturbation or with your partner. "But doesn't this distract from the intimacy of the moment?" some people ask. We think not. During the act of making love, you are choosing to share your body with your partner. Using a mental image to heighten your arousal is no different from stroking your own genitals during lovemaking. Intensifying your own excitement doesn't detract from the basic significance of the fact that you are freely choosing to share with your partner one of the most personal and intimate ways of experiencing pleasure.

As we have discussed earlier, sex makes us vulnerable. Egos can be fragile. We wouldn't suggest that after the next act of lovemaking, as you lie with your partner in a brief postorgasmic glow, you say, "That was great! Between you and Brad Pitt, that was one incredible experience!" Your sexual fantasies belong to you. Fantasies are not wishes or intentions. Some couples enjoy sharing fantasies; others wisely agree to respect boundaries in each other's private world. You can certainly discuss with your partner how you want to handle talking about sexual fantasies.

Like any resource, you can use fantasy in an adaptive or maladaptive way. When it comes to sexual fantasy, we think there's a big difference between lusting after every warm body that walks by and making use of thoughts and visual imagery to enhance a moment of shared pleasure with a sexual partner. In Chapters 12 and 14 we present suggestions for enriching your sexuality with fantasy.

Some professionals have questioned whether encouraging people to use fantasies will leave them dissatisfied with the real thing. It's similar to the fear that if a woman uses a vibrator, she might end up preferring it to the real thing. We don't believe either possibility is a realistic concern, with one important caveat. If a couple has good communication, works hard at developing a relationship characterized by mutual respect and sensitivity for each other, and approaches sex in a loving way without hidden agendas, neither fantasies nor vibrators will ever compare to the real thing.

Foreplay

This is probably not the type of foreplay you're thinking of—we're not talking about the hugging, kissing, and stroking that precedes intercourse. Instead we're talking about what occurs before the clothes come off—the intellectual and emotional stroking that can precede lovemaking.

One colleague described foreplay as "offering to take the garbage out after dinner." Foreplay is two lovers taking the time to talk, and listen, about each other's day. It's laughing over some silly occurrence. It's doing a favor, offering praise, saying thank you. Foreplay is breaking out of the daily routine long enough to share a quality moment together; foreplay is any moment that heightens the couple's sense of connectedness. When this type of sharing and caring occurs, the mind and emotions are stimulated, and any physical contact that follows is all the more likely to be exciting and fulfilling.

That's why so many couples find sex more enjoyable when they run off on a lovers' weekend. Yes, part of the reason is that they're escaping the stress of their daily routine, but an even bigger part is that they have the time to reconnect with each other and rediscover the qualities that first brought them together. Both find themselves saying, "Oh, yeah, *this* is why we fell in love."

Unfortunately, there can never be enough run-away weekends in our lifetime. Foreplay allows us to create at least run-away moments, which serve as a great prelude to loving sex.

Positions for Intercourse

Experimenting with positions for intercourse is a valuable way of stimulating both the mind and the body. Being on top, underneath, or beside your partner; facing him or away from him—each of these options affords variations in what you see, where you can touch and be touched, and how your body is stimulated.

Missionary Variations

The most familiar position for making love is the "missionary position," in which the woman lies on her back with her partner positioned over her—the epitome of conventional sex. Its very name reflects Western restrictions in regard to sex: it was the only position that missionaries would condone for their unenlightened converts. (Today, one might question who the unenlightened ones were.)

There are variations of the missionary position that can be quite pleasurable. In the normal missionary position, the woman typically spreads her legs wishbone style. Placing pillows under her hips and buttocks can be a nice variation, allowing deeper penetration and additional stimulation to the front wall of her vagina. The woman can also bring her legs up and wrap them around her partner. This movement repositions the pelvis, creating both a variation in stimulation and the sense of being physically entwined with each other. Finally, for those yoga-esque women who are sufficiently limber, bringing their knees up to their chest and looping their ankles over the partner's shoulders can permit deep penetration and intense vaginal stimulation. If the man kneels when his partner is in this position, the G spot can receive exquisite stimulation.

A nice feature of the missionary position is that it allows partners to make eye-contact during lovemaking. If you haven't tried it before, the next time you're about to orgasm, look directly into your lover's eyes. There can be an intense feeling of shared union when eyes are locked at the moment of climax.

Female Superior

The female superior position, in which the woman and man switch positions so that the woman is on top, allows the woman to take a more active role during intercourse. She can position her body to maximize stimulation and control the tempo of thrusting so that it matches her growing arousal. With the woman riding atop her partner, the man's hands are free to caress her breasts, face, arms, and buttocks. An equally arousing advantage is the visual stimulation this position provides. Not only can the lovers admire each other's naked bodies, but also they are able to make eye contact.

The female superior position can also take on subtle but enjoyable variations. The woman can either kneel over her partner or, with her feet flat on the surface, crouch over him. Kneeling is more common and comfortable, but crouching and rocking up and down can be great exercise and provide a subtle variation in vaginal stimulation. The woman also has the option of facing her partner or having her back to him. In the latter position, the woman's hands are free to stimulate both her clitoris and her partner's scrotum. Finally, with all the options above, the woman can further modify the position by remaining upright, leaning forward, or arching backwards. Each option varies the stimulation, makes different body parts available for caressing, and provides different visual perspectives of your bodies.

We've had a number of our cancer and heart transplant patients, both men and women, report that a variation of the female superior is particularly helpful. The man lies in a semi-reclining position with pillows propping up his back. The woman then kneels astride and upright. The couples report that this position maximizes accessibility for penetration while minimizing pain and discomfort.

Rear Entry

With the rear-entry position, the man approaches the woman from behind (not to be confused with anal sex). In this position, the woman is on her hands and knees or lying with her head and shoulders on the bed and her buttocks in the air. The position allows deep penetration and intense vaginal stimulation. Also, if her shoulders and head are resting on the bed, the woman has a free hand and can reach back and stimulate both her clitoris and her partner's scrotum. This position minimizes any visual stimulation for the woman, but she may enjoy her partner caressing her buttocks. This position is particularly valuable when the woman has back problems or other physical difficulties that would make it painful to have her partner lying on top of her.

Spoons

The spoon position is an option when both partners are tired and looking for a nice, leisurely-paced coupling. In this position, both are lying on their sides with the woman's back to her partner. If they were upright, they would look like the woman was sitting on the man's lap. Lying on their sides demands minimal energy. The couple can gently rock in a mutual rhythm that's pleasurable for both. The man has at least one free hand to caress his partner. The woman can reach down between her legs and stimulate her clitoris, her partner's scrotum, or both. Women often find this position emotionally appealing because it creates the sense of being held or cuddled during lovemaking.

The spoon position may require some practice, flexibility, and good humor. One difficulty is that the man's penis can slip out easily, and alignment must be done by touch—neither the man nor the woman is in a position to view the genitals. Heavier couples may have to improvise if they find it difficult for their bodies to fit together like spoons. As a variation, they can position their upper torsos into a V-shape, with their penis/vagina connection being the base of the V.

The four positions described above are hardly an exhaustive list. Feel free to experiment. Depending on your physical flexibility, turn and twist, rise up and lower as you search for new variations that might lead to a different angle of penetration, a different view of your partner, or a better vantage point for caressing both your and his genitals. Enjoy the variety!

New Ways to Make Love

Another way to stimulate the mind as well as the body is by experimenting with new ways to make love. We're not merely referring to different positions for intercourse but to a broader definition of lovemaking, one that's not synonymous with intercourse. Contrary to popular thinking, lovemaking without intercourse is not second-rate, incomplete, or flawed. Once a couple understands and accepts this premise, a whole range of options opens up for them. They are no longer shackled by a rigid formula involving mandatory groping, penetration, thrusting, orgasm, and sleep. They become more open and eager to experiment. Even couples with sexual problems such as erectile difficulty or pain with penetration, can still have dynamite sex when they follow this broader notion of lovemaking.

> "It was a nice evening," Lloyd said as he removed his tie.
>
> "And it's not over yet," Carla answered with a coy smile.
>
> Lloyd looked surprised. "With that medication I'm on, I don't know if I can do the job." He tried to appear matter-of-fact, but his awkwardness was apparent.
>
> "Oh, I don't want to screw," Carla said. "I've got other ideas."
>
> Seductively, she pulled him toward the bed and removed his shirt. Lloyd's reluctance melted away as Carla's tongue traveled from his lips to his nipples. Finally she looked up. "Undress me, handsome," she said playfully.
>
> Lying naked together, Carla took Lloyd's hand to her mouth and then guided his moistened fingers to her vulva. Satisfied that he would follow her cue, she shifted her attention to his penis. They explored each other's mouths with their tongues and pressed against each other in every conceivable way.
>
> Lloyd slid his hands along her vulva, fingering her labia and clitoris. With his other hand he touched her breast, circling it with his fingertips. When his teeth pressed firmly but gently against her swollen nipple, Carla felt a warm wave of pleasure wash over her.

She reached down and took his scrotum and penis in her hands. His penis was swollen, but lacked hardness. As she continued to stroke and caress him with her hands, she reveled in his moans of pleasure. *They had made love*, she thought, *such beautiful love*.

KEEP AN OPEN MIND

There are a number of erotic practices that some people find to be enjoyable enhancements to their lovemaking repertoire, but others find disagreeable. We've made frequent reference to the sexual negativity that exists in our society. There's a widespread tendency to label any form of sexual variation as being abnormal or perverted. The longstanding assumption going back more than a thousand years in Western culture is that sex, and all pleasures of the flesh, for that matter, is essentially immoral. Early philosophers and theologians were faced with a dilemma, however. Even though they were inclined to condemn sex as the number one evil of the flesh, the future of humanity would be short-lived without it. Their solution was to condone sexual intercourse for procreation. Any sexual activity not directed to that end (masturbation, oral sex, anal sex, protected sex, homosexuality) was considered evil. Times change. Or do they?

More than a thousand years later remnants of this thinking continue to subtly, and sometimes not so subtly, influence our beliefs and attitudes about sex. For many, anything that hints at being sexually unconventional leads to feelings of awkwardness and shame. People are often quick to use labels like *perverted* and *sick* for anything that falls outside their comfort zone. As a counterpoint, we would like to suggest that *any consensual sexual practice among adult participants that does no harm and provides mutual pleasure is fine*.

As we discuss how to expand one's sexual horizon in the next few sections, we remain respectful of people's individual preferences and moral beliefs. We do not advocate engaging in any sexual activity that you find to be distasteful or morally objectionable. What we do advocate is openness and a nonjudgmental attitude. It's one thing to say, "I'm not comfortable with masturbation because I believe it's morally wrong"; it's a whole different "ballgame" to say, "Masturbation is disgusting, and anyone who does it is sick!"

Let's look at common sexual practices that may add variety to a sexual relationship.

Oral Sex

Oral sex refers to stimulating your partner's genitals with your lips, mouth, and tongue. *Cunnilingus* is the Latin word for when a woman's genitals are stimulated orally; *fellatio* is the Latin word for oral stimulation of a man's genitals. Oral sex can lead to orgasm, or it may be used to heighten arousal before switching to intercourse or some other variation of lovemaking. It's a common sexual practice; studies report that as many as 90% of all couples have engaged in oral sex as a part of their lovemaking experience.

Some people fear that oral sex is unhealthy. They assume that the genitals are somehow less clean than the rest of the body. Because sexual matters are often labeled dirty (as in dirty pictures, dirty movies, the dirty deed, etc.), the genitals end up taking the same rap. Another common objection is, "I'm not going to put that thing in my mouth—he pees out of it." Assuming that neither partner has a sexually transmitted disease and that both practice good hygiene, oral sex should not present a health concern. The genitals should be as clean as any other part of the body, and unless there's an infection, urine is sterile. Still, some people find that they are more comfortable with oral sex if their partner showers prior to lovemaking.

Women often have many questions about fellatio before deciding whether or not to try it. Here are some of the more common questions and their answers:

- *Will it make me gag*? If the penis hits the back of the throat, it can trigger a gag reflex. The woman can prevent gagging by positioning her hand on the shaft of the penis, which gives her control over how much of the penis enters her mouth.
- *How much semen is ejaculated*? On average, a man's ejaculation will produce between one and three teaspoons of semen. The amount varies depending on genetics, age, and the recent frequency of sex. A man ejaculates less semen as he grows older. If he ejaculates more than once over the course of a few hours, the amount of semen will decrease with each successive ejaculation.
- *What does it smell and taste like*? The smell makes many people think of ammonia. Taste varies from man to man and can be affected by diet, but in general, it will be salty and mildly acetic. One woman compared its consistency to a light white sauce she makes by mixing flour, milk, and butter.
- *Does it have calories*? Semen contains about five calories per teaspoon, hardly a diet buster.
- *Can the force of ejaculation make me gag*? Although the force of ejaculation is not enough to make a woman gag, if she's not prepared, the sudden squirt of semen can startle her. Some women enjoy orally stimulating their partner's penis but dislike swallowing semen or being caught off guard by the ejaculation. If this is the case for you, share your preference openly and tactfully and ask your partner to signal you when he's about to climax. You can then stroke his penis with your hand until he ejaculates or take the ejaculate in the front of your mouth and spit it out.

Many women and men highly value oral sex as part of their lovemaking. Some women report that their most intensive sexual arousal occurs when their partner's tongue strokes their clitoris and probes the opening of their vagina. Many men not only enjoy the physical sensation of their penis being orally stimulated but also find great psychological satisfaction from the act. Often men have been conditioned to interpret fellatio as evidence that they are attractive and that they excite their partner. They figure, *if she's willing to do this for me, I must really turn her on.*

Although most women understand men's interest in fellatio, many wonder why some men put great emphasis on cunnilingus. *As long as I'm satisfied*, they reason, *what difference does it make whether or not he performs oral sex on me*? What these women fail to take into account is that it feels good to some people to perform oral sex, especially if their partner is aroused by it. It makes them feel valued as a lover.

This does not mean that a woman must perform fellatio to prove that she's attracted to, or in love with, her partner. Nor should she feel pressured to receive cunnilingus simply to soothe her partner's ego. There are numerous other ways for partners to pleasure each other. In healthy sexuality, choices such as whether or not to practice oral sex are made through open communication and by partners' honesty with each other, and with themselves.

Oral sex, when performed out of desire for mutual pleasuring, can introduce an exciting variation in lovemaking.

Anal Sex

Anal sex involves any stimulation of the anus. This particular form of eroticism not only carries the cultural bias against sex but also collides with our cultural fetish for cleanliness. Nevertheless, anal eroticism is a popular form of sexual stimulation in mainstream America; 30–40% of American women have experimented with anal intercourse, and about 10–12% of American women regularly engage in it (Reinisch, 1991).

What's the attraction to anal sex? One factor is physical pleasure. For men, stimulation of the prostate gland, which is next to the rectum about two inches past the anus, is highly arousing and can quickly trigger orgasm. Inserting a finger in the anus and rubbing or applying gentle pressure on the front wall of the rectum can stimulate the prostate gland. In both women and men, the anus has abundant nerve endings that make it an exquisitely sensitive area of the body for sexual stimulation.

In addition to the physical pleasure, anal sex can also create psychological stimulation. First of all, there is the novelty of making love differently. Perhaps even a greater factor than novelty, however, is the stimulation that comes from doing the forbidden. Forbidden fruit has always held a strange lure for people, and because anal sex has long been considered in polite circles to be dirty and unthinkable, it easily qualifies in the minds of many as forbidden. Another source of psychological stimulation is the sense many people have that the more unconventional the sexual act is, the more exclusive the relationship. The man might reason, *Not only am I the only person she will have intercourse with, but I'm so special to her, she's even willing to allow me to penetrate her in the most private of places*. The woman might think, *There's no part of my body I'm unwilling to share with him.* For both of them, this sense of exclusivity might be highly erotic and satisfying.

Unlike oral sex, anal sex does present some health issues that should be considered. Bacteria reside in the anal area as well is in the rectum. Unprotected sex exposes the man's penis to these bacteria, which can enter the body either through breaks in the skin of the penis or through his urethra. This danger can be minimized but not eliminated by thoroughly washing the anus prior to lovemaking. Using a condom during anal sex is the best way to avoid the risk of infection. Because of the bacteria, the penis should never be moved directly from the anus to the vagina. Following anal activity, the penis should be thoroughly washed and a new condom applied before any vaginal contact. Otherwise, the woman will very likely develop a vaginal infection.

Unlike the vagina, the anus does not secrete natural lubrication. Small tears in the rectum are particularly worrisome if the rectum houses a sexually transmitted disease. When attempting any form of anal penetration, precautions must be taken to prevent tissue damage. The use of saliva, or even better, a good water-soluble lubricant, can make anal penetration far more comfortable and less harmful to the rectal lining. And, most important, penetration needs to be slow and unforced.

So much has been said about AIDS being transmitted through anal sex that the two—AIDS and anal sex—have become synonymous in the minds of many. Anal sex itself does not cause AIDS—HIV can only be transmitted if one of the partners is already infected with the virus. Because anal sex has been shown to be the easiest way for an infected partner to spread the virus, however, this sexual behavior should be reserved for long-term monogamous relationships, or at least for relationships where safer-sex practices are followed (see Chapter 9).

Anilingus and digital penetration are two additional variations of anal eroticism. Anilingus is the stimulation of the partner's anus with the tongue. Proper hygiene, which includes a thorough washing of the anus and the surrounding area, is essential to minimize the risk of infection during this activity. When both individuals are comfortable, anilingus can be a highly personal, intense form of pleasuring. A more commonly accepted form of anal stimulation is digital penetration—the insertion of a finger in the partner's rectum. Both women and men report that during sexual arousal, touching the anus or having a finger inserted can greatly intensify arousal and often trigger orgasm.

Although many men are fascinated with anal sex, some are quite threatened by allowing penetration by the woman's finger. Many men in our society are phobic about anything resembling homosexuality. Because anal eroticism has been associated with male homosexuality, some men are afraid to acknowledge that they find pleasure in anal stimulation. It's important to note that anal stimulation is pleasurable regardless of gender or sexual orientation. Because a man enjoys stimulation of his anus implies nothing about his sexual orientation.

Masturbation

Although masturbation implies a solitary act, it has relevance when discussing sexuality and relationships. Masturbation can be either a source of conflict and misunderstanding for a couple or a practice that enhances sexual satisfaction in a relationship.

Masturbation is another one of those sexual practices that has long carried a social taboo. People often blush when the topic is raised, yet as many as 94% of all men and 70% of all women have masturbated to orgasm at some point in their life. And the practice of masturbation isn't restricted to adolescents who have hormones bursting out of their ears. Research has suggested that a third or more of all women and men over the age of 70 masturbate (Reinisch, 1991). We're therefore talking about a very common practice, despite a history of social and religious condemnation.

Even though masturbation is so common, many people are troubled if they learn that their partner is doing it. Perhaps priding themselves on being open-minded, they concede that masturbation is okay for adolescents, single adults, and even married adults when separated from their spouse. But, they argue, masturbation shouldn't be necessary if you're in a satisfying sexual relationship. *If my wife's happy with our sex life*, a man might reason, *why would she want to masturbate*? *Why settle for a substitute*, a woman might argue, *when he can have the real thing*? Yet despite these common misgivings, anywhere between 40 and 70% of married women and men masturbate even though they have sexual partners.

It's unfortunate that masturbation has such a bad name. We believe that self-pleasuring is a positive thing in our lives and should be enjoyed and valued. Consider the fact that we feel no shame when taking delight in any of our senses. We relish the aroma of fresh bread baking in the oven, the melody of a musical score, the feel of silk against our skin, the subtle aftertaste of a fine wine, the eye-pleasing hues of a sunset. How fortunate we are as human beings to experience these simple pleasures in life. And, we would argue, isn't it also wonderful that we can touch certain parts of our body and produce immense pleasure? Why should this pleasure be considered differently from any other pleasure we derive from our bodies?

We also believe that masturbation shouldn't be viewed as a consolation prize for when a partner isn't available. Many people report that masturbation produces a very powerful orgasm. If you think about it, masturbation represents the perfect touch—you know exactly where to touch, how to touch, and how much to touch. The amount of pressure and the speed of the stroking are continuously adjusted to match your growing level of excitement until you climax. Emotionally, masturbation may not compete with the joy of making love to your partner, but that doesn't mean that masturbation can't be enjoyed in its own right.

Mutual masturbation involves partners masturbating in each other's presence.

Initially this practice can seem awkward and embarrassing. Most of us are accustomed to viewing masturbation as highly personal and private. When we were younger, the act was done quickly and quietly to avoid detection. The thought of being caught by anyone—parent, sibling, or playmate—was horrifying. Yet despite these initial inhibitions, many couples find mutual masturbation exciting and informative. They report feeling a unique intimacy that results from watching each other engage in what has traditionally been such a highly personal act. By watching each other self-pleasure, couples can learn how to more effectively stimulate their partners during lovemaking.

Finally, masturbation can serve as a creative solution for couples when there is an ongoing discrepancy in sexual desire.

"Good night, darlin'," Patrick said as he kissed Kathleen on the forehead. Reaching for the lamp, he turned the lights off and settled back to fall asleep.

"Tired?" Kathleen asked in the darkness.

"Yeah, it's been a hell of a day."

"Too tired to make love?" she asked.

After a moment of awkward silence, Patrick answered, "The way I feel tonight, it would be more like work than fun."

"Do you mind helping me?" she asked.

"Not at all," Patrick answered, rolling over toward Kathleen.

Laying her head on his shoulder, Kathleen cuddled against her husband. Through the thin cotton of her nightgown, Kathleen lightly traced the lines of her labia.

With his free hand, Patrick stroked her cheek. Kissing the top of her head, he whispered, "I love you, darlin.' Enjoy."

By now, she could easily feel the fullness of her vulva as she became more aroused. When she felt moisture coming through the material, shivers of excitement began racing from her vulva and up her spine.

Reaching to touch herself, Kathleen spread open her labia and slid her fingers along the shaft of her clitoris with short, rapid strokes. Still aware of Patrick holding her next to him, she slowly, rhythmically rocked against her lover's body.

Her breathing quickened as excitement continued to build. Her pelvis felt full and her vulva was wonderfully sensitive and swollen. She could sense that her orgasm was coming. She changed her pace of self-caressing, her strokes now longer and more deliberate. Finally, as the sensations and excitement built, she felt the spasms of her orgasm.

She lay against Patrick, completely content. Patrick hugged her and kissed her hair, then rolled over on his side. Within moments, he was asleep. Kathleen lay silently, feeling spent but invigorated, relaxed but wide awake. *How wonderfully different tonight turned out*, she thought, *compared to what would have happened just a few years earlier.*

Kathleen's sex drive had always been stronger than Patrick's. This discrepancy often resulted in tense moments, especially when she wanted to make love and he didn't.

Fortunately, things were different now. A few years ago, Kathleen asked Patrick if he would like to watch her masturbate. Even though she was comfortable with self-pleasuring, it had always been something she had done in private. She was fearful that Patrick might be shocked by her question, but to her pleasant surprise, he agreed. Dim lights and soft music helped her to overcome her initial embarrassment. After coming to orgasm, she was pleased to find Patrick aroused rather than disgusted.

In later discussions, Kathleen asked Patrick how he would feel if she masturbated on those nights when she was turned on and he wasn't in the mood. She explained that having him present would make it feel much more special than if she went off by herself in another room.

Fortunately, he was open to the idea. After the first few times, he told her that he was enjoying being part of her self-pleasuring. He appreciated no longer feeling pressured or guilty. And best of all, on those occasions when he was an active partner, the sex was wonderful. He no longer felt conflict and resentment hanging over their lovemaking.

Since that time, Patrick and Kathleen have continued to enjoy intercourse once or twice a week, but to both of their satisfaction, they now make love almost daily.

Sexually Explicit Videos

It is not an uncommon Friday night ritual in many homes for Dad to go to the local video store and rent the most recent Disney release for the kids and an X-rated movie for Mom and Dad to view after the kids go to bed. The practice is so common that clerks at video stores have learned to carefully check to make sure renters don't accidentally return the videos in the wrong cases.

Before we wade into the controversy involving pornography, a clarification of terms might be helpful. First of all, when we talk about material being sexually explicit, we're talking about the graphic depiction of sexual activity. When considering sexually explicit videos, some people will use the terms *soft porn* and *hard porn* to distinguish just how graphic the sex is. With hard porn, nothing is left to the imagination—the viewer sees the erect penis and swelling clitoris. Soft porn, on the other hand, involves frontal nudity and depicts couples having sex, but actual genital contact is not shown.

There are critics who insist that all sexually explicit material is obscene and should be banned from the marketplace. Legally, however, material is considered obscene only when it intends to arouse the reader or viewer by depicting actions that most people find offensive and shameful. In other words, obscene material attempts to sexually excite by glamorizing behaviors most of us would find to be unacceptable and disgusting. Examples of obscenity would include children being sexually abused, graphic rape scenes, and sex with animals.

Erotica is the artistic depiction of love and sex. Erotica can be quite explicit, but unlike obscenity, the intent is not to use lewd material to arouse its audience. It attempts to inspire its audience by capturing in word or image the sensual quality of our existence. Although some might argue that X-rated videos are erotica, anyone who has viewed much of this material would have to agree that we're definitely not talking about art.

Pornography is a drawing, song, book, or movie that attempts to sexually excite its audience through the graphic depiction of "socially acceptable" sexual activity. Under the law, there is a wide range of behavior that is considered "socially acceptable" but may not be acceptable to a particular individual or couple. What one person finds acceptable may not be acceptable to another. Some people find pornography to have erotic power while others do not. For some, pornography is disgusting and unacceptable; for others, it is the graphic depiction of actions in which they have engaged or about which they have fantasized.

The issue of pornography is certainly complex. From the papers to the pulpits, from courtrooms to coffeehouses, it is hotly debated. In this book we have no intention of offering the final word on this controversy. We believe that there are sexually explicit videos that couples can view as an enjoyable source of variety for their sexual relationship. We also believe that there are sexually explicit videos that are degrading and negative to both women and men.

Does erotica or pornography have any merit? For some couples, viewing sexually explicit material is exciting. Other couples feel that watching sexually explicit videos with their partner objectifies sex and dilutes the intimacy between them. It's entirely personal. If you do decide to watch a tape and find it offensive, turn it off.

Sexually explicit material is not for everyone, and your values, attitudes, and beliefs should be respected. If you're curious, consider experimenting with sexually explicit material. If you're not interested in hard core, find a sexy, R-rated movie. Have a movie night with your partner. Enjoy the raw eroticism depicted on the screen. Enjoy the fantasies and desire the movie might conjure up within both of you.

Erotic Power Play

Bondage and discipline, sado/masochism, and fetishistic activities aren't just for the guys. Many women enjoy dominance/submission play in the bedroom. This may vary from talking dirty to acting out fantasies. If you're interested in trying and want to keep it fun, we suggest that you learn about the basics. There are several books describing erotic power play in the "Suggested Resources" list at the end of the book.

Erotic power play can be aggressive or gentle; the line between pain and intense sensation is different for everyone. Many couples engage in occasional "light bondage" by gently tying hands or feet. They find the novelty exciting and feel that it increases their erotic focus. Because household items like scarves or neckties can cut off circulation, we suggest investing in Velcro ties made for the occasion and sold through the companies listed under *sex toys* in the "Suggested Resources" list. Remember to establish a word for *stop* and another for *lighten up*. Most people don't mean stop when they say it in erotic power play. Find a different word that is guaranteed to slow down the action if you need to.

People who are involved in "heavier" sado/masochism usually find an S/M group or club and meet regularly. If you decide to get involved, remember that you need to set up careful boundaries with others and avoid being exploited by anyone. It's important that you have the freedom to choose the type of activities and the pace that works for you.

Most people use the rule "safe, sane, and consensual" when engaging in erotic power play. If your partner is pressuring you and you're not interested in this kind of thing, tell your partner no. Sex has to be consensual, especially sex that flirts with aggression.

Toys and Other Props

Vibrators, dildos, sexy lingerie, body oils, and a host of other sexually oriented items are now part of a multimillion-dollar industry. Many couples find that such toys and props bring a touch of novelty to their lovemaking. We've already made the point that lovemaking can be playful and that making use of fantasy and creativity can heighten pleasure for lovers of all ages.

The only point we wish to add when considering toys and props is the importance of not being taken in by the myth that "natural is best." Somehow many people have gotten the idea that an orgasm should come only from a penis or vagina, or if they're very progressive, perhaps also from a finger and a tongue. *Heaven forbid*, they reason, *that an orgasm ever be triggered by something inanimate or mechanical. And if love is not enough to stimulate passion*, they conclude, *the relationship must be in trouble*.

Why? If your partner stimulates you to climax with an electric vibrator, is his desire to pleasure you any less than if he had used his finger, his tongue, or his penis? Is the mood set by your partner wearing sexy briefs or you wearing flimsy lingerie any less legitimate or meaningful than the mood set by candles and music? If you suggest a sensuous massage with body oil, are you implying that your partner is a lousy lover and you need more to be satisfied? If you want to wear six-inch heels into the bedroom to excite your partner, are you turning yourself into an object? We think not. Sex provides the opportunity for two people to play, to harmlessly indulge their own and each other's fantasies. When toys and props are used playfully by a couple, they can provide novelty, excitement, and fun.

PART V

Overcoming Sexual Difficulties

This final section is devoted to problem solving. If you have determined that you have low sexual desire, low arousal, or orgasm difficulties, you'll find practical help here. We talk about how medical and psychological factors can cause these problems and what kinds of treatment options exist. We also present a series of exercises that many women have found helpful in overcoming sexual problems caused by psychological issues. At the end of Part V, we offer guidance for determining when sex therapy might be helpful and how to find a qualified therapist. For those who would like to augment the suggestions in Chapters 13–17 with more self-help, the Appendix offers additional exercises.

In Part V you'll find answers to these common questions:

- Isn't my problem all in my head, like my partner says?
- When my healthcare provider gives me only 10 minutes to ask questions, how can I bring up embarrassing sexual problems?
- I want to feel desire for my husband—why can't I?
- How can I focus on making love when I feel like I live in the middle of a three-ring circus?
- Could my medication be causing the problem?
- Is there a female version of Viagra?

- Isn't there something wrong if I don't orgasm every time we have intercourse?
- Why do I orgasm on vacation but rarely at home, and what can I do about it?
- What is sex therapy all about, and how do I know if it can help me?
- How do I find a good sex therapist?

CHAPTER THIRTEEN

What to Do When Sexual Problems Arise

Throughout this book, we have discussed factors that influence our sexuality, including childhood events, cultural messages, relationship issues, previous sexual experiences, life stressors, and physical health. When these influences don't encumber us—when our bodies are working normally and our minds are able to focus on eroticism without distraction—nature is free to take its course and we should be able to respond normally to sexual cues. On the other hand, when a medical problem exists or when psychological issues distract us from the eroticism of the moment, our bodies will often fail to function normally in a sexual situation.

There are many ways the body can fail to function sexually; that is, there are many different types of sexual dysfunction. You may have lost interest in sex or hate sex. You may feel your sex drive is excessive or compulsive. Perhaps you can't lubricate or find you can't stay focused on your sexual feelings. Maybe you're unable to orgasm or can orgasm only in very specific situations, like when you're alone or drinking. You may have pain before, during, or after sex. Or you may have nongenital pain, such as cramps, headaches, or back pain, that occurs during or after sex.

> "I thought my low sexual desire was due to working and having a baby, but I asked my doctor and she found out that I have a thyroid problem and needed medicine."

"I was sure that my sexual pain was some awful disease, but my gynecologist did a careful exam and there was nothing wrong with me physically. She did a good job of explaining how my body can have a real physical problem, like muscle spasms and pain, but not have a medical cause for that problem. She was the first person to tell me about sex therapy."

"I was never able to get aroused even though I wanted to want sex. Every time I talked to a physician about my problem, I felt like he or she was telling me that it was 'all in my head.' I was so ashamed."

Before discussing specific sexual problems and ways to overcome them, we outline general steps that all women should take when they have sexual difficulties, regardless of the problem. We talk about how to self-assess a sexual problem, how to get a medical evaluation, the importance of finding accurate information, and the value of including your partner in any effort to overcome a sexual problem. We also introduce a valuable technique to combat the distracting and negative thoughts that are present in almost all sexual dysfunctions. Finally, we give some suggestions for getting the most benefit from the self-help exercises in the next three chapters.

CHECK IT OUT: DOING A SELF-ASSESSMENT

Some women know right away that something has gone wrong sexually, but for others the awareness dawns gradually. We think you should do a self-assessment of your sexual functioning as soon as you become concerned that something might be wrong. You'll notice that the self-assessment gives you valuable information that will help you make decisions on how to address the problem and whether or not to get help.

"When I discovered I couldn't even do the self-assessment, I realized I had another problem besides sexual pain. I'm going to see a counselor because I'm scared to even think about sex."

"It wasn't until I wrote down my answers to a self-assessment that I realized I had low sexual desire only at home. I felt great about sex when we were away."

Take a look at the list of questions that follows. If you're comfortable expressing yourself in writing, you may want to write your answers on a piece of paper or in a journal. You'll be amazed by what insight you can gain when you go through the effort of trying to capture thoughts, feelings, and experiences into written words. Recording your thoughts will also give you something to refer to when you see your healthcare provider.

• *What is the problem*? Give a full description of what happens or doesn't happen for you in sexual situations.

• *Is the problem physically painful, or does it cause bleeding, chronic itching/soreness, or infection*? If your sexual problem has immediate medical implications like the ones suggested in the question, make an appointment with a healthcare provider as soon as possible.

• *When does the problem occur*? All the time? Only in certain situations? These questions are designed to help you determine what might be triggering the problem, such as stress, fatigue, disagreements, interest in someone other than your partner, shame about being sexual, or resentment over being pressured to have sex.

• *When did it first happen*? Has the problem been lifelong? If not, what was going on in your life when the problem first appeared? These questions may also help you understand what is causing your sexual problem. For instance, if you lost your sexual interest around the same time that you were going through a marital crisis, perhaps the low desire is related to a lack of trust in the relationship.

• *If the problem is lifelong, can you write down why you want to address the problem now*? Is it because you want to correct the problem, or is someone else pressuring you to change? We have found that change is very difficult when we're not doing it for ourselves but to please someone else.

• *What thoughts go through your head when you're being sexual*? This is a great question because it helps you gain an insight into your current feelings about sex. For instance, if you discover that your thoughts during sex involve self-criticism for being overweight or unattractive, then you have a good idea about what is preventing your erotic focus during sexual activity. More important, you also have an idea about where to direct your attention when trying to resolve your sexual problem. Strategies for overcoming negative thinking are presented later in this chapter as well as in the next three chapters.

• *How comfortable are you with sex*? If you're not comfortable, where is the discomfort coming from? Are there things in your past that might make sex a problem? Look back through Part I, "Knowing Your Sexual Story," and try to pinpoint a time when you were comfortable with sex. For instance, some women say they felt good about sex until they had kids. From that point on, they felt self-conscious and more like a "mommy" than a sex partner.

• *Do you avoid relationships that have the potential to become sexual?* Here again is a place to examine your reactions to Part I, "Knowing Your Sexual Story." By reflecting on your sexual story, you may come up with insights into why a sexual relationship might be threatening. Upon reflection, you may discover that past abuse prompts you to avoid sexual relationships. In that event, reading Chapter 10 may be helpful.

• *Do you have certain beliefs and attitudes about sex that might not be helpful?* Think about what sexual messages you have been exposed to, both now and in the past. Pay particular attention to the stereotypes for your age and stage in life. Do you believe that there is something wrong with you if you're 21 and not oozing raw sexuality all of the time? Are you expecting yourself to be over the hill sexually just because you're over

40? Part I, "Knowing Your Sexual Story," and Chapter 6 can help you identify many of the common myths and stereotypes that follow us throughout our lives.

- *Do you have accurate information about sex in general and about your problem in particular?* If you are like most women, you've been given few specifics about how your body functions sexually. This would be a good time to review Part II, "Understanding Your Body," which provides a wealth of practical and useful information.
- *What impact does this problem have on your partner and your relationship?* Review the suggestions in Part IV, "Creating a Better Sexual Relationship," to gain general information about couples and sex. Although you might think the problem is "just yours," we have found that a sexual difficulty always affects both the partner and the relationship, making it a shared problem.
- *How are things going in your relationship, both sexually and nonsexually?* This is a further elaboration of the preceding question and encourages you think about your overall relationship. Couples have challenging times together. Is this one of those times for you right now? How much are you enjoying each other? Do you spend quality time together? Do you have a sense of good will toward each other? When you argue, are you both trying hard to resolve the problems? Have you considered specific strategies to help your relationship, like reading self-help books or going to couples counseling?
- *How are things going in your life in general?* Are there current major stressors in your life? Do you escape from problems by drinking or taking drugs, reasoning that you "deserve" a drink or must have a drink to have a good time? Do you chronically yell at people you love and then have to apologize later? Are you continually worried about money or upset about your work? Have there been serious problems with your children? If you answer yes to any of these questions, we recommend that you contact a counselor and discuss these stressors in your life. A counselor will be able to do an in-depth evaluation with you and can recommend strategies to help you cope.
- *How's your health?* Are there any health problems that could be contributing to your sexual problem? Are you worried about your health? When was your last physical? Do you feel healthy? Are you getting exercise, sleeping well, and following a healthy diet? Your lifestyle is fundamental to taking care of yourself. It may be time to contact your healthcare provider and share your concerns about your health or lifestyle.

TELL ME IT'S NOT IN MY HEAD

As sex therapists we encourage every woman we see to stay current in her healthcare. We encourage our patients to get yearly physical exams and to see their healthcare provider more frequently if they experience any medical difficulty. Good healthcare is essential for good sexual health. Failure to detect and treat medical conditions such as thyroid problems, diabetes, or high blood pressure can affect your sexual functioning. A healthcare provider should always be consulted when there is a sexual dysfunction, both to determine whether or not there is a medical cause and also to make sure that the dysfunction is not signaling the presence of a potentially serious health problem.

If you don't have a healthcare provider, you will need to choose one. Many women have a "primary care" physician or nurse practitioner. These are professionals trained in the comprehensive care of the patient. Some women also have a gynecologist, a physician who cares for the woman's reproductive system and hormonal balance. Many women ask their friends for advice about how to find a good healthcare provider. If you don't know whom to ask, call a local hospital for names of healthcare providers in your community.

In choosing your healthcare provider, you'll need to find out whether you can use your health insurance or will have to pay "out of pocket." Ask what the normal fees and lab test expenses will be for a general physical or gynecologic work-up and how long you'll have to wait for an appointment.

When making the appointment, the receptionist will probably ask why you want to see the healthcare provider. If you are not comfortable providing details over the phone, you can simply answer, "I have some sexual concerns that I would like to discuss with the doctor." You may be asked if you want a full physical examination or just a gynecologic (pelvic) exam. If you've recently had a complete physical, you can opt for the pelvic exam only. Ask the receptionist if the healthcare provider will have time on the day of the exam to discuss your questions or whether you should schedule a separate appointment.

When you go for your appointment, have your questions written down. Mention to the medical assistant who puts you in the exam room that you have several important questions for the healthcare provider and would like to ask them while you're still dressed in street clothes. Remaining dressed until you've discussed your questions helps you feel more comfortable while discussing your sexual concerns; lets the healthcare provider know, right from the start, that you have concerns you wish to discuss; and prevents you and the healthcare provider from dashing over the questions because they were left to the final moments of the appointment.

Begin your discussion with the healthcare provider by saying, "I have some questions about my health—in particular, my sexual health." Some women find it helpful to use the following outline in succinctly presenting their problem:

- Description of problem
- Onset of the problem (when and under what circumstances the problem started)
- Your understanding, if you have one, of the problem
- What, if anything, you've done to try to correct the problem
- What your expectation is

Using this outline, some women may write a script for what they want to say when they meet with the healthcare provider. Here's an example:

"Doctor, I wanted a chance to talk to you at the beginning of the appointment. I have a problem that seems to happen only during sex. I get pain in my abdomen [description]. It started about three months ago and happens every time [onset] I have sex. I don't know why it happens [understanding], but I have tried relaxing more and using different positions [past experiences in trying to help yourself]. I want to have sex without pain [expectation].

If your healthcare provider is not helpful, you have to decide whether you want to find another provider or want to try to work things out. If you decide to try to work it out, you may find it helpful to take your partner or a close woman friend with you to the next appointment. Your friend or partner can be an objective observer and give you valuable feedback following the session. His or her presence in the room will demonstrate to the healthcare provider your seriousness about getting help for your problem. Some women have found it helpful to make statements like the following to an unhelpful healthcare provider:

"I realize that you're quite busy today. Why don't I make an appointment for a different time? I really need your expertise."

"When you say 'There's nothing wrong,' can you tell me what possible medical problems you've already considered?"

If you continue to be dissatisfied with the healthcare provider, ask to speak to another provider in the group or ask for a referral elsewhere.

Experiencing a sexual problem can be distressing and confusing. If you go for a medical evaluation, you may be like many women who hope that a straightforward and easy-to-treat medical condition will be found. If you're told that everything is medically normal, you may feel that the implication is that the problem is "all in your head." Nothing could be further from the truth. Regardless of whether or not a medical diagnosis is made, your sexual difficulty is real, not imagined. As we've pointed out throughout this book, powerful social influences from the earliest days of our lives impact our sexual knowledge, attitudes, and self-esteem. It's this impact, not the problem, that ends up in our head, and as we discuss later in this chapter, so is the solution.

INFORMATION/EDUCATION

Accurate sexual information is critical for overcoming sexual difficulties. After our many years of clinical work, we continue to be impressed by how often sexual problems develop as a result of misinformation or the lack of information. Most adults today, even young adults, received sexual education that was far from stellar. Discussions at home were likely to be rare and painfully awkward or infuriatingly condescending. Little practical information was provided in the classroom. In church, temple, or mosque we were told what not to do rather than how to do it successfully. For most of us, our primary sex educator was a girlfriend who claimed to be experienced; an older sister; or a nameless, faceless writer of an advice column for a teen magazine. As a result many, perhaps most, of us were deprived of basic information necessary for healthy sexual growth and adjustment. If we don't know what a normal sexual response is, what sexual wishes and behaviors are common in the general population, or how we can make lovemaking more satisfying, we are susceptible to developing sexual problems.

The problem, of course, is finding good sources of information. Frank discussions with family and friends can sometimes be helpful, but there is always the danger of people merely sharing their own misinformation. Articles in popular magazines may help, but they vary in quality. Some magazine articles are superb, but others end up being mostly hype with little substance. Beware of syndicated radio and television programs that focus on sex. Some provide a true public service, but far too many place entertainment and ratings ahead of solid education. Internet websites and self-help books like the one you're reading right now can be an important source of adult sexual education, but be sure the authors have solid credentials in the area of human sexuality. Things to look for in so-called sexperts are advanced degrees in relevant fields like medicine, nursing, psychology, social work, or counseling; professional certification as sex educators or therapists; and/or affiliation with a reputable university. Adult education classes or sexuality courses at a local community college are additional sources of valuable information. For still more ideas, consult the resources at the end of this book. The important message here is to seek accurate information. What you don't know can hurt you.

THE SOLUTION, NOT THE PROBLEM, MAY BE IN YOUR HEAD

Do any of the following statements sound familiar?

- No one could ever love me with this body.
- The only way I can keep a partner is by being good in the bedroom.
- Sex is dirty.
- Women shouldn't enjoy sex too much.
- I'm just not a sexual person.
- I could never learn to be sexual.
- I have to keep control at all times.
- Sex is for the young and beautiful.
- No one is sexy after menopause.
- Everybody has better sex than I do.
- If he's ready, I should be.

Can you imagine the effect that these beliefs might have on a woman's sex life? There's an old saying in mental health circles: "How you think, so shall you feel."

This adage applies not only to conditions like depression but also to sexual dysfunctions. Negative thoughts and misinformation can, in the short term, distract us during sexual activity and, in the long term, cause chronic problems with desire, arousal, and orgasm. Fortunately, we have found that by helping people challenge these negative thoughts and replace them with more positive, reality-based ones, called "positive cognitions," we can often help them overcome their problem.

Negative thoughts that affect sexuality can range from self-criticism to unrealistic expectations to outright misinformation about sex. Sometimes the problematic thinking during sex may be more distracting than negative. For example, thinking about work or unpaid bills during lovemaking can have a disastrous effect. Remember, for normal sexual functioning, the mind must be free to focus on the eroticism of the moment. If the mind is preoccupied with mundane or critical thoughts, is it any wonder that the person has difficulty experiencing a hunger for sex, arousal during sex, or the contentment that comes with orgasm? That's why cognitive work is so important for overcoming sexual dysfunctions: your mind has to be free of distraction to enjoy erotic sensations.

In the next few pages, we describe three steps for overcoming distracting and negative thoughts. If your self-assessment uncovered distracting or negative thinking, you may want to try these steps to change or revise the thoughts. In the next three chapters we frequently refer you back to these steps as a way to help overcome difficulties with sexual desire, arousal, and/or orgasm.

Step 1. Identifying Distracting and Negative Thoughts

You need to identify what goes through your head when you encounter sexual cues. What messages are you hearing in the background when you see yourself naked, when your partner touches you, or when you feel a warm tingling in your genitals? Although there are a multitude of possible distractions, here are five of the most common varieties.

- *Distractions of daily life*. Some distracting thoughts are the result of the challenges of daily living. Parenting concerns, deadline pressures, the long-term illness of a parent, the threat of job loss, and financial worries are examples of daily life issues that can preoccupy, follow you into the bedroom, and distract you from responding sexually.
- *Performance pressure*. You might feel pressure to please your partner. If you think your partner views your orgasm as a measure of his or her success as a lover, you may feel a strong obligation to orgasm. Natural body responses can be disrupted when you feel pressure to perform. The harder you try to do something, the more difficult it can be to accomplish.
- *Self-esteem issues*. As we have discussed earlier, sexuality has a powerful ability to bring our insecurities to the surface. Sex tends to highlight issues about com-

petence and desirability that can trigger distracting thoughts and worries. Sexual behavior puts your body at center stage; if you're not happy with your body, sex can be intimidating.

• *Sex-negative thoughts and beliefs*. For most of us, sex-negative messages were plentiful during our upbringing. Even though sex is glamorized in the media and exploited in advertising, the messages that sex is shameful, that sex is dangerous, and that sex is impure can remain ever present in your psyche. The media can also portray sex as suitable for a certain few—the beautiful people. Ignoring these messages, especially in the midst of sexual activity, can be very difficult.

• *Reliving past trauma*. Have you ever heard a song from the past and immediately been flooded with images, sounds, and even smells from that era? The song served as a memory link; it was a common denominator between the present moment and some moment in the past when you were listening to that song. Just like hearing an old song, sex too can serve as a potent memory link.

Consider a woman who was sexually traumatized in the past. Years later, in a wonderful relationship, she becomes confused by her negative reactions to sex. When she makes love, she tenses up. Images from the past assault her. *Why is this haunting me?* she wonders. *My partner is kind and gentle, nothing like the man who abused me. I shouldn't feel this way. What's wrong with me?*

What this woman doesn't realize is that sex, like an old song, has become a bridge linking her past with the present. Unfortunately, as long as the resulting thoughts and recollections remain in the forefront of her mind, a natural sexual response will be very difficult to achieve.

Step 2. Sidestepping Distracting Thoughts

Once you've identified distracting thoughts that pop up during sex, the next step is to take a close look at them to judge their accuracy and validity. Some distracting thoughts may accurately reflect current life issues. "I can't forget to pick up the kids," "There's a rumor about layoffs at work," and "Right now I'm furious with my partner" are examples of thoughts that may accurately reflect reality. When that's the case, your task is either to change the reality or improve your ability to cope with it. Having a backup plan for the kids, researching new job opportunities, and heavy-duty communication and problem solving with your partner are examples of trying to minimize the impact of distracting worries.

When you have little control over stressful issues, your task is to come up with strategies for checking troublesome thoughts at the door before entering the bedroom. Unfortunately, putting such thoughts aside is easier said than done. If you realize that you're putting pressure on yourself to perform during sex, it won't be enough to simply decide *I won't think that way!* Most people don't have that kind of control over their thinking.

Picture a beautiful sun-swept beach with white-capped waves crashing against the shore. Make the image as vivid as possible. Got the picture in your mind? Now get rid of it—don't think about or imagine the beach.

What happened? If you're like most people, an image or thought is not easily willed away. More likely, the more you tell yourself not to think about the beach, the more resilient the image becomes. So how do you get the image of the beach out of your mind? Thought substitution. Odds are that as you read on, by the time you finish the next paragraph or two, you'll no longer be consciously aware of the beach. The beach image will be gone, not because you told yourself to stop thinking about it but because other thoughts will have replaced it.

Freeing yourself of distracting thoughts is a paradoxical process. Rather than directly trying to rid yourself of the thoughts, you are more likely to be successful if you go about this indirectly. In the example of being plagued by performance worries, rather than thinking, *I won't think about trying to perform well*, you'd be better off thinking, *I'm going to focus on the great sensations in my body.*

Step 3. Challenging Unhealthy Thinking

While some distracting thoughts are accurate reflections of reality, more often self-defeating thoughts, when placed under the light of scrutiny, prove to be unfounded, unfair, and irrational. "I look hideous," "Sex is disgusting," and "I'll never be able to enjoy sex" are examples of thoughts usually based on emotion rather than reason. Because they pop up so easily and "naturally," we rarely challenge them. We often conclude, *Because I've felt this way for so long, it must be true.* When you're burdened by inaccurate and unhealthy thoughts, it's not enough to sidestep them. It is important to challenge these thoughts with healthier and more accurate alternatives.

Hardly an impartial judge in this area, how can you determine whether your thoughts are accurate reflections of reality or self-defeating distortions? One simple approach is to write the thoughts down on paper, and next to them to list facts supporting the thought. If you're still not convinced that the thought is irrational, play devil's advocate and write down alternative positions for what you've been thinking.

As an example, say you are tense and ill-at-ease during lovemaking. Upon reflection, you realize that whenever you're undressed in front of your partner you think, *I look disgusting.* Is that accurate? Highly unlikely. But at first glance you may insist it's true. Going through the exercise described above, you might write, as "proof" of the accuracy of your beliefs:

- I'm 35 pounds overweight.
- My breasts are sagging.
- I have stretch marks.

Your reasoning has been contaminated by many of the cultural influences we've discussed earlier in this book. After writing down supporting arguments for your belief, you may feel even more strongly that your self-criticism is accurate. But is it?

The next step is to challenge this distorted logic. If you make an honest attempt to play devil's advocate, you can come up with statements like the following:

- A model's figure is not essential to being worthwhile.
- Sensuality goes far beyond body type.
- There are parts of my body that bring me great pleasure, parts that if I choose to share, should make my partner feel privileged.
- There are parts of me as a person that, if I choose to share, should make my partner feel even more privileged.

Left unchallenged, self-defeating thoughts like *I look disgusting* can have a devastating impact on both you and your sex life. Upon examination, however, the bedrock of negative and irrational convictions can begin to crumble. This may take time to change, especially if you've practiced unhealthy thinking for years. But we have seen many women learn to steadily dismantle their negative thoughts and replace them with more positive ones.

If you need additional guidance for doing this kind of cognitive work, check out *The Feeling Good Handbook* by David Burns (1999), an excellent resource to help you identify and change unhealthy thinking.

BRINGING YOUR PARTNER "UP TO SPEED"

It has been our experience that people can best address a sexual problem when they feel that they have their partner's support. Even when only one person in a relationship has a sexual problem, both people are involved. Without realizing it, the partner may be reinforcing the problem or making it worse. Certainly the partner will be affected by the symptom; he or she will often feel disappointed, resentful, inadequate, or insecure. The attitude *It's your problem, so you fix it* doesn't help anyone. It's important for you and your partner to approach a sexual difficulty as a shared problem needing a shared effort to resolve it.

When your partner participates in the healing process, you both become a source of support and encouragement for each other. If you decide to attempt the behavioral exercises, knowing that your partner understands what you are doing and why can be a positive support. By making the healing process a joint project, both of you are less likely to feel that either one of you is somehow defective or solely responsible for the sexual problems in the relationship. Your partner's participation also makes it possible for both of you to openly discuss ways to make sexual encounters more relaxed and arousing.

There are a number of ways your partner can be an active participant in resolving a sexual dysfunction. First, by discussing sex in general and the sexual problem in particular, both you and your partner can become sensitized to each other's sexual issues, needs, and concerns. Second, by reading this book, your partner can become better educated about female sexuality. People need to know not only more about their own sexuality but also about their partner's sexuality. Third, some of the behavioral exercises in this book are designed for couples. By doing these exercises together, both of you may find it easier and less awkward when making the transition into an active sex life. Finally, you can work together in strengthening the nonsexual dimensions of your relationship. It's not uncommon for a relationship to take some hits when facing a sexual problem. Taking time to work on better communication, to ensure that there is quality time together, and to resolve areas of disagreement can be valuable ways to help the relationship grow and to counteract the strain created by the sexual problem.

If your partner is unaware of or uninterested in your sexual concerns, here are some suggested ways to bring him or her "up to speed":

- At a nonstressful and nonsexual time, tell your partner you'd like to discuss your sexual relationship.
- Begin by describing the problem as you see it. Avoid blaming ("It's all your fault") or generalizing ("You've never been a good kisser").
- Ask your partner to repeat what you have just said. This allows for early corrections of any misunderstandings.
- Explain what you've learned from your self-assessment and medical evaluation.
- Ask your partner for feedback as you discuss your concern and answer any questions.
- Explain this book and the self-help exercises.
- Suggest that your partner might want to read this book to find out more about women's sexuality (this applies to lesbian couples as well).
- Explain that there are some exercises that will require your partner's cooperation and participation.
- Ask your partner directly for respect and emotional support in this process.
- Tell your partner what steps you plan to take to address the problem, and when and how you would like to involve him or her.
- End the discussion by assuring your partner that you will talk about this concern again and set a date for the next discussion, if that feels comfortable.

INSTRUCTIONS FOR SELF-HELP EXERCISES

In the next three chapters we provide detailed self-help exercises for overcoming low sexual desire, low sexual arousal, and orgasm difficulty. Each exercise begins with an *introduction* that explains the rationale for the exercise, followed by *directions* for you, and in some cases, for you and your partner. After you follow the directions, a *reflection* section will help focus your attention on the key outcomes and possible sticking points of the exercise. We also suggest the *next steps* to be taken following the completion of the exercise.

The self-help suggestions offered in the next three chapters have been effective for many women. But a few cautionary notes must be made.

- If you have a physical problem, all the self-help exercises in the world won't correct that medical condition. Psychological intervention can help you increase your sexual satisfaction but cannot substitute for proper medical care. Review the suggestions offered earlier in this chapter for seeking a medical evaluation.
- These self-help suggestions, by themselves, will not benefit everyone. You may find you need assistance beyond the suggestions offered in this book. If this is true for you, it doesn't mean you have grave, deep-seated problems. It simply means that your problem requires a more customized intervention. In such a case, sex therapy may be very helpful in resolving your problems and improving your sexual functioning. The final chapter will help you find a sex therapist if you need one.
- Once you've made the commitment to do these exercises, try to stick with them even if you feel you're not having much success. Simply attempting the exercises is a positive step toward sexual health because, at the very least, they will leave you with a better understanding of where the problem lies and whether it's a problem that will require additional help.
- If you find the exercises to be challenging, you might benefit from setting aside a routine time to work on them. Also, discuss them with your partner, making them a shared project. If any of the instructions make you feel overly uncomfortable or violate your personal or moral values, feel free to modify them to make them acceptable.
- Try to be positive and not approach these exercises as drudgery. This can be a good opportunity to practice the cognitive work described above: rather than focusing on the negative, try to view these exercises as an opportunity to do something positive for yourself, something that can continue to enrich your life for years to come.
- Even though a sexual dysfunction can have a negative impact on a partner (hurt ego, feelings of deprivation, etc.), it's a mistake to do these exercises solely for the benefit of the partner. To do so can result in resentment at a later time ("Look what I was willing to do for him"; "Look what he made me go through"). Instead, first and foremost, do these exercises for your own benefit. Focus on how your efforts can lead to your own sexual growth, comfort, and satisfaction. Take care of your sexual needs, and you'll find that your partner's satisfaction will naturally increase as a result of your sexual growth. As you become more comfortable experiencing sexual pleasure, you will become more comfortable pleasuring your partner.
- Finally, remember that growth is not without risk. Whenever we attempt to tackle a problem, we face the danger of opening a Pandora's box. As you focus on

your sexuality, you may come up with insights that are hurtful or embarrassing. You may suddenly see flaws in your relationship that, until now, you have managed to avoid acknowledging. Before proceeding with these exercises, you should be prepared to take such risks. You must decide whether sexual growth is worth the awkwardness that can come from self-discovery or the tension that might arise if you and your partner become truly honest with each other. For many people, these risks are outweighed by the potential benefit of sexual growth. But you will have to decide for yourself. If you do go ahead with these exercises and suddenly feel that you're in over your head, don't hesitate to seek professional help.

CHAPTER FOURTEEN

Overcoming Low Sexual Desire

"I used to love sex. Now it seems like nothing can make me horny."

"Everyone makes such a big deal about sex, but in all honesty, I could easily live without it."

Low sexual desire is one of the top two reasons that people seek help for sexual concerns. In a national survey, researchers found that 33% of women reported that they lacked sexual interest (Laumann et al., 1994). Low sexual desire isn't the same as having difficultly getting aroused or experiencing orgasm. In fact, you may find that even though you lack desire, you can still get turned on and even orgasm when you're sexually active. Low sexual desire isn't the same thing as being afraid of, or disgusted by, sex. With low sexual desire, it's not that you find sex scary, bad, or distasteful; you simply have no interest in it. You don't seek it, don't fantasize about it, and wouldn't miss it if sex disappeared from your life altogether.

HOW DO I KNOW IF I'VE GOT LOW SEXUAL DESIRE?

Have you wondered if a drop in the frequency of intercourse means you've got low sexual desire? Some researchers and clinicians have used frequency of intercourse as the criteria for diagnosing low sexual desire. Using the "numbers game," however, distorts our understanding of sex and sexual desire. Sex is more than just intercourse; you don't have to be active in the bedroom to be a sensual, sexual person. Overburdened schedules, a health problem, or even the lack of a partner could make the frequency of sexual intercourse very low, yet you may have a very normal sex drive.

Maybe you've suspected that you have low sexual desire because it seems like you don't think about sex anymore. Or maybe you think about sex, but you don't have any interest in having sex with your partner. Perhaps you start thinking about sex but can't stay focused on it because of competing thoughts about shopping you need to do, the sleep you don't get enough of, or the great dinner out you are craving.

If you find it confusing trying to figure out if you have low sexual desire, join the club. Sex therapists and researchers think it's one of the hardest sexual problems to measure. What we suggest as a helpful way to assess your sex drive is to ask yourself two questions:

- Do I ever have sexual thoughts?
- Do I have an interest in being physically aroused, either by myself or with my partner, *if the circumstances are favorable*?

If you've answered yes to these questions, you may not have low sexual desire but another problem, like too much going on in your life. Normal sexual desire doesn't mean wanting to have sex every waking minute of the day. It doesn't mean wanting to have sex simply because someone else makes an offer. It does mean that you have sexual thoughts on occasion and that when you're rested, when the surroundings are private and relaxed, and when the distractions are at a minimum, you may on occasion want to experience sexual pleasure, either by yourself or with a partner.

What if you have a normal sex drive, but because your interest is less than your partner's, you worry that something may be wrong with you? In fact, you're fine—you don't have a sexual desire problem. Rather, you and your partner have a sexual desire discrepancy or sexual frequency discrepancy in your relationship. See Chapter 12 for information on this common challenge, including ways that you and your partner can work through it.

IN THE SYMPTOM LIE THE CLUES

Low sexual desire comes in different varieties. For example, it can be a lifelong problem or a recent one. It can also be a global problem (you have no interest in sex regardless of the partner, circumstances, or timing) or a situational one (it only occurs in certain situations).

> "I have zero interest in having sex with my partner. I feel guilty because I masturbate frequently and I notice I get turned on by looking at other guys at the gym

where I work out. I can't seem to feel any desire for my partner! I know we have our ups and downs, but honestly, I'm not trying to sabotage our relationship!" [This woman is describing a *recent situational* problem.]

By determining whether your low sexual desire is lifelong or not, and whether it is global or situational, you gain valuable clues about its cause and possible solution. If the problem is lifelong, sex-negative influences dating back to your childhood may be contributing to your low sexual desire. If, on the other hand, the problem appeared after you started taking medication for depression, there is a good chance that your low desire is a medication side effect. If your problem is situational, you can probably learn a great deal by carefully analyzing the circumstances associated with the symptom. You can also be fairly confident that if there is a medical problem, it is not the sole or major cause for the low sexual desire. If it were, your desire would probably always be low, not just under special circumstances. When low sexual desire is global, we will often find general, pervasive difficulties like depression, chronic fatigue, disillusionment, sexual conflict, or a medical problem.

In the self-help exercises found later in this chapter, we provide suggestions for using these discoveries to overcome your low sexual desire.

IS SOMETHING PHYSICALLY WRONG WITH ME?

Certain medical conditions and drugs can directly affect sexual desire by altering hormone levels or disrupting the normal function of the limbic system, sometimes referred to as the sex-center of the brain. Table 14.1 provides a list of conditions and medications that are known to have a direct impact on sexual desire.

Having one of the illnesses or taking one of the medications listed in this table doesn't mean you'll necessarily have low sexual desire. And to make matters more complicated, even if a medical condition or drug isn't on the list, it doesn't mean that it can't affect sexual desire. The stress and fatigue that often accompany illness can dampen or shut down the sexual drive, even if the illness does not directly affect hormonal or limbic functioning. (We discuss illness and disability in detail in Chapter 7.) Some medications are highly idiosyncratic—that is, they can affect certain people in unique ways, unlike their effect on most other people. If you're experiencing low sexual desire and have a medical problem or are taking medication, regardless of whether or not the medication or illness is listed in the table, discuss your symptoms with your healthcare provider. Review the suggestions in Chapter 13 for talking with your healthcare provider about sexual concerns.

COUNTERACTING DRUG EFFECTS

If you're taking a medication that is affecting your sexual desire, your healthcare provider may have a number of options for correcting the problem. In some cases,

TABLE 14.1. Medical Conditions and Drugs That May Decrease Sexual Desire

Medical conditions

- Addison's disease
- Chronic renal failure
- Cushing's syndrome
- Depression
- Estrogen-producing tumors
- Head trauma
- Hepatitis
- Hypothyroidism
- Menopause
- Parkinson's disease
- Pituitary diseases
- Stroke
- Temporal-lobe epilepsy

Drugs

Blood pressure and heart medication
- Aldactone (spironolactone)
- Aldomet (alpha-methyldopa)
- Catapres (clonidine)
- Digoxin (lanoxin)
- Hygroton (chlorthalidone)
- Inderal (propranolol)
- Ismelin (guanethidine)
- Lopressor (metoprolol)
- Minipress (prazosin)
- Oretic (thiazide)
- Prinivil, Zestril (lisinopril)
- Serpasil (reserpine)

Cancer medication
- Nolvadex (tamoxifen)

Minor tranquilizers
- Ativan (lorazepam)
- Tranxene (clorazepate)
- Valium (diazepam)
- Xanax (alprazolam)

Major tranquilizers
- Compazine (prochlorperazine)
- Haldol (haloperidol)
- Mellaril (thioridazine)
- Navane (thiothixene)
- Prolixin (fluphenazine)
- Risperdal (risperidone)
- Thorazine (chlorpromazine)

Mood medications (antidepressants and medication for bipolar disorders)
- Anafranil (clomipramine)
- Asendin (amoxapine)
- Effexor (venlafaxine)
- Elavil (amitriptyline)
- Eskalith (lithium)
- Nardil (phenelzine)
- Paxil (paroxetine)
- Prozac (fluoxetine)
- Tofranil (imipramine)
- Zoloft (sertraline)

Sedatives
- Dilantin (phenytoin)
- Luminal (phenobarbital)

Ulcer medication
- Tagamet (cimetidine)
- Zantac (ranitidine)

Recreational drugs/abused substances
- Alcohol (chronic use)
- Cocaine (chronic use)
- Methadone (dolophine)
- Narcotics

changing the dosage of the medication can lessen the side effects without compromising the medication's effectiveness. Substituting medications is another possibility. For example, while some antidepressants may decrease sexual desire (Prozac, Zoloft, Paxil), other antidepressants tend to leave sexual response intact (Wellbutrin, Serzone, and Desyrel). Another possibility to counteract a medication side effect is the addition of a medication as an antidote. For example, preliminary research findings suggest that the addition of Wellbutrin or BuSpar may eliminate or minimize sexual side effects caused by popular SSRIs (selective serotonin reuptake inhibitors) antidepressants (Prozac, Zoloft, or Paxil).

DRUGS FOR DESIRE: WHAT'S OUT THERE?

For thousands of years people have sought out aphrodisiacs, which range from oysters and ground beetle shells to vitamin E and ginseng. Despite all the hype and dramatic claims made by herbalists and health food stores, we still lack scientific evidence that any vitamin, herb, food substance, or drug is the perfect aphrodisiac. Researchers are finding some substances, however, that show promise in certain cases.

Testosterone

If you experience a drop in sexual desire with menopause, the inclusion of a small dose of androgen (a naturally occurring testosterone in women) as part of your hormone replacement therapy (HRT) may be helpful. Testosterone can be administered as a pill, a patch, or a cream that is applied topically to the vulva, wrists, or thighs. If you've entered menopause prematurely due to illness or surgery, androgen replacement can be especially helpful. Chapter 5 provides additional information about menopause, hormones, HRT, and sexual desire.

Wellbutrin

Unlike many antidepressants that cause low sexual desire as a side effect, Wellbutrin has been proven to be effective in treating depression without sexual side effects. Recent studies suggest that nondepressed women with low sexual desire may also benefit from this medication. Further research is necessary, but the preliminary findings are encouraging.

Herbal and Other Remedies

Some women report being helped by herbal remedies like *Ginkgo biloba*, ginseng, DHEA, *dong quai*, or L-arginine. Researchers are reporting promising results from their initial investigation of DHEA, a hormone that is transformed into testosterone and estradiol. Currently DHEA is considered to be a herbal supplement and is sold at health food stores. It's important to realize that, with the exception of DHEA, to date there is little or no scientifically controlled research on these remedies and no real understanding of their safety or effectiveness over long-term use. If you're considering any over-the-counter product, be cautious and educated in your decision-making and be sure to discuss your decision with your healthcare provider.

You may find that the most effective medical intervention for low sexual desire is optimizing your health. Many women report that they experience increased sexual desire when they get enough rest, eat a healthy diet, and exercise regularly.

IF IT'S NOT PHYSICAL, THEN WHAT?

> "I followed the self-assessment and went to see a doctor. Guess what? Nothing wrong physically, and no medication that will take the rap. That left me with my relationship and myself. Because I didn't think I had the time, the ideas, or maybe even the interest to fix it, I put my low desire back on the shelf and ignored it for a long time."

If, after a medical evaluation, it appears that your problem is due to psychological rather than physical factors, don't panic. Many women face this problem at some point in their lives, and most find ways to increase their sexual desire. In this section we present examples of psychological causes for low sexual desire, ranging from deeply hidden issues that have been around for a long time to issues of a more recent vintage that are fairly apparent and easy to identify. We encourage you to think about these examples and consider whether any might apply to you. With this insight, you'll be in a better position to make good use of the self-help exercises at the end of this chapter.

Self-Protection

Sometimes the mind unconsciously decides that, for reasons of safety and self-preservation, sex must be avoided at all costs. For example, if you were sexually molested in the past, avoiding sex in the present may serve as a way to avoid a repeat of the past trauma. Because these efforts at self-protection are often unconscious, it may be very difficult to figure out what's going on. It may be helpful to pay close attention to thoughts that go through your head when encountering sexual situations, for they may provide clues to why you're avoiding sex. But there is a good chance that you may never know whether or not your lack of sexual interest has an unconscious or hidden origin.

The good news is that we can often overcome an unconscious barrier, even if we don't know what that barrier is. In many cases doing exercises like the ones you'll find at the end of this chapter can help make sex feel more comfortable and less threatening, which in turn lessens the unconscious mind's need to self-protect. If you find that doing the exercises makes you feel uncomfortable and anxious, however, consider seeking professional help to explore your low sexual desire more closely and find ways to overcome it.

A Stranger to Pleasure

Some people are raised in such a way that they have a very difficult time experiencing pleasure. We see this most often in people who come from emotionally constricted backgrounds. If you were taught from early childhood to ignore sensory pleasure, you may not be accustomed to enjoying the beauty of a sunset, taking time to appreciate beautiful music, or reveling in the fragrance of a fine wine. In short, you've been programmed to live life in as conservative, modest, unassuming a manner as possible. You've been taught that if you expect little, you'll seldom be disappointed.

This way of approaching life can influence your sexuality. You can become so successful at ignoring the simple pleasures of the body that you end up minimizing the pleasure of sex.

If you're a stranger to pleasure, begin with the sensory journey exercise in the Appendix. Try a facial, pedicure, manicure, or massage as a way of experiencing pleasure in your body. Next, focus on the exercises in this chapter, reminding yourself to stay in your senses.

If, despite your best efforts, you can't seem to awaken pleasure in your body, consider seeing a sex therapist who can help you uncover other conflicts that may be getting in the way of pleasure.

Competing Priorities

Sometimes you can get so caught up with all the challenges and responsibilities in your life that you let sex drop to the bottom of your priorities. For instance, you may be juggling your career and parenting obligations and feel so overwhelmed that you put all thoughts of sex on the back burner. If you have a sexual stirring, you dismiss it, telling yourself, "Some other time—I'm too busy right now." After doing this time and time again, you may become insensitive to any sexual stirrings. It isn't that you make a conscious decision to become nonsexual; instead, your loss of sexual interest happens by default.

Fortunately, recognizing competing priorities is the gateway to overcoming low sexual desire. Start by listing what your priorities are and looking carefully at how you spend your time. Do you have time for sex? If not, how can you make time? Rather than trying to radically change your lifestyle all at once, try starting slowly. Begin by inserting small segments of "pleasure time" into your schedule throughout the day—two extra minutes of touching your body in the shower, two minutes of deep breathing and massaging your temples at midday, three minutes of sitting quietly in your car and relaxing tensed muscles before driving home from work. These snippets of time will help you refocus on your body. Once you can accommodate these time-outs in your schedule on a regular basis, you'll be ready to carve out the 20- to 30-minute segments necessary to do the exercises.

Fatigue

This is another outcome of a busy and complex lifestyle. It's difficult to think about sex when you feel sleep-deprived or sapped of all your energy. Sex is a basic instinct, but it waits in the background until other bodily needs, including rest, are met. If you find that you're interested in sex when you're on a restful vacation, you may have low sexual desire that is situational due to fatigue.

There are a number of things you can try to overcome this difficulty. Start by setting realistic expectations. For instance, plan sex for the weekends, when you have more time to rest. Start exercising. Sometimes exercise actually reduces fatigue. Even a brisk walk for 10 minutes can infuse you with new energy. Try walking before you do the self-help exercises at the end of this chapter and see if that helps your energy level.

If your fatigue is linked to having young children, you'll have to tailor your downtime to the needs of your situation. Make sure you involve your partner in finding solutions, because fatigue can be caused or amplified by feeling isolated and overburdened. Arranging a few hours away from the kids on a regular basis can be very important. Some women find that it works best for them to get a sitter during the late afternoon and early evening rather than at night. Other women arrange for childcare at someone else's home so they can occasionally enjoy having the house to themselves. Get a sitter for a late Saturday afternoon and go with your partner to an inexpensive motel. If you take a picnic dinner, it may cost no more than going to a restaurant and a movie. When you're at the motel, start with a nap before making love. You can be back by 11:30, early enough to get your sitter home before curfew. Who says you have to go away overnight to enjoy a sexual rendezvous with your partner?

Fatigue can be physical, like sleep deprivation, or it can be emotional, like being exhausted from caring for the kids. You'll need to experiment with solutions that work for your situation.

Lack of Attraction

If you're no longer attracted to your partner, your motivation for sex has probably diminished. Lack of attraction is more complex than simply how good a person looks. Negative changes in attitude or behavior can have a far greater impact on a person's attractiveness than changes in appearance. Insensitivity, crudeness, incessant faultfinding, emotional lability, and obnoxious behavior can make a person less attractive and serve as a powerful turn-off.

If you're disgusted with your partner's behavior, have you considered telling him or her how you are feeling? Honest and open dialogue, though at first difficult, can often break down barriers. Check the resource list at the end of the book for suggested readings on improving relationships. In some cases, couples therapy can be very helpful to address resentment and communication problems in the partnership. Lack of attraction won't just "go away" on its own. Tackling the problem head-on is essential.

> "When I realized that I was getting nowhere with all my resentments, things began to change. We got into couples therapy and I felt supported in addressing

his negativity and self-absorption. He really hadn't realized how unattractive he'd become."

Relationship Problems

A troubled relationship is the most common psychological cause for the loss of a previously normal level of sexual desire. If you're angry with your partner, unable to trust, or feel betrayed, you won't be enthusiastic about jumping into bed with him or her. Strong negative emotions can override your sexual appetite even though it's a basic biological drive.

Relationship problems can impact sexual desire in different ways. Your loss of interest may be restricted to just your partner. You may still have sexual fantasies, get turned on by romantic books and movies, and masturbate. But your sexual feelings turn cold when you're confronted by the prospect of having sex with your partner. Or you may find that your disillusionment spills beyond the relationship so that all sexual interest is lost, regardless of the circumstances. In this latter case, because your partner was the center of your sex life, when he or she fell from grace, so did all of your sexual interest.

In either case, you'll need to take charge of your sex life. Begin by reviewing your self-assessment. Can you pinpoint when you began to lose your sexual interest? Does the timing coincide with other problems occurring in your relationship? Next, review the steps you've taken to try to correct your relationship problems. Sometimes couples continue to use negative patterns of interacting with each other and don't look for, or try, new ways of relating. What strategies have you used to improve your relationship in general and sex in particular? You may benefit from concentrating on improving your relationship before addressing the sexual relationship. Take a look at the "Suggested Resources" list for self-help books that deal with relationships. If necessary, consider couples therapy. Once you feel that the relationship is improving, you may want to review suggestions in Chapter 12 and the exercises in the Appendix for ways to reconnect sexually to each other.

WAYS TO INCREASE YOUR SEXUAL DESIRE

Reading through this chapter has required that you take an honest look at yourself, your relationship, and your thinking about sexual desire. The following exercises build on what you've learned and help stimulate your sexual interest. To get the most from these exercises, try the following suggestions:

- Review your self-assessment and the general instructions in Chapter 13.
- Pay particular attention to the caveats listed at the end of Chapter 13.
- Make sure you have privacy for doing the exercises.
- Allow yourself time. Each exercise may take about 25 to 30 minutes. Don't try to do them all at once.

EXERCISES FOR OVERCOMING LOW SEXUAL DESIRE

SELF-ASSESSMENT

Introduction

In this exercise you'll build on the self-assessment that you started in Chapter 13. The answers to these questions can give you important insight into your low sexual desire. It's helpful to figure out whether your low sexual desire has been a lifelong condition or a problem that's emerged in response to a personal or medical event; whether changes in your life could account for your lack of desire; and whether your lack of desire is global or only in response to certain situations.

Directions

Spend time reflecting on the questions listed in the self-assessment section of Chapter 13 and on the questions listed below. Consider taking the time to write down your answers on paper or in a journal.

- Are there health issues I need to discuss with my healthcare provider?
- Has there been a time in the past when I've wanted sex, looked forward to sex, missed sex, or just downright felt horny?
- What's different now (job, relationship, life challenges, health, etc.) compared to what was going on in my life the last time I felt the desire for sex?
- Are there still moments during the day when sexy thoughts cross my mind?
- Do I wake up at night sexually aroused?
- Do I find I have sexual urges when I can't act on them?

Reflection

If you decided that this has been a lifelong problem, can you identify any early experiences that made sex something to be avoided? People are not merely born without a sex drive. The intensity of a sex drive can vary from person to person, but normally everyone should have at least a minimal appetite for sex. If that appetite never existed, something early on must have accounted for its absence (early negative messages about sex, faulty sex education, etc.). Review Part I, "Knowing Your Sexual Story," for ideas about what in your background might be inhibiting your sexual interest.

If this is a problem that developed later in life, did you identify life events that may be contributing to the low sexual desire? Consider making a list of action steps you could take to modify the influence of these events (e.g., address relationship problems, learn stress management skills, seek counseling, etc.)

Do you lack desire all the time? If your low desire only happens under certain circumstances, it's more likely due to psychological and relationship factors than to medical factors. Review the psychological factors described earlier in this chapter to see if any apply to you. In the discussion of psychological factors, we have given you specific recommendations that may help.

Next Steps

- If appropriate and you haven't done so already, schedule an appointment with your healthcare provider.
- Follow through on any action steps you came up with to modify the impact of life events that contributed to your loss of desire.
- Move on to the next exercise.

MENTAL EAVESDROPPING

Introduction

Sometimes overcoming low sexual desire merely requires getting back into the routine of taking time for personal pleasure. Even if at first it seems like a chore, having scheduled sexual experiences can at least serve as a beginning framework for constructing a routine for a meaningful sex life.

More importantly, the sexual activities give you an opportunity to eavesdrop on your thoughts when you're confronted with sex. This allows you to identify the distracting and self-defeating thoughts that may be dampening your sexual interest. Listen carefully. Your reactions to scheduling sexual activity will help you decide what direction to take in overcoming low sexual desire.

Directions

Plan and schedule at least one or two sexual activities each week. The activity can be by yourself (masturbation) or with your partner (intercourse, mutual masturbation, oral sex, nongenital massage, etc.). If you want to involve your partner, make sure he or she has had a chance to read this chapter and Chapter 13. Be honest about your concerns and your goal of increasing sexual desire. Make sure that he or she is supportive of this goal.

After each sexual activity, take time to reflect on what thoughts and feelings occurred before and during the activity. Consider writing them down on paper or in a journal. Ask yourself:

- Was I able to initiate sexual activity and feel good about it?
- Did I stay focused or did my mind wander?
- Can I identify any actions I took—like fantasizing, self-caressing, creating a romantic mood—that made me feel more sexual desire?

Reflection

Was finding time for the sexual activities difficult? Was it difficult because you were so busy or because the activity seemed distasteful? What thoughts crossed your mind as the time approached? What thoughts did you have as you were going through the activity?

If your thoughts and feelings were strongly negative (e.g., *I hate doing this,* or *This is disgusting,* or *I just can't do this*), were they prompted by anger or disgust with your partner? If so, that's where the major work needs to be done. If your thoughts were very negative about sex but weren't due to negative feelings about your partner, we may be talking more about a sexual aversion than low sexual desire. Thoughts associated with low sexual desire are more often neutral, such as, *I can do this, but it feels like I'm just going through the motions,* or *I can take it or leave it, but mostly, I'd just as soon leave it.*

Next Steps

- If you're having a major problem with your partner, consider ways of addressing it, including the possibility of counseling. Reread Chapter 12, "Taking Care of Your Sexual Relationship." Also, consider reading at least one self-help book on relationships (see the "Suggested Resources" section for ideas).
- If the prospect of being sexual, regardless of the partner, seems distasteful, read about sexual aversion in Chapter 10.
- If you've discovered that you had some pleasant reactions to this exercise, you're beginning to rekindle your desire. Remember that your motivation is key, and now that you're making time to focus on sexual pleasure, you've taken an important step toward your goal of increasing your sexual desire.

MODIFYING AND REVISING

Introduction

What goes through your head can have a significant impact on your sexual response. By decreasing distractions, improving your circumstances, and revising inaccurate, negative thinking, you can help remove the barriers that have been preventing nature from taking its course. Remember, sex is a natural biological drive.

Directions

Study the thoughts you identified in the previous exercise. Reread the section on cognitive work ("The Solution, Not the Problem, May Be in Your Head") in Chapter 13. Sort your thoughts into the following categories:

- Distractions of daily life
- Performance concerns
- Self-esteem issues
- Sex-negative thoughts and beliefs
- Reliving past trauma

For thoughts that reflect distractions of daily life (job, parenting responsibilities, family illness, relationship problems, etc.), list concrete steps you can take to minimize the distraction or resolve the problem. Try to keep the steps small and doable rather than attempting giant changes.

For other thoughts, challenge the logic of each and try to revise the cognitive text so that it reflects reality more accurately and fairly. For instance, if you thought, *I'll never get turned on,* a more accurate self-reflection would be, *I'm not turned on now, but I'm working on getting more turned on.* (Remember to refer back to the cognitive work section in Chapter 13.)

Reflection

Identifying the thoughts that get in your way is a difficult task, one that you may not fully accomplish on the first attempt. You may have to continue to do this on an ongoing basis. In the process, you will likely fine-tune your ability to mentally eavesdrop.

Revising negative thinking also takes time. Don't expect longstanding negative thoughts to disappear easily. Usually they fade away in time as you continue to refocus on reality and succeed with new behaviors. For example, if for years you kept telling yourself, *Sex is not important,* that thought will probably linger even after you identify and challenge it. To alter this thinking, you might tell yourself that even though sex is not a life and death issue in your existence, it can add an exciting dimension that has been missing in your life. More importantly, ensuring that you take time to be sexual and taking steps to increase sexual satisfaction will create positive experiences that, over time, will replace your negative thoughts.

Next Steps

- Put into action any concrete steps you came up with to resolve daily distractions.
- Continue to review the challenges and revisions in your thinking that you identified.
- Move on to the next exercise.

PRIMING THE PUMP

Introduction

Even when you're successful at finding and removing barriers to sexual desire, by force of habit, you may find it difficult to get back in touch with erotic feelings. The exercises that follow are designed to help you to (1) tap into things from the past that had the power to arouse you, and (2) discover new fantasies and behaviors that can help whet your appetite. In addition, if you can get caught up in a sexual fantasy, you will have succeeded in escaping the distracting and dampening impact of negative cognitions.

Directions

If you've had normal sexual desire in the past, make a list of things that used to turn you on (clothes, music, fantasies, movies, books, etc.). Pull them out of storage and experiment with them.

Explore your capacity for fantasy. (If you feel any discomfort in response to this suggestion, reread the section on fantasy in Chapter 12.) Try the following:

- If you ever had a stimulating sexual experience in the past, recall it in vivid detail. Write about it in your journal. Embellish the details to make it even more dramatic, romantic, or sexy.
- Read examples of other women's sexual fantasies. There are many excellent books and magazines featuring women's sexual fantasies and erotica. See the "Suggested Resources" list at the end of the book.
- Take a shot at writing your own sexual fantasy. Remember, just because you fantasize about someone or something doesn't necessarily mean that you would ever act out the fantasy in real life.
- Try the self-pleasuring exercises found in the next chapter.

Reflection

If you read samples of female erotica, you may find that many of the fantasies have little effect on you. That's fine. Fantasies are highly personal and can be incredibly diverse. Even if you find only one or two intriguing or exciting examples of fantasy when reading these books, your time will have been well spent. The object is to expand your horizons and to come up with imagery that can excite and arouse rather than depress and discourage you.

Next Steps

Go on to the next exercise.

GETTING BACK TO BASICS

Introduction

Do this exercise if you have a sexual partner. Otherwise, skip to "Next Steps" for this exercise.

Discovering or rediscovering sexual feelings and desires can be complicated if you're not allowed to make a comfortable transition back into sexual activity. Structured exercises like the one that follows help you and your partner overcome residual awkwardness and develop a comfortable sexual rhythm with each other.

Sex therapists call this exercise "Sensate Focus" because, in part, we're trying to help the couple focus on their sensory experience without being distracted by fears associated with sexual performance or failure. The steps of the sensate focus exercise are practiced over a number of weeks, which allows you to gradually phase in sexual behavior that has been difficult or threatening

You'll notice that bringing your partner to orgasm is introduced early in the process. We do this to help decrease some of the sexual tension that might have developed while you were experiencing a lack of desire. Your partner may have felt sexually deprived, which may have led to feelings of hurt or resentment. We all tend to be more reasonable and cooperative when our needs are being met. If your partner reconnects with you sexually now and realizes that you do care about his or her sexual experience, then it will be easier for him or her to participate in these exercises in a supportive and enthusiastic manner.

Directions

If you have a partner, suggest that for the next two or three weeks, sensate focus will be your only form of lovemaking. For the first week, follow these directions:

- Schedule in advance one or two lovemaking sessions for the upcoming week.
- Set a comfortable mood with music, lighting, etc. Be sure privacy is assured and that you both have enough time so you won't feel rushed.
- Undress each other. Take your time, be sensual.
- Have your partner lie face down. Begin a slow, sensuous body massage. Experiment with body oil. Pay attention to all of your senses. Smell the scent of the burning candles. Feel the texture of your partner's skin. Hear the music; listen to your partner's sighs and moans. Look at your partner's face, hair, and body, appreciating the curves and shapes that make him or her unique.
- After slowly moving from head to toe, have your partner roll over. Repeat the massage, starting with the facial muscles and working your way down to the feet. Avoid genital contact.
- When finished, switch roles and allow your partner to massage you, back and front. Give yourself permission to relax and indulge yourself in pleasure. This is not the time to worry about whether your partner is enjoying him- or herself—these are a few moments for you to be selfish.
- When your partner has finished, take a few more moments and hold each other. Enjoy the silence together or talk about your reactions to the experience you just shared.

During the following weeks, introduce further elements into the sensate focus exercise.

- Unless it makes you uncomfortable or awkward, introduce genital stimulation for your partner, helping him or her to get sexually aroused (and even orgasm) during the sensate focus exercise.
- For yourself, during the next session or two, have your partner add "casual" genital stimulation. The object isn't to produce an orgasm but for you to merely enjoy genital sensations without the pressure to perform or orgasm.
- In later sessions, when you're ready, have your partner increase the genital stimulation. Gently provide guidance and feedback so that he or she can help you get intensely aroused and, if it comes spontaneously, orgasm.
- You can include intercourse when you feel comfortable.

Reflection

If your partner is unwilling to go along with the sensate focus exercises, it will be important to find out why. Sometimes the intention behind the exercise is poorly understood by the partner and needs to be reviewed. When trying to understand your partner's refusal to participate in the sensate focus exercise, avoid blaming and accusing. Explain that this process is important to you, and that you want to understand how these exercises might make your partner feel uncomfortable. Sometimes the reason the partner is unwilling to participate is related to the reason the woman is having a sexual problem. For example, you may be reacting to tension in the relationship or to your partner's negativism about sex. If there are problems in the relationship, it's important to bring them out into the open so that you can work toward their resolution.

Pay attention to your thoughts and reactions during the sensate focus exercise. One type of thinking to watch for, particularly when going through sensate focus, is *I wonder if I'm too slow; I better move faster; It doesn't really matter if I don't feel anything.* Use the cognitive techniques we discussed in Chapter 13 for analyzing, challenging, and modifying distracting or self-defeating thinking.

Next Steps

If your sexual desire has not improved yet, consider additional help. Be sure, however, that you have given yourself enough time to do all of the preceding exercises. If you need to consult with a therapist, remember that it's not a negative reflection on you, and it doesn't mean that you have a bigger problem than the other 30% of American women who have low sexual desire. It merely means that you need a more customized approach than can be provided by a book like this.

If you've noticed an improvement in your sexual desire, move on to the next set of directions.

RELAPSE PREVENTION

Introduction

Whenever we break old habits and change behavior, setbacks are inevitable. Continuing to make sexuality a valued priority in your life helps to minimize such setbacks. The knowledge that the above techniques helped you to claim or reclaim your sexuality can reassure you when periods of low sexual desire recur in the future.

Directions

Continue to find time each week to explore and enjoy your sexuality, whether it's taking a warm, sensuous shower, musing over erotic images and fantasies, stimulating yourself to orgasm, or making love with your partner.

Periodically review your work on the above exercises. Review progress on your action plans and continue to monitor for new and old negative thinking.

Anticipate setbacks and don't panic when they occur. By now you know the routine for increasing sexual desire, and you know it works. If there's a setback, repeat the basic steps described above.

CHAPTER FIFTEEN

Overcoming Low Sexual Arousal

"I used to get turned on whenever I wanted. I just had to think about sex and I'd get wet. Now I feel like the juices never flow, the heat never happens. Even though I want to be excited, I'm frustrated. I can't get a fire started."

"I can get aroused, but it's flat, like drinking soda without the fizz."

HAVING DESIRE BUT NO FIRE

What is sexual arousal for women? "Turned on." "Hot pants." "Getting naked." "Wet." A woman has her own language for sexual excitement, and it tends to be highly individual. A man might equate arousal with an erection, but a woman relies on more diverse and subtle cues to signal that sexual desire is turning into something physical.

"When I'm aroused, I feel it in my nipples. They get a little swollen and hard and I love to have them sucked. My lips and skin are sensitive. I feel like rocking my pelvis."

"Turned on is when I feel fullness in my whole crotch. My clitoris becomes sensitive to touch and my labia seem more swollen. Sometimes I get wet right away, but other times I'm aroused but not very wet."

It's frustrating for a woman when she wants to feel arousal but can't. As one woman described it, a lack of sexual arousal is "having desire but no fire." In medical textbooks low sexual arousal is called "female sexual arousal disorder" and is defined as an "inability to attain or maintain . . . an adequate lubrication-swelling response of sexual excitement" (American Psychiatric Association, 1994, p. 502). Inadequate lubrication is a common problem; in a large sample of American women between the ages of 18 and 59, 19% reported having this difficulty (Laumann et al., 1994).

Lubrication is an important part of a woman's sexual arousal, but we think that a narrow medical definition of arousal that only considers the presence or absence of lubrication overlooks important realities about a woman's sexuality. Sometimes medical factors prevent vaginal lubrication, but other parts of the body can still respond to the sexual activity. And just because a woman lubricates doesn't necessarily mean she's turned on. A woman can lubricate yet find the sexual activity unsatisfying, unpleasant, or even traumatic (Laan, Everaerd, Bellen, & Hanewald, 1994). Being aroused or sexually excited means that not only your body but also your mind is responding to the sexual activity. Feeling the "fire" is not necessarily feeling wet, but it is *always* exciting and pleasurable.

Rather than using the medical criterion of inadequate vaginal lubrication, in this chapter we consider situations where a woman has sexual desire and doesn't experience pain, but neither her body nor her mind becomes excited. This is a common problem—research suggests that more than a fifth of American women do not find sex pleasurable.

WHEN ILLNESS OR MENOPAUSE STEALS THE FIRE

"I came through a major depression, and with medication I've gotten my life back on track. Everything but my sex life, that is."

"I thought I was lucky because the only chemotherapy side effect I had was not being able to get turned on. Then one day I realized I was sick of being grateful for being alive. I wanted something more."

Rarely will an illness or medical condition directly suppress a woman's ability to experience sexual pleasure. Indirectly, however, the pain, vaginal dryness, worry, and fatigue associated with many medical problems can sufficiently distract a woman so that she either is unable or finds it difficult to focus on sexual cues and enjoy sexual feelings. Many women also find that hormonal changes due to menopause lower their sexual arousal. Part of what we discuss in this chapter is how to minimize the distracting effects of illness and menopause and focus directly on sexual cues so that you can better enjoy the sexual feelings in your body. But first let's look at the medical conditions and drugs that can cause low sexual arousal.

The most common biological cause for vaginal dryness is estrogen deficiency. The lubrication in your vagina and swelling in your pelvis are caused by an increased blood flow to your genitals when you're turned on. Estrogen keeps the process working smoothly by making sure that tissue stays supple and the blood supply to the genitals is steady. At menopause or with an illness that causes estrogen deficiency, you may notice much less lubrication. Without sufficient estrogen levels, the endothelium—the tissue through which lubrication passes to the vagina—and the network of small blood vessels that provide the fluid for creating lubrication will atrophy (shrivel up).

Menopause is the most common cause for estrogen deficiency. The impact of menopause on vaginal lubrication varies dramatically among women. Although it appears that the effects of menopause are less severe for women who remain sexually active, this is not always the case. Research continues to seek explanations for why some women experience greater vaginal atrophy during menopause than others. If you've experienced this difficulty, the medications and exercises we suggest later in this chapter may help you.

Table 15.1 lists the common medical conditions and drugs that decrease sexual arousal.

Although these are the most likely culprits to affect arousal, they do so only rarely (except for menopause). If you have one of these illnesses or take one of these medications, chances are that you don't experience any side effects at all. It's also possible that some other illness or drug could cause arousal difficulties, because some medications and medical conditions affect certain people in unique ways. So whether or not your medication or illness is listed in the table, if you're experiencing vaginal dryness during sex, discuss your symptoms with your healthcare provider.

Hormone Replacement Therapy

If you have an estrogen deficiency, hormone replacement in the form of either an oral medication or a vaginal cream may be prescribed if you are at a low risk for developing cancer. Increasing the estrogen supply to vaginal tissue helps reverse the effects of atrophy and improves lubrication. If you are at a greater risk for developing cancer, there are new hormone replacement therapies that do not appear to increase the risk of cancer. In Chapter 5 we discuss hormone replacement therapy and suggest additional resources for you to consult so that you can make an informed decision on this important issue.

Lubricants

Lubricants are another remedy for vaginal dryness. Many different types of lubricants are available over the counter at your local pharmacy. You'll find them where the spermicidal jelly and condoms are kept. You can also order lubricants online

TABLE 15.1. Medical Conditions and Drugs That May Decrease Sexual Arousal

Medical conditions

- Adrenal disease
- Alcoholic neuropathy
- Amyotrophic lateral sclerosis (ALS)
- Diabetes
- Epilepsy
- Hepatitis
- Herniated lumbar disk
- Kidney disease
- Menopause
- Multiple sclerosis
- Oophorectomy
- Pituitary disease
- Postradiation treatment of the vagina
- Radical pelvic surgery
- Severe malnutrition
- Stroke
- Thyroid deficiency
- Vaginitis
- Vascular disease
- Vitamin deficiency

Drugs

Blood pressure medication
- Aldactone (spironolactone)
- Catapress (Clonidine)
- Inderal (propranolol)
- Oretic (thiazide)

Cancer medication
- Nolvadex (tamoxifen)

Minor tranquilizers
- Valium (diazepam)
- Xanax (alprazolam)

Major tranquilizers
- Prolixin (fluphenazine)
- Risperdal (risperidone)

Mood medications (antidepressants and medication for bipolar disorders)
- Asendin (amoxapine)
- Nardil (phenelzine)
- Paxil (paroxetine)
- Prozac (fluoxetine)
- Tofranil (imipramine)
- Zoloft (sertraline)

Antihistamines and decongestants (Drugs that can dry up nasal passages can also inhibit vaginal lubrication. You may hear them referred to as "anticholinergic" medications.)

(both www.goodvibes.com and www.babeland.com have many products to choose from). Water-based lubricants like Astroglide and K-Y have been popular for many years. There are newer silicone-based lubricants that some women like because they last longer and don't dry out and get sticky. Some women prefer vitamin E oil or vegetable oil because either is easy to find and completely natural. There are also commercial lubricants that are totally natural. Sylk, for example, is a natural extract from the kiwi fruit plant. Avoid petroleum-based lubricants (like Vaseline or Johnson's Baby Oil) because they break down the latex in condoms and can trap bacteria in your vagina, which increases the risk of irritation or infection.

Most lubricants are applied to the vulva and up into the vagina right before sexual activity. They differ in how thick, gooey, and slippery they are. Lubrin is different from most traditional lubricants because, as a vaginal suppository, it's inserted into the vagina about 30 to 60 minutes before sexual activity. It melts slowly and, mimicking the way your body works, slides down the walls of your vagina and over your introitus. Vaginal moisturizers (for example, Replens) are also available. Unlike traditional lubricants that are only used during or immediately before sex, products like Replens are used daily to help the vaginal walls retain moisture, which makes the tissue more resistant to irritation and damage during sexual activity.

You'll need to become a lubricant connoisseur and find the one that is right for you. In Chapter 4, we provide additional information about sexual response and lubrication.

Drugs for Arousal: What's Out There?

Researchers are trying to find drugs that will help women with arousal difficulties just as Viagra was successful in helping many men with erectile difficulties. Currently, there is no magic blue pill, but there are a number of promising developments. We'll give a brief overview of possible treatments and encourage you to seek the most current information from your healthcare provider.

Testosterone

We know that androgen levels decrease for women as they age and that testosterone supplements are helpful in some cases. Testosterone can be administered as a pill, patch, or a cream that is applied topically to the vulva, wrists, or thighs, depending on the medical situation. Testosterone patches are applied for shorter periods of time by women than when used by men.

In research studies testosterone has been shown to increase arousal and genital responsiveness in women. Side effects of testosterone include secondary male sexual characteristics, enlargement of the clitoris, acne, weight gain, and liver damage. In the very low dosages prescribed for women, however, these side effects are very unlikely to occur and can be controlled additionally by reducing the dosage further when necessary, taking "drug holidays," and working closely with your healthcare provider.

Viagra and Other Vasodilators

It seems reasonable to assume that vasodilators (chemicals that dilate blood vessels) could increase arousal by increasing pelvic blood flow during sexual stimulation. Because Viagra (its pharmaceutical name is sildenefil) has proved so helpful to men, it was hoped that it would have the same effect on women's arousal. So far, research studies have produced mixed results, and though it may be helpful for some women, Viagra is certainly not the "Holy Grail" for all women with low arousal. Scientists are pursuing research on prostaglandin E-1, phentolamine, pentoixifylline, vasoactive intestinal peptide (VIP), and other chemicals as possible vasodilators that will enhance arousal. Because vaginal tissue is highly permeable, many of these chemicals are being developed for topical application, which will result in a more rapid response compared to medicine in pill-form. Ask your healthcare provider about what medications are currently available. Remember, however, that if psychological factors are causing your arousal problem, it's unlikely that any medicine is going to fix it.

Herbal and Other Remedies

The herbal remedies discussed in Chapter 14 for low sexual desire (*Ginkgo biloba*, ginseng, DHEA, *dong quai*, or L-arginine) also have been reported to help with problems of low sexual arousal. In addition, some women have had success with yohimbine, an oral medication that has been shown to enhance arousal in men. Yohimbine, however, can have many side effects, so remember when considering any over-the-counter product to be cautious and educated in your decision-making and be sure to discuss your decision with your healthcare provider.

Counteracting Drug Effects

If you're taking a medication that is affecting your sexual arousal, your healthcare provider may have a number of options for correcting the problem. The options discussed in Chapter 14 for low sexual desire (changing medication, decreasing the dosage, or combining with an antidote) also apply for women with low sexual arousal. For women who experience arousal difficulties as a result of taking SSRI antidepressants (Prozac, Zoloft, Paxil, and others), the addition of Viagra may help reverse the unwanted side effect.

Gadgets

Mechanical devices for increasing sexual arousal are not new. Many women find that vibrators help increase their arousal and frequency of orgasm. A new device (EROS-CTD) has recently been approved to increase clitoral sensitivity. A small, hand-held, battery-operated device is placed over the clitoris and, by creating a vacuum, draws additional blood into the organ. Because of the increased blood flow, the clitoris is more sensitive to stimulation. Preliminary data suggest that lubrication, satisfaction, and orgasm increase for many women when using this device.

Vibrators can be ordered online (see the section on "Sex Toys, Videos, and the Internet" in "Suggested Resources"). The EROS-CTD requires a physician's prescription.

WHEN YOUR MIND PUTS OUT THE FIRE

> "It's so much work to stay tuned in to arousal that I check out. I work too hard during the week to want to work on Saturday night. Just let me read a good book or get the laundry caught up."

"I try to get aroused. I'll take a warm bath. I'll drink some wine. Maybe I'll feel a little twinge of turn-on, but frankly, my heart's not in it."

From time to time your ability to lubricate can be affected by worry, stress, or mental distraction. But if you experience vaginal dryness regularly, it's most likely due to medical factors. On the other hand, the lack of "subjective" arousal—that is, not enjoying the experience—will often be the result of psychological factors.

Where Your Head's At

One common psychological barrier to subjective arousal is mental distraction. Focusing on the eroticism of the moment is critical for sexual arousal. Anything that distracts you from an erotic focus can prevent sexual arousal, especially your subjective arousal. Examples of common distractions include:

- Tension in the relationship
- Job stress
- Financial concerns
- Health worries
- Performance pressure
- Feelings of sexual inadequacy
- Poor body image
- Demanding schedule
- Fear of being discovered or interrupted

Learning, biology, and culture influence your ability to focus on sexual cues and achieve sexual arousal. These factors appear to have a different impact on women and men. A closer look at these gender differences will help you understand common barriers to your arousal and will suggest possible steps to overcome arousal difficulties.

One important way to focus on eroticism is by tuning in to your body's response to sexual stimulation. This ability to tune in to bodily cues is not innate but largely learned. A number of writers have suggested that masturbation serves as an ideal learning opportunity for people to explore how their bodies respond to stimulation. Masturbation is a common behavior for adolescent boys that allows them to become comfortable with their genitals and sexual feelings. As we've discussed in the first part of the book, society's double standard has prevented many women from having the same opportunity to learn how to become attuned to sexual feelings. Not only are women discouraged from masturbating, but they are often taught to avoid looking at, or touching, their genital area except for necessary hygiene.

Whether masturbating or having sex with a partner, a man has an advantage over a woman in being aware of how his body is responding to sexual cues. He can easily feel, perhaps even see, his penis harden. There is no mistaking when his desire is becoming fire. A natural feedback loop develops. The unmistakable presence of his erection captures his attention; it draws him to the eroticism of the moment, which further increases his arousal. For you as a woman, the swelling of your labia, a feeling of fullness in your genitals, and lubrication in your vagina are much more subtle than an erection. The presence or absence of lubrication is not nearly as noticeable, unless (of course) penetration is attempted when your vagina is dry. As a result, you will find it more difficult than men to identify when you are beginning to respond physically to sexual cues. You won't have nearly as strong a feedback loop to quickly intensify your arousal.

Even when you are aware of growing sexual arousal, you may notice that it's easy to be distracted by non-sexy thoughts. You may wonder why you can't stay focused on the sexual cues around you. As we discussed in Part I, "Knowing Your Sexual Story," you were exposed to many cultural and family influences regarding your sexuality. In most cultures, there's a sexual double bind for women. From early childhood, you were warned about dangers associated with sexuality. You could be sexually exploited. You could be the victim of sexual violence. You could get pregnant by accident, and it's certain your parents warned you that you would carry the major burden of an unwanted pregnancy, whether that burden was shame, financial hardship, restricted freedom, medical risk, or physical discomfort. For all of these reasons, you developed a self-protective vigilance, a watchfulness in sexual situations. When you tune in to sex, part of your brain is still tuned in to those "be careful" messages.

For a guy, if his partner's willing and his penis is hard, life is good. For you, much more is at stake sexually. You learn to monitor for signs of danger and risk. The tendency toward vigilance can become so routine that even when you're in a trusting, loving, equal relationship, you may, through force of habit, still monitor nonerotic cues. During sex, you'll be more much likely than your male partner to notice the furnace rattling or a light coming from underneath the bedroom door.

> "I've given up trying to have sex at home. Our youngest talks in his sleep. Our oldest keeps strange hours. We get calls on the answering machine. The icemaker clunks, the water softener chugs, and somebody over on the next street must own a Harley."

> "It bothers me to have sex before I finish my lists. I can't concentrate on sexual feelings because I'm dreading having to get up early to do the things that I didn't get done before going to bed."

> "I know why women have low sexual arousal: it's called kids and work."

The exercises at the end of this chapter offer a number of strategies to help you overcome mental distractions, pick up on body cues, and remain focused on the eroticism of lovemaking.

The Wrong Script

Not only what you think about during sex but also what you do during sex will have an important impact on your sexual arousal. Certain ways of making love can be a real turn-on, while other ways can be a turn-off or just not hit the mark. Things that usually turn men on during sex are often different from the things that turn women on. For men, because of how they've learned to think about sex and how their bodies respond, they tend to see getting and keeping an erection as the essential objective for intercourse. Their script for lovemaking tends to be simple and unswerving—genital stimulation, penetration, and ejaculation. Anything else may seem unnecessary.

As a woman, you may be more turned on by holding, touching, and bonding emotionally. If you're like many other women, however, you may think you're supposed to comply with a man's sexual script. Masters and Johnson (1979) demonstrated this tendency in a study in which they compared sexual behavior of heterosexual and lesbian couples. The researchers found that lesbians spent considerably more time engaging in nongenital touching and caressing during lovemaking than did heterosexual women; the heterosexual women focused more on direct genital stimulation. This finding demonstrates that when women have male sex partners, they tend to go along with the male script for lovemaking.

Whether you have mistakenly assumed that the male sexual script was a "universal given" or felt that your needs didn't matter, you are probably cheating yourself of what turns you on. Rather than just pleasing your partner or trying to "get it over with," think about putting yourself in the sexual driver's seat. To increase arousal, you'll need to create a sexual script of your own. No time? Too much effort? It's not somebody else's responsibility to rev up your sex life, any more than it's somebody else's responsibility to pick up your kids or work your job. Think about how you handle other parts of your life—even when you're pressed for time and burdened with responsibilities, you probably do your best to figure out how to accomplish your priorities. Making sexual arousal a priority means becoming purposeful and focused about finding ways to craft a sexual script that brings you pleasure and satisfaction.

> "I felt terrific when the last minivan pulled out of the driveway. Three kids, and every one of them at a friend's for the night. I've got a whole night alone with my partner. If I can plan the rest of my life, I can make this happen too."

The exercises at the end of this chapter will help you revise your script for lovemaking to help increase your sexual arousal.

Choosing Anger over Arousal

Some women complain and even brag to each other about how sexually unresponsive they've become since having children. They treat low sexual arousal like the red badge of courage for motherhood. If you are chronically complaining about sex being unfulfilling but do nothing to try to correct it, perhaps you need to look at your relationship with your partner. Are you relying on complaints about sex as a way of expressing dissatisfaction with your relationship or anger toward your partner? Are you choosing self-righteous anger as your arousal of choice? If you are getting back at your partner through sexual complaints and indifference, then you're giving up the pleasure of sex for the pleasure of martyrdom. If so, perhaps it's time to consider counseling. Chapter 17 explains how to find a qualified sex therapist.

HOW TO LIGHT THE FIRE

Because male and female arousal scripts are different, increasing sexual arousal is not merely learning how to touch the right spots at the right time. It takes much more than a moist vagina for you to find pleasure in a sexual situation. Increasing sexual arousal requires self-knowledge, self-esteem, increased body awareness and comfort, meaningful sexual stimulation, and a relationship with your partner that works for you.

In the self-help exercises that follow, we begin by helping you first address physical arousal concerns, then how to increase your subjective arousal. Before starting the exercises, you may find it useful to review the general guidelines for self-help listed in Chapter 13. Pay particular attention to the material in the sections titled "Instructions for Self-Help Exercises."

EXERCISES TO INCREASE SEXUAL AROUSAL

SELF-ASSESSMENT

Introduction

In this exercise you'll build on your self-assessment that you started in Chapter 13. The answers to these questions can give you important insight into your sexual concerns and where to begin addressing them.

Directions

Spend time reflecting on the questions listed in the self-assessment section of Chapter 13 and on the questions listed below. Consider taking time to write down your answers on paper or in a journal.

- Are there health issues I need to discuss with my healthcare provider?
- In recent months have there been times when I've wanted sex, looked forward to sex, missed sex, or just downright felt horny? (If the answer is no, read Chapter 14.)

- When I'm stimulated or aroused, does my vagina usually become moist?
- During sex, can I relax and let go, or do I tense up?
- During sex, do I usually get turned on and feel pleasurable feelings? (If the answer is yes, you probably don't have an arousal disorder. If you have difficulty lubricating, consult with your physician. If, despite your arousal, you usually can't orgasm, read the next chapter.)

Reflection

If low arousal is due to a lack of interest in sex, the low desire should be addressed first. You can begin by reading Chapter 14.

Difficulty with orgasm does not necessarily mean that a woman has an arousal disorder. If you find sexual activity physically and psychologically pleasurable, and in the absence of medical factors, you're able to lubricate during sex, you probably don't have an arousal disorder.

If low arousal is not a lifelong problem, can you identify life events that may be contributing to your lack of arousal? Consider making a list of action steps you can take to modify the influence of these events (e.g., address relationship problems, learn stress management techniques, seek counseling, etc.)

If you're uncomfortable in sexual situations, can you identify reasons for this discomfort? Make a list of action steps you can take to minimize the discomfort (e.g., read more books about sex, share sexual concerns with your partner, seek information and suggestions from your healthcare provider, etc.).

Did you identify distractions that prevent you from relaxing during sex (thoughts, life circumstances, etc.)? Make a list of steps you can take to minimize the distractions (e.g., plan in advance, make use of fantasy, focus on body sensations, etc.).

Next Steps

- If appropriate, schedule an appointment with your physician.
- If you came up with any action steps, follow through with them.
- Move on to the next exercise.

BODY WORK: INTRODUCTION

Introduction

To enjoy sexual feelings, it's important to be firmly rooted in your body—not a perfect body but *your* body. All too often women become alienated from their bodies because they don't conform to Madison Avenue's definition of beauty. If they don't dwell on their bodies, they decide, they won't feel ashamed or disgusted. Other women are alienated from their bodies because of upbringing. They learned at an early age that nakedness was bad and sensual pleasure was shameful. This exercise is designed to introduce you to your body, and if necessary, to make peace with your body. The more often you look at your body, the less foreign it will be to you. What at first you considered to be flaws or imperfections should become, to you, aspects of your uniqueness. By becoming more accepting of your body, you'll feel less self-conscious during lovemaking; you'll be less distracted and more capable of focusing on erotic cues.

Directions

Find time alone when you have privacy and no concerns about being interrupted. First take a leisurely bath or shower to unwind and relax. Afterward, stand before a full-length mirror and study your naked body. Talk out loud to yourself, describing what you see, what you like, and what makes you feel awkward.

Highlight and let yourself feel good about features that please you—perhaps the shape of your calf, the curves of your breast, the profile of your face, the muscle tone of your arms, the softness of your thighs, or the texture of your nipples.

Note your negative reactions and recognize that these reactions are probably based on society's obsession with the perfect body. Refer to the cognitive work section ("The Solution, Not the Problem, May Be in Your Head") in Chapter 13 for guidance on challenging and revising any negative thoughts you have.

Reflection

If you find it difficult looking at yourself nude, perhaps try the exercise in your underwear or fully clothed. Start by restricting your focus to just one part of your body. Repeat the exercise over a number of days, carrying on a healthy dialogue with yourself. Identify the thoughts that make nakedness threatening and process them by using the suggestions provided in the section "Challenging Our Thinking: Moving from Punitive to Positive Awareness" in Chapter 6.

It can be difficult to downplay the constant hype about perfect bodies. It's important to confront Madison Avenue's beauty bias and not allow it to rob you of the pleasure you can feel in your body.

Next Steps

- Work on analyzing and revising negative and inaccurate thinking.
- Move on to the next exercise.

BODY WORK: PELVIC FLOOR MUSCLE EXERCISES

Introduction

Pelvic floor muscles are very important source of sexual pleasure and arousal for women. Contracting and relaxing the pelvic muscles can actually promote lubrication and increase arousal. The sensations of sexual activity can be heightened by consciously pulsing these muscles. When your partner inserts a finger or penis into your vagina, she or he can feel the sensation of those muscles gripping and relaxing. Some people find this very pleasurable.

Gaining voluntary control over the pelvic floor muscles can have additional benefits to increasing sexual satisfaction. As women age and lose estrogen, the elasticity of the muscles can be affected. Strengthening these muscles not only counteracts this loss of elasticity but also can help with involuntary urine loss that some women experience.

Directions

Identify the pelvic floor muscles and how you control them. As a first step, when you are urinating, start and stop the flow of urine. When you have accomplished this, you have begun to isolate control of the pelvic floor muscles.

- Find a comfortable place and time where you can lay back and use a hand mirror to see your vulva. Contract and relax your pelvic floor muscles. You may be able to see the perineum (the area between your vaginal opening and your anus) move in and out as you are contract and relax these muscles. Your buttocks may squeeze together, but the goal is to notice the sensation of contracting the muscles around the vulva rather than the butt muscles, stomach, or thigh muscles. Depending upon your body size and flexibility, you may not be able to see much, but you should be able to feel whether your muscles are appropriately contracting. Place your hand gently against your vulva and contract your muscles. You'll feel them move.
- Moisten a finger with saliva or a water-soluble lubricant and try inserting it in your vagina. With your finger inserted, contract your pelvic muscles. Note the pressure of the muscular contractions around your finger.
- Experiment with the sensation of contracting and relaxing the pelvic muscles. Exercising the pelvic muscles can be sexually arousing. Focus on your arousal. Try contracting the muscles in brief, short pulses and in longer, more concentrated contractions. See which is the most satisfying and arousing to you. This exercise may remind you of the description of Kegel exercises in Chapter 8.

Reflection

The goal of this exercise is to learn about how the pelvic floor muscles contribute to higher sexual arousal and how you can control their response. Many women have weak control of these muscles and have never attempted to increase voluntary control of them. At first it may seem like these muscles have a mind of their own, but don't become discouraged.

Begin again with the exercise of starting and stopping a stream of urine. When you are doing this exercise, note which parts of your pelvic region are contracting. Don't just tighten the muscles: alternately push out, as if you were trying to expel a tampon. Notice the differences in the sensation of contracting and relaxing the muscle. Practice the tightening and relaxing exercises frequently during the day. You can do pelvic floor muscle exercises anywhere without anyone being aware of what you are doing. Just as with any exercise program, don't expect that you will gain dramatic control or feel the sexually arousing aspects of pelvic muscle exercises immediately.

Next Steps

- Continue practicing pelvic floor muscle exercises frequently every day.
- Try lying on your back while tensing and relaxing your pelvic muscles several times. Then proceed to rock your pelvis up and down, as if mimicking intercourse in the missionary position. Try 10 "rocks" followed by 10 pelvic floor muscle exercises.
- Do the exercise above and add a sexy fantasy. If you can't think of a fantasy, read through self-help exercises in Chapter 14.
- Move on to the next exercise.

BODY WORK: UP CLOSE AND PERSONAL

Introduction

Comfort with your body, including your genitalia, is important in allowing you to become more responsive to sexual stimulation. Many women have been conditioned to have negative or even phobic reactions to their genitals. Familiarity, up close and personal, can help desensitize these reactions.

Directions

Undress from the waist down and make yourself comfortable on your bed or sofa. Prop pillows behind your back. Spread your legs apart, and with a small mirror, study your vulva. Have this book alongside you, opened to the illustrations in Chapter 3.

- Identify your clitoris, labia majora, labia minora, perineum, and anus.
- After propping the mirror to free your hands, spread the labia apart and look for the urethra and examine the introitus (vaginal opening). Take your time, paying attention to the texture of the skin and whether the opening of your vagina is moist or dry.
- Slide back the prepuce (clitoral hood) and examine the exposed clitoris.
- Moisten a finger with saliva or a water-soluble lubricant and insert your finger in your vagina. Explore the interior of your vagina. Notice its ridges and wetness. If you have the physical flexibility to do so press the upper wall of your vagina (about two inches inside) toward your pubic bone. Try rubbing back and forth. You may feel some pressure to urinate, and you may feel pleasant sensations. If you continue the stimulation, you may experience sexual arousal. The level of arousal will be different for different women and will be somewhat dependent upon how much experience you have had with stimulating your G spot. The goal is to be aware of the different areas of arousal of your body, not to achieve a specific level of stimulation. You can also reread descriptions of your G spot in Chapters 3 and 4.

Reflection

For many women this exercise will be the first time they have closely examined their genitals, or perhaps the first time they have touched their genitals directly without using a towel, washcloth, or tissue. This can be a big step, and initially it may feel threatening or embarrassing.

If you find yourself becoming anxious, stop for a few moments, close your eyes, do some deep breathing, and remind yourself that this exploration and touching is really no different from examining your nose or ear. Remember, this is *your* body.

If you find this exercise overwhelming at first, break it down into steps that seem more manageable. For example, the first time simply study your vulva in the mirror until you feel more comfortable. Perhaps the next time you repeat the exercise, add touch, but only touch your pubic hair and surface skin. Later, when you feel ready, you can explore the opening of your vagina. By slowly phasing in all the steps as you repeat the exercise over time, you will probably reduce your uncomfortable feelings.

As you perform this exercise, pay close attention to your thoughts, emotions, and physical reactions. Consider recording your reactions in a journal and spend some time writing about the possible origin of these reactions. Use the cognitive restructuring techniques you learned in Chapter 13 for any negative or inaccurate thinking that you uncover. You may want to review Part II, "Understanding Your Body."

Next Steps

- Work on analyzing and revising negative and inaccurate thinking.
- Move on to the next exercise.

FANTASY

Introduction

Fantasy can serve as a wonderful aphrodisiac. The mental imagery not only helps to excite us but also competes with distracting thoughts that can so easily intrude upon our sexual experiences. Remember, women are often conditioned to be much more attentive than men are to the little distractions that can pop up during sexual situations. Sexy thinking and imagery can help a woman maintain the erotic focus that is critical for sexual arousal.

Directions

Explore your capacity for fantasy. Reread the section on fantasy in Chapter 12 and the self-help exercise on fantasy in Chapter 14. Try the following:

- If you ever had an exciting sexual experience in the past, recall it in vivid detail. Write about it in your journal. Embellish the details to make it even more dramatic, romantic, and arousing.
- Read examples of other women's sexual fantasies. (There are many excellent books and magazines featuring women's sexual fantasies and erotica. See the "Suggested Resources" section at the end of the book.)
- Take a shot at writing your own sexual fantasy. Remember, just because you fantasize about someone or something doesn't necessarily mean that you would ever act out the fantasy in real life.

Reflection

If you read samples of female erotica, you may find that many of the fantasies have little effect on you. That's fine. Fantasies are highly personal and can be incredibly diverse. Even if you find only one or two intriguing or exciting examples of fantasy when reading these books, your time will have been well spent. The object is to expand your horizons, to come up with imagery that can excite and arouse rather than depress and discourage you.

Next Steps

Move on to the next exercise.

MASTURBATION

Introduction

Masturbation is an ideal learning environment; it provides a safe, private, relaxed opportunity for you to explore your body and how you respond to stimulation. Most men benefit from this learning opportunity during adolescence. Many women don't have this advantage. From an early age they're taught that good girls don't touch themselves "down there." Because early in life many women are told that menstruation is "the curse," their genitals become guilty by association.

Contrary to popular opinion, the clitoris and vagina are not your only sex organs. Your mind and your skin, whether on your face or the soles of your feet, function as vital sex organs, capable of producing intense sexual arousal.

Directions

Before attempting this exercise, read and reread the following set of instructions to minimize any distractions such as wondering, *What am I supposed to do next?* Once you understand the steps, go ahead and enjoy.

Find a time when you're home alone and won't be interrupted. Consider taking the phone off the hook. If you want, start with a leisurely bath or shower. Set a comfortable, sensuous mood with lighting and music. For this exercise you can either be nude or wear underwear or lingerie that makes you feel sensual. Lie down and make yourself comfortable. The following steps are suggestions—feel free to improvise:

- Lightly touch your face with your fingertips. Lightly stroke your cheeks and draw your fingers across your forehead. Rub your temples; massage your scalp. Slow down, take your time. Notice the texture and the temperature of your skin. Pay attention to your breathing. Take long deep breaths and tell yourself to relax; try to make your entire body go limp each time you exhale.
- Now move your hands up and down your arms, across your shoulders, and behind

your neck. Note your muscle tone, especially any sign of tension or tightness. Vary your touch by rubbing, lightly stroking, and kneading your muscles. Continue to slow your breathing; take long, deep breaths and tell yourself to relax.

- Move your hands to your breasts; cup them, stroke them, play with them. Lightly roll your nipples between your fingertips. Gently pinch them, pull on them, stroke them.
- Continue down, massaging your abdomen, hips, and thighs. Slow down; vary your touch; keep your breathing slow and even. If you want, you can sit forward and massage your calves and your feet. Whatever you do, don't rush.
- When you're ready, move back up your body to your pelvis. Place both hands over your vulva and apply gentle pressure. Barely move your hands in small, slow circles as you again tell yourself to relax.
- Position your hand so you touch your clitoris, rubbing it gently between your thumb and fingertips. Now stroke the shaft of your clitoris, the part that is below the surface of your vulva; lightly stroke the entire length of your clitoris with slow up-and-down movements. Experiment with speed and the amount of pressure.
- While stroking your clitoris, with your other hand explore your labia, rubbing and stroking gently. Touch your introitus. Experiment with pressing your thighs together as you stroke your vulva to apply more pressure. Try gently rocking your hips up and down as you stroke. Using a lubricant may make it easier to glide your fingers along your clitoris, over your vulva, and into your vagina.
- If you have the flexibility to reach two inches or so inside of your vagina, stroke along the front wall. It may take some minutes of direct stimulation and firm pressure in this area before the stimulating effects are evident. Experiment with speed and amount of pressure.
- From here you're on your own. Self-stimulation is a highly personalized experience in self-loving. Experiment by searching for movements and touching that create the most pleasurable sensations. Give yourself permission to abandon yourself to your sensations. Indulge yourself in fantasy to help heighten your focus and arousal. For a few moments forget about your scrutinizing self—there will be time later for that.
- Stop when you feel satisfied. Don't wait for an orgasm. If one comes, fine. If you don't orgasm but find the stimulation pleasurable, that's equally fine.

Reflection

Were you able to relax enough to allow yourself to experience the sensations? If no, look for possible reasons and distracting thoughts. Write them down and speculate on any steps you can take to overcome these challenges. As before, make use of your cognitive restructuring skills.

Don't expect any specific outcome on your first attempt. For some of you, the above exercise may seem quite radical and may take a number of times before you become sufficiently relaxed to enjoy the experience.

As you repeat the above exercise, don't be restricted by our instructions. The steps are not meant to be a cookbook recipe for sexual arousal. Experiment, follow your instincts, do what feels good.

If this exercise seemed overwhelming, break it down into more manageable parts.

Perhaps start fully clothed, wearing loose-fitting, comfortable garments. The first few times you do the exercise, restrict your focus to nongenital stimulation.

If masturbation is an unacceptable behavior for you, consider making use of this exercise by restricting it to nongenital touching to learn more about deriving pleasure from your entire body. Even if religious or personal reasons prohibit you from performing this exercise, don't worry. These steps can be incorporated later in an exercise with your partner. That way, you will still have an opportunity to explore ways of arousal without using masturbation.

Next Steps

- Follow through by cognitively restructuring any negative or self-defeating thinking.
- Repeat this exercise, modifying and customizing the steps until you become comfortable and find the experience pleasurable (not necessarily orgasmic, but pleasurable).
- Move on to the next exercise.

DESIGNING THE IDEAL ENCOUNTER

Introduction

One of the factors exerting a negative influence on women's sexual arousal is that lovemaking is often based on a male rather than female script. Men are often more genitally focused than women are, and all too often, women comply with their partner's script. It is important for you to identify aspects of lovemaking, especially at the emotional level, that can intensify your sexual experience.

Directions

On a pad of paper or in your journal, write a script for the ideal sexual encounter with your partner. Pay close attention to the setting and activities leading up to lovemaking. Choreograph the lovemaking in detail and write the dialogue. If you can't think of a script, try reading women's erotic stories. Check the list of suggested readings at the end of the book.

Reflection

- How similar or different is your ideal script compared to your actual lovemaking activities?
- If reality is very different from your ideal script, how do you explain the difference?
- What can you do to make your sexual experiences more closely resemble the spirit of your ideal script?

Next Steps

- Work toward implementing your script.
- Move on to the next exercise.

PARTNER WORK: CAN WE TALK?

Introduction

If you don't have a sexual partner, skip down to "Next Steps" at the end of the "Partner Work: Sensate Focus" exercise. Otherwise, read on.

For women, sexual arousal depends on more than genital stimulation. Despite the fact that communication and emotional intimacy are tremendous turn-ons for many women, couples often leave far too many of their thoughts and feelings unspoken. This exercise can serve as a valuable first step in verbalizing affection and openly communicating about sexual preferences and concerns.

Directions

Make two copies of the following questions:

- The thing I most admire about you is ____________.
- The sexiest thing about you is ____________.
- You make me feel special when ____________.
- The thing you do sexually that turns me on the most is ____________.
- If you weren't a part of my life, I'd feel ____________.

Make a date with your partner for a quiet, romantic dinner at home or at a restaurant where there'll be enough privacy to do some serious talking. Before the dinner date, give your partner a copy of the five questions and ask for the answers to be written out beforehand and brought along to dinner.

Be sure to write down your answers to the questions, too.

On your date, after both of you have had a chance to relax, pull out your answers. Read the first question aloud and then your answer. Allow your partner to respond; be prepared to elaborate. Then ask your partner to read his or her answer. Before moving to the second question, be sure both of you have had ample opportunity to talk about the answers.

For the remaining questions, alternate who reads his or her answers first.

Reflection

Honest communication is critical for a successful relationship, yet it can be difficult and scary. The communication sparked by these questions should be nonthreatening—the questions were designed to elicit flattering feedback, not criticism. You and your partner will also have to talk about the rough spots in the relationship, but for right now, enjoy hearing and giving positive feedback.

If you and your partner find it difficult to do this exercise, you may have an answer to your sexual arousal problem. If as a couple you can't discuss issues raised by these five simple questions, you probably don't have much communication or mutual expression of affection as part of your lovemaking. Working on the relationship will probably be productive, as is the case if this exercise leads to criticism rather than compliments. You may want to review Chapter 12 on relationships.

Next Steps

- If problems become obvious, consider steps to help improve and strengthen your relationship (e.g., counseling, marital enrichment weekend, communication course, etc.).
- Keep talking, honestly but lovingly.
- Move on to the next exercise.

PARTNER WORK: SENSATE FOCUS

Introduction

Do this exercise if you have a sexual partner. Otherwise, skip down to "Next Steps" in this exercise.

Sex therapists call this exercise "Sensate Focus" because, in part, we're trying to help partners focus on their sensory experience without being distracted by fears associated with sexual performance or failure. The steps of the sensate focus exercise are practiced over a number of weeks, which allows you to gradually phase in sexual behavior that has been difficult or threatening.

In the traditional lovemaking script, a woman often fails to receive meaningful sexual stimulation. For many women, arousal depends on more than genital stimulation; holding, touching, and caressing are critical ingredients for female sexual arousal. The sensate focus exercise helps a couple rewrite their script for lovemaking, so that partners have a new script that is responsive to both their needs.

The sensate focus exercise also helps you apply the lessons you've learned during the earlier exercises to the actual experience of making love with your partner.

Abstaining from intercourse after the sensate focus exercise, even if for an hour, helps the couple experience physical touch and caressing as powerful ways of connecting in their own right, not merely as warm-up routines for intercourse.

Directions

Suggest to your partner that for the next two or three weeks, sensate focus will be your only type of lovemaking. If the two of you would prefer not to abstain from intercourse, agree that you will do the following exercise at least twice a week for the next couple of weeks and that you will not have intercourse for at least one hour after completing the exercise.

Start by reading the introduction to the "Getting Back to Basics" exercise in Chapter 14. Follow the directions that are provided for the first week.

During the next week, introduce the following elements to the sensate focus exercise:

- Before starting the exercise, tell your partner that you want to share what you've learned about your body during the earlier exercises. Suggest that when it's time for genital stimulation, you'll guide your partner's hand or give some verbal cues on how to help heighten your arousal. Make these suggestions with gentleness and tact—you certainly don't want to communicate the message that your partner is incompetent as a lover.

- During the sensate focus, if you both agree, end your partner's massage by pleasuring his or her genitals and helping him or her to orgasm.
- When your partner is pleasuring you, guide him or her during genital stimulation or demonstrate by stimulating yourself while he or she observes. Enjoy the genital sensations without putting pressure on yourself to perform or orgasm. End the genital stimulation when you orgasm or feel satisfied and comfortable.

For women who skipped the self-stimulation exercise:

- If you opted to skip the masturbation exercise due to personal or moral objections, this second week of sensate focus exercises can provide you with another opportunity to learn more about how to pleasure your body. Together with your partner, read and follow the masturbation instructions.

Reflection

To help focus on the key outcomes and possible sticking points of this exercise, review the "Reflection" section of the "Getting Back to Basics" exercise in Chapter 14.

Next Steps

If you're still not experiencing pleasure during sexual activity, consider getting additional help. Be sure, however, that you have given yourself enough time to do all of the exercises. If you need to consult with a therapist, remember that it's not a negative reflection on you, and it does not mean that you have a bigger problem than the other 20% of American women who do not find sex pleasurable. It merely means that you need a more customized approach than can be provided by a book like this.

If you've noticed an improvement in your sexual arousal, move on to the next set of instructions.

GOING ON FROM HERE

Directions

Continue to find time each week to explore and enjoy your sexuality, whether it's taking a warm, sensuous shower, musing over erotic images and fantasies, stimulating yourself to orgasm, or making love with your partner.

Periodically review your work on the above exercises. Review progress on your action plans and continue to monitor for old negative thinking so that you can replace it with your new ideas, perceptions, and insights.

CHAPTER SIXTEEN

Overcoming Orgasm Difficulties

Did you come? Was it good for you? Do you have multiple orgasms? Questions like these reflect what we call the "tyranny of the orgasm": society's insistence on placing the orgasm at the center of female, as well as male, sexuality. From an evolutionary point of view, men need to ejaculate as part of their sexual response for the purpose of procreation. Female orgasm, in contrast, is not essential for conception. Neither is a woman necessarily sexually dysfunctional if she's not orgasmic.

When we say that *sex matters*, we mean your entire sexual experience. Many women don't orgasm regularly and think their sexual experiences are just fine. Many don't even think that orgasm is essential for positive sexuality; instead, they value sex that is emotionally and physically satisfying. In a large magazine poll of women in the Netherlands, for example, only 20% of the women felt that orgasm was the most important source of their sexual pleasure (de Bruijn, 1982). Because women are so different from men and because sexual satisfaction for both women and men is so subjective, we think it's a mistake to assume that orgasm—or any other single factor—is critical to positive sexuality.

So when is lack of orgasm a problem? It's a problem when you think it's a problem. If you're enjoying sex unequivocally, then everything is just fine. Do you have a sexual difficulty because you've never had an orgasm? Not if you're okay with this. Do you have a sexual difficulty because you don't orgasm every time you have sex? We don't think so. If your partner has a bruised ego because you don't orgasm, is this your problem? It's a problem, but not yours.

We think of orgasm as a sexual choice, and it's yours to make. You have a right to make your own decision about your orgasms and when, where, and how you will have them. If you've decided that orgasms are something you'd like to have, or have more reliably, the exercises in this chapter will help you improve your experience of orgasm. Remember, however, that this is your choice. In our experience, orgasms pursued to keep a partner happy aren't really sexual orgasms; they're just muscle spasms.

WHERE DID MY ORGASM GO?

If you've decided that you want to orgasm more frequently or more easily, read on. We start with a description of different types of anorgasmia (inability to orgasm), explain the causes of orgasm difficulty, and then describe methods you can use to become orgasmic.

The inability to orgasm can be lifelong or develop after a period of normal orgasmic response. Probably one of every 10 women has never experienced an orgasm (Reinisch, 1991). Almost one out of every four women has orgasm difficulties at some time (Laumann et al., 1994). Orgasm problems can be global or situational. We call the problem global when a woman is unable to orgasm regardless of the circumstances: whether she is alone or with a partner, whether the method of stimulation is intercourse, oral sex, or a vibrator, she can't orgasm. Anorgasmia is situational when a woman can orgasm only under certain circumstances. For example, a woman may be able to orgasm when she masturbates but not with her partner.

A common form of situational anorgasmia is the inability to orgasm during intercourse. While some authorities have maintained that the inability to orgasm during intercourse is abnormal, the majority of experts disagree. Intercourse is highly effective in stimulating men to orgasm, but it can be inefficient in providing necessary physical stimulation for women. Depending on the position for intercourse, stimulation of the front wall of the vagina (location of the G spot) may be minimal or nonexistent. Stimulation of the clitoris, an important source of most women's arousal, is also minimal during intercourse. The total amount of clitoral stimulation during thrusting is far less than when the clitoris is stimulated directly during masturbation, oral sex, or manual stimulation. As a result, less than 30% of women report always experiencing orgasm during intercourse (Laumann et al., 1994); many of these women probably orgasm during intercourse only because they or their partners apply direct clitoral stimulation.

We have often had women come to our offices with complaints of not being able to orgasm during intercourse, even though they were otherwise quite orgasmic and sexually satisfied. In many of these cases, we found that they were seeking help because this was more of a problem for their partners than for themselves. The men mistakenly believed that it was normal for women to orgasm during intercourse. The men felt sexually inadequate because their partners weren't having wild and dramatic orgasms at the time of their penile thrustings. In most of these situations, rather than trying to help the women orgasm during intercourse, we have provided education and reassurance to the couple about the normalcy of their experience.

If orgasm is not always essential for sexual satisfaction, and the inability to orgasm during intercourse is not abnormal, when would an orgasm difficulty warrant a closer look?

If the inability to orgasm is lifelong and global, we need to consider the possibility of a medical problem, a sexual inhibition, or a lack of critical sexual learning. If you stopped having orgasms after years of being orgasmic, a medical problem, relationship difficulties, depression, or stress may be the cause. If you can orgasm by yourself but not in the presence of your partner, you might have a sexual inhibition or relationship concern. For any of these situations, you may want to explore possible causes for the orgasm difficulty and ways to resolve it.

COULD THIS BE A MEDICAL PROBLEM?

> "I stopped being able to orgasm after I took medication. I'd get very excited, feel the readiness to come, but then my body would slide right past the orgasm, like missing an exit on the highway. I'd still be aroused, but I knew I wasn't going to get off."

Normally for an orgasm to occur, your nerve impulses have to be able to travel back and forth between your genitals and spinal cord, and between your spinal cord and brain. This two-way communication allows genital stimulation to register in your brain and mental activity in your brain to enhance the physical response in your genitals. When physical stimulation is sufficient and mental activity is conducive, a signal is sent to your pelvic musculature that triggers a series of pleasurable, involuntary contractions that mark the beginning of your orgasm. When a drug, injury, or medical condition interferes with the communication process along the spinal cord, achieving an orgasm can be difficult.

Table 16.1 lists medications and medical conditions that can inhibit orgasm.

You may find that you continue to orgasm after illness or injury. Even women with serious spinal cord injuries have reported experiencing orgasm. Many women report that they retain their capacity for orgasm but experience changes in its physical sensations. You may be experiencing orgasm difficulties associated with an illness or medication we've not listed. Make sure you check with your healthcare provider about your concerns.

While lifelong and global orgasm problems may have a medical cause, situational anorgasmia is almost always due to psychological factors. If you are unable to orgasm regardless of circumstances and you have a medical condition or take a med-

TABLE 16.1. Medical Conditions and Drugs That May Inhibit Orgasm

Medical conditions

- Adrenal disease
- Alcoholic neuropathy
- Amyotrophic lateral sclerosis (ALS)
- Epilepsy
- Diabetes
- Hepatitis
- Herniated lumbar disk
- Kidney disease
- Multiple sclerosis
- Pelvic surgery
- Pituitary disease
- Severe malnutrition
- Spinal cord injury
- Thyroid deficiency
- Stroke
- Vitamin deficiency

Drugs

Blood pressure medication
- Aldactone (spironolactone)
- Aldomet (alpha-methyldopa)
- Catapress (clonidine)
- Ismelin (guanethidine)
- Serpasil (reserpine)

Minor tranquilizers
- Klonopin (clonazepam)
- Valium (diazepam)
- Xanax (alprazolam)

Major tranquilizers
- Compazine (prochlorperazine)
- Risperdal (risperidone)

Mood medications (antidepressants and medication for bipolar disorders)
- Anafranil (clomipramine)
- Asendin (amoxapine)
- Aventil, Pamelor (nortriptyline)
- Effexor (venlafaxine)
- Nardil (phenelzine)
- Paxil (paroxetine)
- Prozac (fluoxetine)
- Tofranil (imipramine)
- Zoloft (sertraline)

Sedatives
- Luminal (phenobarbital)

Recreational drugs/abused substances
- Alcohol
- Amphetamines
- Cocaine (high dosage)
- Methadone (neptazane)
- Narcotics (high dosage)

ication listed in the table, discuss your difficulty with a healthcare professional. Even if you're in good health, if you have been orgasmic in the past but now you're unable to orgasm and there are no psychological factors in your life to explain this loss of ability, seek a medical consultation. Sometimes the emergence of sexual symptoms can signal the early stages of a medical condition that has not yet been diagnosed.

Medical interventions may include diagnostic testing, changes in prescribed medications, the addition of medications that increase blood flow to the pelvic area, or a more aggressive management of your medical condition. Because orgasm usually requires adequate sexual arousal, the same factors that can interfere with arousal can also inhibit orgasm. Read about medication adjustments and devices to increase sexual arousal described in Chapter 15. Much of this information will also apply to orgasm difficulties that are the result of medical conditions and medication side effects.

COULD THERE BE SOME PSYCHOLOGICAL REASON?

Again, you may want to review Chapter 15 to understand some of the common reasons for not being able to get turned on, because arousal difficulties can lead to orgasm difficulties.

You may find that you do get physically and emotionally aroused during sexual activity but that you reach a plateau and can't get beyond it. It may feel like some invisible barrier is preventing you from "going over the top." This can be very frustrating. Here are some common causes for, or contributors to, this barrier.

Insufficient Learning

Sexual response is natural in that everyone has the inborn potential to experience it, but learned behaviors can—and do—have an impact on it. Even though you have a natural capacity to experience orgasm, you may need to first learn how to realize this inborn potential. If not, you could experience the contractions and spasms of orgasm, perhaps weakly, but fail to interpret these feelings as signals of orgasm. As a result, you could ignore the sensations or fail to focus on them in a way that would embellish and strengthen the orgasmic response.

Culture greatly influences sexual learning. Anthropologists studying various tribes and societies around the world have noted that women coming from cultures encouraging sexual exploration and assertiveness experience orgasm more readily and with greater satisfaction than women coming from cultures that encourage modest, passive behavior. These observations highlight the importance of taking care of your sexual self: learning about your body, learning to experience sexual pleasure without shame or guilt, and learning to take responsibility for your sexual satisfaction rather than relying on your partner to take care of you.

Orgasm Watching

Even if you're aroused, obsessive self-observation can prevent you from achieving an orgasm. If you become obsessed with watching for any sign of a pending orgasm, you're likely to shut yourself down. Perhaps you feel self-conscious about taking what you feel is too long to orgasm or you may be worried that the orgasm will never come. You can get so caught up in monitoring your sexual response that you become a spectator rather than a participant in the sexual activity. At these times, your erotic focus, which is critical for heightening and sustaining arousal, is replaced by anxious vigilance. By wanting the orgasm so badly, you can end up preventing it from happening.

"Just like Meg Ryan in *When Harry Met Sally,* I can fake my orgasm. I start out with the best of intentions. I promise myself: *not this time.* But my partner won't leave me alone till I come. Even if I've enjoyed myself and want to stop, I can't until I've done my orgasm-thing."

A common variation on orgasm-watching is feeling pressured to orgasm to please your partner. As we discussed earlier, some partners feel that their sexual prowess is in doubt if the woman doesn't orgasm. If you dread disappointing your partner, you may try too hard to manufacture a response that should emerge naturally. Trying to force a natural orgasm response is like trying to force a laugh when you're under pressure. You know it's not from your heart. Orgasms require you to focus on your genuine sense of pleasure, not worry about your partner.

Fear of Losing Control

An orgasm, as brief as it may seem, is nevertheless a powerful experience. In addition to the involuntary muscular contractions in the pelvis, the body experiences sudden changes in heart rate, breathing, blood pressure, and brain-wave activity. Your body may spasm. Uncensored words and sounds may blurt out. Even the clarity of your thinking is affected for a brief moment. Researchers have suggested that one of the reasons people have difficulty accurately describing what an orgasm feels like is that at the moment of orgasm, your observing thought processes are temporarily suspended.

Although for many women the brief moments of total surrender to these powerful body reactions feel like ecstasy, some women are threatened by the prospect of not being in control at all times. Women are often conditioned to be vigilant in sexual situations, to be wary of manipulation, exploitation, or violence. This wariness can be so strong that the unconscious mind will put a cap on arousal when a loss of control seems imminent.

Feeling Self-Conscious

Moaning, thrashing, and screaming may make for hot literature in romance novels, but you may balk at the prospect of such behavior for yourself. We're not saying that uninhibited orgasm has to be that dramatic; orgasm can be quiet yet intense. But you might be afraid that the gyrations of orgasm, dramatic or subtle, will make you look ridiculous. You may find it difficult to ignore your childhood lessons about acting like a lady or being a good little girl. While worrying about image and propriety, you may find it difficult, if not impossible, to throw yourself into lovemaking with abandon.

Holding Back Feelings

Sometimes people find it necessary to hold back intense feelings. Perhaps you harbor rage at your partner but dare not express it. Perhaps you feel grief over the death of a loved one, a grief so great that you keep it buried far away from conscious thought. Efforts to hold back strong emotions can spill over into your sexual life. It's difficult to keep strong emotions submerged; the task can easily become an all-or-nothing proposition. Giving free reign to any emotion creates the risk of other emotions surfacing at the same time. In such cases, the mind becomes the jailer, conscientiously guarding against the escape of unwanted emotions. Out of self-protection, all intense emotions, including sexual feelings, become suspect; they're discouraged, denied, controlled, or avoided.

The exercises at the end of this chapter encourage you to experiment with "letting go" during sexual activity. If the exercises don't help, we encourage you to try sex therapy. If you are holding back your feelings without even realizing it, your therapist can help you unblock them in a safe and constructive way.

A Battleground for Your Relationship

Sometimes the inability to orgasm is a reflection of problems in your relationship. You may be angry with your partner but haven't acknowledged it, or perhaps you don't know how or don't want to express these feelings directly. Whether unconscious or conscious, you might engage in what is called passive–aggressive behavior: you may hold back at the moment of orgasm, not wanting to give your partner the satisfaction of feeling sexually potent or competent. Conversely, your partner may engage in his or her own passive–aggressive behavior by subtly sabotaging your orgasm. By emotionally holding back or perhaps acting moody or disappointed during lovemaking, your partner can sufficiently distract you so that you don't orgasm. Your disappointment, frustration, or sense of failure would be your punishment. This holding back can be intentional and premeditated, but more often it's an example of the unconscious mind at work. At the conscious level, both partners remain puzzled; their only awareness is that a certain level of excitement is attained and then things level off and go no further. Unconsciously, however, someone is getting even.

Control issues are another example of how relationship problems can inhibit your orgasm. If you feel powerless in your relationship, you may jealously guard the few areas in which you still have control. One of those areas can be sexuality. At an unconscious level, you can find satisfaction in the fact that you, and you alone, have the power to bring yourself to orgasm. You may be reluctant to share this power with your partner, preferring instead to exert control over one of the few areas in which you have power in the relationship.

The reasoning from these two last examples may seem illogical, but remember, the unconscious mind is not governed by the normal rules of logic. As irrational as unconscious motivations may seem, they can be powerful determinants of behavior, until they are explored and understood.

As you work on the self-help exercises at the end of this chapter, you may become aware of similar relationship problems affecting your sex life. If so, this could be a valuable discovery—and hopefully you and your partner will decide to address these problems before they do serious harm to your relationship.

TAKING CHARGE OF YOUR ORGASMS

If you find it difficult or impossible to orgasm, the following exercises may help you increase your sexual satisfaction. These exercises are designed to increase arousal and to help you overcome barriers to orgasm. Even if sexual arousal is not a problem for you, consider going through all of the exercises. When you pick and choose exercises, you run the risk of inadvertently missing an important building block for constructing a solution to your sexual difficulty.

Before starting the exercises, you may find it useful to review the general guidelines for self-help listed in Chapter 13. Pay particular attention to the material in the section titled "Instructions for Self-Help Exercises."

EXERCISES FOR LEARNING TO ORGASM

SELF-ASSESSMENT

Introduction

The answers to these questions can give you important insight into your sexual concerns and pinpoint where to begin addressing them.

Directions

Spend time reflecting on the questions listed in the self-assessment section of Chapter 13 and on the questions listed below. Consider taking the time to write down your answers on paper or in a journal.

- Are there health issues I need to discuss with my physician?
- In recent months have there been times when I've wanted sex, looked forward to sex, missed sex, or just downright felt horny? (If the answer is no, read Chapter 14.)
- During sex, do I usually get turned on and feel pleasurable feelings? (If the answer is no, read Chapter 15.)
- Are there times when I can reach orgasm? What makes those times different from times when I don't orgasm?
- How does my partner feel about my orgasm difficulty?

Reflection

It can be difficult to orgasm when a person has low sexual desire. Usually for an orgasm to occur, a person must reach an intense level of sexual arousal. If sexual desire is low or if it is difficult for a person to become sexually aroused, these issues should be addressed before focusing on orgasm.

If the only time you cannot orgasm is during intercourse, many experts would tell you that you don't have a sexual dysfunction. More than two-thirds of American women do not regularly orgasm during intercourse. The important distinction is: if the stimulation is appropriate, can you orgasm when your partner is present? If you can't, you probably have a relationship issue or inhibition that you may choose to work on.

If you're feeling pressured by your partner's reaction to your difficulty with orgasm, are you talking about it? Discussing the self-help steps you're about to begin could be a valuable way to start a constructive dialogue with your partner about sexual issues.

Next Steps

- If appropriate, schedule an appointment with your physician.
- Move on to the next exercise.

BODY WORK: INTRODUCTION

Directions

Complete the "Body Work: Introduction" exercise in Chapter 15.

BODY WORK: PELVIC FLOOR MUSCLES

Directions

Complete the "Body Work: Pelvic Floor Muscles" exercise in Chapter 15.

BODY WORK: UP CLOSE AND PERSONAL

Directions

Complete the "Body Work: Up Close and Personal" exercise in Chapter 15.

FANTASY

Directions

Complete the "Fantasy" exercise in Chapter 15.

AN ACADEMY AWARD PERFORMANCE[1]

Introduction

Orgasm can be a powerful experience involving involuntary sounds and movements. Some women are fearful of losing control during an orgasm and appearing foolish. Play-acting can help to loosen you up and desensitize you so that the prospect of a dramatic orgasm won't seem so threatening.

Directions

When the house is empty, lie back and relax. To help create a sensual mood, you may want to read erotic literature or fantasize about a sexy scene. You may want to listen to music. Some women prefer quiet music, others prefer high-energy, get-the-body dancing music.

Role-play the most dramatic, violent orgasm imaginable. Pull out all of the stops. Start by moving your hips, rocking them up and down or side to side. Press your thighs together and tense your muscles in your feet, legs, and arms. Try quickening the pace of your breathing. Begin making sounds—moaning sounds, groaning sounds, sounds of unendurable pleasure. Try to let go and roll and thrash about; claw the sheets or pillow with your fingernails; moan, groan, and yell in fake ecstasy.

Reflection

Most women who do this exercise at some point start laughing at themselves, feeling ridiculous going through such dramatics. Laughing at yourself is great; sex needs to be more playful. More importantly, succeeding in this exercise, despite feeling mildly embarrassed and self-conscious, serves as good practice for loosening up internal control over your behavior.

If propriety and a sense of decorum prevented you from doing this exercise, even though you were alone and no one could observe you, you have highlighted a possible barrier to reaching orgasm. You may choose to do further work to loosen up, to allow yourself to feel freely and express your pleasure and joy without fears about appearance or criticism. Take some time to analyze your hesitation. Try to identify self-defeating thinking and experiment with the cognitive restructuring techniques described in Chapter 13.

Next Steps

- Keep working on cognitive restructuring until you feel more comfortable role-playing a dramatic orgasm.
- Move on to the next exercise.

[1]This exercise has been adapted from the work of Julia Heiman and Joseph LoPiccolo (1988) in their book, *Becoming Orgasmic: A Sexual and Personal Growth Program for Women.*

MASTURBATION

Directions

Read the introduction to the "Masturbation" exercise in Chapter 15, and after following the directions, read the "Reflection" section below to help you focus on the key outcomes and possible sticking points of this exercise.

Reflection

What did you learn about your body's responses? Were you aware of small waves of sensation that might have been orgasmic sensations that you have not yet learned to interpret? Did you push beyond what you knew was pleasurable to a point of almost uncomfortable overstimulation? Next time, back off at this point.

To process this exercise further, read the "Reflection" section of the "Masturbation " exercise in Chapter 15.

Next Steps

- Follow through by cognitively restructuring any negative or self-defeating thinking.
- Repeat this exercise, modifying and customizing the steps until you become comfortable and find the experience pleasurable.
- If you are unable to experience an orgasm after repeating this exercise a number of times, continue to the next exercise.
- If you're now experiencing orgasm regularly when you self-stimulate (not necessarily all the time, but often), the next exercise is optional. If you decide to skip the "Good Vibrations" exercise, proceed to the "Designing the Ideal Encounter" exercise.

GOOD VIBRATIONS

Introduction

A woman with lifelong orgasm difficulty may have significant barriers erected against experiencing orgasm. Fear of orgasm or sexual inhibition can create an unusually high stimulation threshold for orgasm. In many cases the increased stimulation from a vibrator surpasses this threshold and leads to an orgasm. For some women, once the first orgasm occurs, the level of fear and apprehension is lowered dramatically—which, in turn, lowers the stimulation threshold. Orgasms become easier to achieve and require less stimulation. For other women, intense stimulation may always or frequently be required due to a naturally high threshold for orgasm. For these women, a vibrator becomes a perfectly acceptable aid to help heighten sexual arousal.

Directions

Purchase a vibrator. You can purchase an all-purpose vibrator (the kind that strap on the back of your hand) at major retail stores, or you can mail-order a wide variety of vibrators specifically designed for genital stimulation.[2] A vibrator should be kept clean with soap and water. Consider a vibrator as private and personal as a toothbrush. Do not use a vibrator on the anus and transfer stimulation to the vagina or vulva without thoroughly cleaning the vibrator first.

Before attempting stimulation with a vibrator, take time to relax. Use the masturbation techniques from the previous exercise to become aroused.

Experiment with applying the vibrator to different parts of your body. The guiding principle is: *if it feels good, do it more before moving on.* The type of genital stimulation you get will depend on the type of vibrator you use. All vibrators allow direct and indirect stimulation of the clitoris. Use varying degrees of intensity until you identify what works best for you. Some vibrators not only allow you to stimulate your external genitalia but are designed for vaginal penetration; you can also stimulate the inner walls of the vagina. Using a vibrator in this way makes it easier to reach the G spot and experiment with sustained, applied pressure. As with any sexually pleasuring activity, there may be times when this stimulation is effective for you, and times when you may prefer another type of stimulation.

Reflection

Do you have any concerns about using a vibrator? Some women fear developing a dependency on a vibrator to the point that it becomes the only way that they can respond sexually. No scientific foundation supports this concern; you will not become addicted to your vibrator!

Sometimes a partner can feel threatened by the woman's use of a vibrator and worry that somehow he or she is failing or that the woman is losing interest in him or her in favor of a mechanical lover. In such instances, dialogue and reassurance are important. The partner needs to be reassured that the use of the vibrator is not an indictment against him or her as a lover. It should be pointed out that plastic and batteries can never compete with flesh-to-flesh contact and emotional intimacy.

Next Steps

- If orgasm continues to elude you, don't be disheartened. Remember that orgasm is a learned response, and you are still learning. If you're in a relationship, continue to the next exercise. Perhaps the above exercises will be more potent when they're combined with efforts to enhance emotional and physical intimacy with your partner. If the following exercises are not applicable because you're not in a relationship, consider seeking sexual counseling for additional help.
- If you are now able to orgasm, the following exercises will help you to transfer this ability into lovemaking (not necessarily intercourse) with your partner.

---

[2]Three popular mail-order vendors are Adam and Eve (1-800-293-4654, www.adameve.com), Toys in Babeland (1-800-658-9119, www.babeland.com), and Good Vibrations (1-800-289-8423, www.goodvibes.com).

DESIGNING THE IDEAL ENCOUNTER

Directions

Complete the "Designing the Ideal Encounter" exercise in Chapter 15.

PARTNER WORK: CAN WE TALK?

Directions

If you don't have a sexual partner, skip to "Next Steps" at the end of the "Partner Work: Sensate Focus" exercise. Otherwise, complete the "Partner Work: Can We Talk?" exercise in Chapter 15.

PARTNER WORK: SENSATE FOCUS

Introduction

The previous exercises were designed to help you learn to orgasm in private. The sensate focus exercise provides a safe, structured environment for you to apply what you've learned about orgasm to sexual encounters with your partner.

Directions

Complete the "Partner Work: Sensate Focus" exercise in Chapter 15.

Reflection

To help focus on the key outcomes and possible sticking points of this exercise, review the "Reflection" section of the "Getting Back to Basics" exercise found in Chapter 14.

Next Steps

If at this point you're not experiencing orgasm with some regularity, consider getting additional help. Be sure, however, that you have given yourself enough time to do all of the exercises. If you need to consult with a therapist, remember that it's not a negative reflection on you and it does not mean that you have a bigger problem than the other 25% of American women who find it difficult to orgasm. It merely means that you need a more customized approach than can be provided by a book like this.

In the "Suggested Resources" section, we list books that specifically focus on becoming orgasmic. You may find additional exercises in these books that will help you.

If you've noticed an improvement in your ability to orgasm, move on to the next set of directions.

GOING ON FROM HERE

Directions

Take the techniques that work for you and incorporate them when having intercourse (e.g., stimulating your nipples, fingering your clitoris, etc.). If coital orgasm is important to you, experiment with positions that maximize stimulation of the front wall of the vagina (where the G spot is located) or positions that allow you or your partner to use a vibrator during intercourse. If orgasm remains elusive during intercourse, don't be frustrated. Remember that coital anorgasmia is very common. If you can't orgasm during intercourse, be sure that intercourse is not the only way you're pleasured during lovemaking. Keep working with your partner to ensure that your lovemaking follows a new script that is responsive to both of your needs.

Continue to find time each week to explore and enjoy your sexuality, whether it's taking a warm, sensuous shower, musing over erotic images and fantasies, stimulating yourself to orgasm, or making love with your partner.

Periodically review your work on the exercises above. Review progress on your action plans and continue to monitor for negative thinking so that you can replace it with your new ideas, perceptions, and insights.

CHAPTER SEVENTEEN

Sex Therapy

If you develop a sexual problem, the first question you need answered is whether the symptom has a medical cause. If there is any possibility of a medical problem, always start by consulting your physician or a medical specialist. Chapter 13 offers suggestions for finding a good healthcare professional and for talking to your doctor once you do. If you discover that your symptoms aren't medical, or that in addition to medical treatment your problem requires psychological help, you may find the exercises in the preceding chapters helpful. Sometimes, though, self-help will not be enough. Many sexual problems require professional help by a clinician trained to do sex therapy.

In this final chapter, we talk about what sex therapy is and isn't, what to expect if you go into sex therapy, and how to find a qualified sex therapist.

SEX THERAPY: WHAT IS IT?

Sex therapy, like most forms of therapy, is designed to be both a healing and a growth process. What makes it distinct from other forms of psychotherapy is that what brings the person through the office door is a sexual problem, as opposed to anxiety, depression, or stress. The client is looking for treatment that is designed specifically to correct a sexual problem. Even so, sex therapy doesn't focus solely on sex. Our sexuality is woven into our lives, making it impossible to isolate our focus on sex alone. As we discussed in Part I, "Knowing Your Sexual Story," it's impossible to have an understanding of your sexuality without taking into consideration your upbringing, religious beliefs, health, relationships, self-esteem, psychiatric status, and more. As a matter of fact, it's hard to talk about any of these topics without also talking about sex, because sex is such an important part of life.

Because sex influences so much in our lives, and so many things in our lives influence our sexuality, sex therapy usually begins with a comprehensive review of upbringing, relationships, and current level of adjustment. The sex therapist then makes suggestions about what factors may be contributing to the sexual symptom and, more important, what steps can help resolve the difficulty. In this process, most sex therapists focus on quality of life—preferring to work toward helping the client realize his or her potential to live and love most fully, as opposed to helping the client increase orgasms by 20% or have sex as frequently as the national average.

The sex therapist may treat the client individually, in a group, or, most often, together with the client's partner. In sex therapy we try to downplay the notion of illness or sickness. Instead, we approach the presenting problem as a shared opportunity for the couple to discover ways of increasing emotional and physical intimacy. The client or the couple is encouraged to find pleasure in their sexuality and to become more comfortable giving and receiving pleasure. Treatment will include identifying and examining feelings, gaining insight into reasons for maladaptive behavior, improving communication, learning new ways to approach old problems, and building on the client's or couple's inherent strengths.

WHAT TO EXPECT IN SEX THERAPY

Because sex therapy is often the subject of jokes and parodies, the public has developed many misconceptions about this valuable form of treatment. Be assured that in legitimate sex therapy, you will not be asked to take off your clothes, have sex with your partner in front of the therapist, or have sex with the therapist. You should, at all times, feel that you are being treated in a professional manner and that your values and religious beliefs are respected.

The cost and length of treatment vary. Depending on where you live and your therapist's credentials, sex therapy can range from $80 to $150 a session. Some health insurance plans will cover the cost, or part of the cost, of sex therapy. If you can afford only a limited number of visits, sex therapy can still be helpful and effective. Even a session or two can be enough to explore and correct misinformation, lead you to self-help resources, identify unrealistic expectations that you may have of yourself and/or your partner, and alert you to other problems that might complicate the resolution of your symptoms.

The length of treatment can range from a couple of visits to many months of weekly sessions. If the focus of treatment expands to resolving longstanding, deep-seated problems, therapy can go on for more than a year. Your therapist should be able to give you an estimate of how many sessions will be required to accomplish your treatment goals. Here is a caution, however. Very often in therapy the problem that brings a person in may be defined differently as things move along. For example, a couple may come into therapy insisting that they have a wonderful relationship and that their only problem is that they can't agree on the frequency of sex. At first glance this may appear to be a straightforward case that shouldn't require more than a dozen sessions. But if it becomes clear during the first few sessions that there are significant relationship problems, the focus and projected length of treatment will have to change dramatically.

As we indicated above, if you are in a relationship, your therapist will probably encourage you to include your partner in treatment. If you are seen as a couple, the therapist will likely keep individual sessions to a minimum and focus on helping the two of you work through your concerns together.

Many sex therapists will use "homework assignments" to help both partners discover patterns in their sexual relationship. These assignments also provide opportunities to learn and practice new, more adaptive ways to relate. Assigned reading and the use of instructional videos are often part of treatment.

It's important to understand that, at times, you may feel uncomfortable in sex therapy. The therapist will ask you detailed questions about your sexual history. You will be encouraged to take an honest look at how you and your partner relate. The struggles you have and the ways you avoid intimacy will be discussed with the goal of helping you both grow. You and your partner will be encouraged to be honest about your needs and frustrations in the relationship.

Why, you may ask, would anyone willingly put him- or herself into such an awkward position? Usually it is because a person or couple is no longer willing to accept the status quo and honestly wishes to change things for the better. They accept that meaningful growth doesn't come easily and that if they can tolerate the momentary discomfort that comes from the process of growing, they can achieve deeper passion and intimacy.

FINDING A SEX THERAPIST

Because a therapist is a social worker, psychiatrist, psychologist, or nurse does not guarantee that she or he has the expertise to treat sexual disorders. When considering sex therapy, you will want to look for a skilled mental health professional who has additional training and experience in the area of human sexuality.

With less than an hour of research, you should be able to find qualified sex therapists in your community. The American Association of Sex Educators, Counselors, and Therapists (AASECT) is a national organization that certifies sex therapists. You can contact AASECT by phone (804-644-3288) or at its website (www.aasect.org) for a list of certified sex therapists in your area. There are also many excellent sex therapists who do not have formal certification but are well-trained and highly experienced in treating sexual problems. Ask your healthcare provider if he or she can recommend a qualified sex therapist. If you live near a university, contact the psychology or social work department and ask for recommendations. Call your state psychological association, psychiatric association, or the state office for the National Association of Social Workers (NASW) for recommendations. Check the Yellow Pages under *Psychologists*; *Counselors*; or *Marriage, Family, Child, and Individual Counselors* and look for therapists who specialize in treating sexual problems.

Once you have the name of a therapist, call and ask questions before scheduling your first appointment. Find out about the therapist's training and experience in treating sexual problems. Ask about the cost of therapy and whether the therapist accepts insurance. If the therapist is unwilling to answer these basic questions, you may want to keep searching. As a consumer, you have the right to know what kind of services you're purchasing.

Besides competence, what other characteristics should you look for in a sex therapist? People sometimes wonder whether they should see a female or male therapist. Research shows that sex therapy can be effective regardless of the therapist's gender. What is far more important than gender is your comfort level with the therapist. You need to be able to trust your therapist and feel that he or she is concerned about your well-being and is respectful of your circumstances, feelings, and beliefs.

If you don't feel you have a comfortable rapport with your therapist after a few sessions, discuss your concerns. If you still feel uncomfortable, consider transferring to another therapist. Be careful, though, that by changing therapists you're not "shooting the messenger." As we discussed earlier, in order to grow you will likely have to face things that will make you feel uncomfortable. It can be tempting to blame the therapist for this discomfort rather than asking what it is about yourself, your background, or your relationship that might be creating this discomfort. If you want to change therapists, be sure that you're reacting to "bad chemistry" and not to the pain and embarrassment that is coming from the truth.

CONCLUSION

If your car's engine breaks down, you'll repair it. If your car's cigarette lighter breaks, even if you're a smoker, you'll probably let it slide. Far too many people view their sexuality like the cigarette lighter, an accessory they can live without. We hope that throughout this book we have made a case for just the opposite. Sexuality should be considered as important as a car's air-conditioner in the middle of summer or a car's heater in the frigid months of winter. You can get around without them, but they sure can make the ride much more pleasurable.

Sexual problems should not be ignored. They can harm our self-esteem, place a strain on our relationships, and, in some cases, serve as a warning for undiagnosed medical problems. For these reasons, if you develop a sexual problem, you should not suffer silently. Medical and psychological help are available and highly effective. When in need, make use of them.

Reading this book can be an important step in overcoming a sexual problem. We encourage you to take as many additional steps as necessary to continue your journey to sexual health and satisfaction.

APPENDIX

Exercises for Sexual Growth

The following exercises are designed to enhance your awareness and understanding of your sexuality and to promote your sexual growth. You might be inspired to try them by something you learned about yourself in one of the chapters in this book. Or you might turn to these exercises as part of a regular commitment to developing your sexual potential. Either way, we hope you will stick with it once you decide to try a particular exercise. View the exercises as an opportunity to do something positive for yourself, something that can continue to enrich your life for years to come. Set aside a regular time to work on them. If possible, discuss the exercises with your partner—make this a shared project. If any of the instructions make you feel overly uncomfortable, or if they violate your personal or moral values, feel free to modify them to make them acceptable. The most important thing is that you approach these exercises with a positive attitude. (If you experience a lot of discomfort or come up with disturbing revelations while doing these exercises and suddenly feel that you're in over your head, don't hesitate to seek professional help. Chapter 13 offers suggestions for what to do if problems arise.)

Each group of exercises corresponds to a particular section of the book. You can work your way through the exercises in the sequence in which they appear or choose the ones that are right for you.

Each exercise begins with *directions*. After you follow a set of instructions, a *reflection* section helps focus your attention on key themes and possible areas that need more attention. We also suggest the *next steps* to be taken following the completion of the exercise.

WAYS TO KNOW YOUR SEXUAL STORY

A significant part of our sexual history is the experience of our own bodies. To be oblivious of our bodies is to be insensitive to the pleasures that they can produce. To be alienated from our bodies is to be deprived of a means of connecting with special people in our lives. The beginning of your body awareness will be found in memories. Whether or not you consciously recall these memories, they influence attitudes about your body, yourself, and your sexuality. By recalling and understanding these early memories, you can better understand your adult response and take action to change it.

Your Body's Historical Timeline

This first exercise focuses on the history of your *body's physical changes*. The next exercise focuses on the history of your *sexual experiences*. As your body changed, so did your perceptions of your physical self. Your Body's Historical Timeline is a way of reviewing and recording your personal history. Just as researching and recording a family history can help you understand and take pride in your heritage, writing your body history can help you feel more accepting of, and grounded in, your body. This history is unique to you. It can influence not only how you feel about your body but also how you care for it now and as you grow older.

YOUR BODY'S HISTORICAL TIMELINE

Directions

- You will need paper, a ruler, and a pen. Turn paper to horizontal position for more space. To make a timeline, draw a long line across the center of the paper. You will need to keep expanding this line, possibly across several sheets of paper. Leave plenty of room to write along it.
- At the beginning of the line, write your date of birth, the time you were born (if you know it), and whether your birth was vaginal or Cesarean section. Now think about all the early years of your physical development and how you changed.
- Note as many changes in your physical self as you can remember through the years. If you can't recall something precisely, write down your "best guess" about the time of the physical change.
- Include physical changes that enabled you to master the new skills and abilities that became the milestones in your development. Your personal milestones will be different from anyone else's. The changes you choose to highlight may have meaning only for you, such as learning how to handle a wrench and other tools so you could fix your own bicycle, or learning to swim so you could join the bigger kids at the dock.
- Make sure to include sexual changes in your body, such as when you started your pe-

riod or noticed breast tenderness and pubic hair. Premenstrual symptoms (PMS) and perimenopausal symptoms (if applicable) are also part of your physical self.

- Some changes aren't changes at all but simply the discovery of a quality that had always been present. If you are a woman of color, for example, you may have had an early, dawning awareness that advertisements all around you were geared predominantly toward Caucasian-featured people. If you were taller than your peer group, perhaps you never paid attention to your size until another girl made fun of you.
- Sometimes temporary or permanent changes in the body occur because of decisions you make, such as becoming pregnant or terminating a pregnancy. The impact of these decisions can occupy a unique place in one's history. Sometimes decisions are positive and a matter of personal choice, such as beginning and maintaining an exercise program. Some decisions, such as abusing drugs or engaging in unprotected sex, are self-defeating. Some decisions can be striking in their importance, such as deciding between a mastectomy and a lumpectomy for breast cancer.
- Keep noting the changes up until your present age. The list may take several days to complete. Make additions as you remember them. You may notice that there are clusters of dates that coincide with developmental milestones such as entering puberty, having a baby, or entering menopause.
- Reflect on each change by asking yourself these questions:

  Did I understand that my body was changing?

  Did anyone give me information or talk to me in order to help me cope with the change?

  Was I shamed or treated negatively as a result of my body's change?

  Did I think I was the only one having this change?

  Did I learn to talk to others about the body change at a later time?

  Was I kind to my body as the change occurred?

Reflection

Reflect on your timeline by asking yourself the following questions:

- Have I had unrealistic expectations for my body?
- Have I let social pressure or advertising negatively influence me as my body has changed?
- Have I loved my body as it is?
- Do I want to love my body as it is?
- What will I give up by loving my body just as it is?
- What will I gain by loving my body just as it is?

As you review your timeline, reflect on what the experience was like to move from the body of a child to that of a woman.

- Were there times of happiness as well as times of grieving?
- Have you found positive aspects in your growth and change, or only negative?
- Did you minimize or downplay the changes as you got older?

- Have you given your body credit for carrying you through so much life?
- Can you be proud of your body and your story?

Next Steps

Continue to update your body awareness timeline as you undergo more physical experiences.

If you take the time to do this exercise, you may make some interesting discoveries about your history. Earlier in your life you may have gone through important physical changes alone and without support. At those times, you may have thought you weren't important or didn't matter to other people. Because of your body changes, you may have been treated negatively by others. When this happened, perhaps a part of you believed that there was something wrong with you. By making a timeline, you are able to look at your history more objectively and challenge unfair and hurtful beliefs about yourself. You are taking back your own history and honoring it.

Keeping your timeline current serves as a reminder that you're aware that your body changes and evolves throughout your life and that you don't have to ignore or ridicule those changes. Ultimately, you have the choice about how you feel about yourself and your body.

Sexual History Timeline

Every woman, whether or not she is sexually active with another person, is a sexual being. The Sexual History Timeline focuses on your sexual identity as a woman. As your body changed, so did your awareness of yourself as a sexual person. From childhood, this awareness may have expanded from first noting that touching your vulva was pleasurable, to sexual thoughts and fantasies, to a crush on "the boy next door," to masturbating while dreaming of movie stars, to kissing and fondling your boyfriend, to sexual interaction with your partner. This expanding sexual awareness is a part of a woman's sexual story. Every woman has a sexual story, and each woman's story is unique.

SEXUAL HISTORY TIMELINE

Directions

Turn a piece of paper to the horizontal position and make a timeline by drawing a long line across the center of the paper. On the far left side of the line, write the date you were born. This begins your sexual history. Now note as many experiences as you can remember or were told about. As a child, early sexual awareness might have involved peeking at your baby brother's penis or rubbing your vulva. If you can't remember something exactly, just write down your "best guess" about the time. Check back with your "Body's History Timeline" for reminders about physical changes that might have prompted sexual activity.

The list will take some time to complete and may become lengthy. You can work on it over a period of days or weeks. As the list develops, you may notice that clusters of dates and sexual activities center on developmental milestones. You will not have every experience on this list, nor will you have them in the order listed.

Not all sexual awareness or activity that you remember will be positive. For instance, a woman's first sexual experience with another person could have been sexual harassment or abuse. Rape or other degrading or humiliating sexual experiences may have occurred. These should be recorded on the timeline too.

There are limitless possibilities of what could be added to this list. The following list of possible sexual activities may be useful in remembering your sexual history.

SEXUAL ACTIVITY LIST

- Aware of the differences between female and male genitalia
- First time touching your genitals
- First time you experienced a sexual sensation
- Sex play with same-age peers
- Discussions with parents or other adults about sex
- Discussions with other children about sex

- First time you were told about sexual intercourse and how babies were made
- First time you masturbated
- First time masturbating by slipping your finger into your vagina
- First time you masturbated to orgasm

- Sex education in school or church/temple/mosque
- Reading sex education materials or viewing sex education films
- Seeing a live birth of a baby (animal or human) in person or on TV
- Curiosity about sexual behavior or nudity (e.g., looking at pictures or peeking at others)

- Menstruation discussed with peers or adults
- Learning the words "masturbate" and "intercourse"
- Learning sex slang like "fuck" or "clit"
- Awareness of prepubertal changes in your body (pubic hair, breast buds, breast development)

- First time you fantasized about another person
- First daydreams that were sexual
- Doing something sexual that was considered "wrong" or "bad" in your upbringing

- First time feeling guilty about something sexual
- Worrying about development of secondary sexual characteristics or starting your period

- First time being stared at in a sexual way
- Being sexually molested or exploited as a child or adult

- First romantic feelings stirred by a book, movie, or other person
- Having crushes on members of same sex
- Realization of sexual attraction to a female
- Realization of sexual attraction to a male
- First falling in love
- First awareness of sexual arousal resulting in nipple hardening or "getting wet"

- First handholding and hug
- First kiss
- First French kiss
- First "hickey"
- First touching of another's body
- Learning about birth control
- First intense touching, "petting" with clothes on
- First intense touching, "petting" without clothes
- First touching of another person's genitals in sexually arousing play

- Seeing sexually explicit material not made for sex education

- Being harassed sexually

- Learning about the sex industry, especially about women who make their living as sex workers (strippers, prostitutes, etc.)

- First time masturbating by inserting an object into your vagina
- First use of a vibrator or other sex toy

- First sexual intercourse
- First pelvic examination
- Decision to use birth control
- First time spending the night with a partner
- First orgasm in presence of partner

- Recognition of self as a bisexual or lesbian woman
- Coming out as a bisexual or lesbian woman

- First oral sex given
- First oral sex received
- Masturbating partner to orgasm

- Masturbating to orgasm in front of partner
- Using sexual fantasies while masturbating
- Sharing sexual fantasies with a partner
- First anal intercourse

- Being drunk or high while having sex

- Contracting an STD
- First sexual difficulty
- First experience of low or no sexual desire or arousal
- First experience of not being able to orgasm
- Yeast infection or other vaginal problem
- Unable to lubricate when having sex
- Sadomasochistic (S/M) behavior in a sexual relationship

- Being paid for having sex
- Being paid for making sexually explicit photographs or videos

- Being beaten up while having sex
- Group sex or swinging
- Watched by others while having sex

- Getting pregnant when not in a permanent partnership
- Having sex after decision to terminate a pregnancy—with same partner
- Having sex after decision to terminate a pregnancy—with different partner

- First sexual awareness of permanent partner
- Falling in love with permanent partner
- First sexual experience with permanent partner
- First intercourse with permanent partner

- Sex when trying to get pregnant
- Sex while pregnant
- Sex postpartum
- Having sex when fatigued from childrearing

- Sexual involvement outside your permanent partnership
- Your permanent partner having sex outside your relationship
- Falling in love outside your partnership

- Dating and sexual involvement after divorce
- Dating and sexual involvement after being widowed
- Continuing to masturbate after divorced or widowed

- Having sex after tubal ligation, hysterectomy, or other reproductive surgery

- Perimenopausal symptoms depressing sexual interest
- Having sex after diagnosis/treatment for illness

- Having sex after menopause
- Having sex with problem of urinary incontinence
- Having sex after significant weight loss or weight gain
- Having sex with a new partner, postmenopause
- Masturbating to orgasm after a change in physical arousal, postmenopause

- Purchasing/using vibrator and lubricants in your fifties
- Purchasing/using sexy lingerie in your sixties
- Having sex or masturbating after working out (exercising) in your seventies
- Watching erotic movies in your eighties

- Asking for specific sexual activity from a partner
- Mutually satisfying sex in a relationship

Reflection

Perhaps you've written short phrases and dates. Maybe you've written a longer narrative. Read back over what you've written. Circle positives and negatives in your experiences. Think about the events and messages that influenced your sexual activity throughout your life.

- In reading through your Sexual History Timeline, you may recognize experiences that sadden you. You may need to take time to grieve that these occurrences happened to you.
- Are there other not-so-wonderful experiences in the past that you now see are important learning events in your sexual journey?
- Are there experiences that you can laugh about?
- Do you see a trend toward becoming more assertive, surer of yourself, more interested in mutual and reciprocal sexual relationships?
- Do you like the sexual self you're becoming? Are you continuing to value yourself sexually?

Next Steps

- The timeline can be used in many ways; it's a journal that can be added to over time.
- You could share your timeline with a friend who has been creating her own Sexual History Timeline. If you're in a relationship, you can encourage your partner to make a timeline. Consider talking about the timelines together. Have you had similar or different experiences? Can you each listen to the other's sexual experiences?
- If you have questions about your sexual orientation, or if you want to look more closely at your orientation, go on to the next exercise, "Your Sexual Orientation." If

you're comfortable in your orientation, move on to the "Living in Your Skin: Ethnicity and Color" exercise.

- If there are aspects of your sexual journey that concern you and affect your ability to have sexual pleasure, you may want to reread the material in Part V, "Overcoming Sexual Difficulties."

Your Sexual Orientation

In Chapter 1 we discussed how many women have memories of loving and being physically expressive with other women. These may be memories of childhood, adolescence, or adulthood. If you are seeking to understand more about your sexual orientation, you may find it helpful to look back over the Sexual History Timeline you've just made and ask yourself the following questions. Write out your responses in a journal or as a letter to yourself.

YOUR SEXUAL ORIENTATION

Directions

Write your responses to the following questions. You can refer to your Sexual History Timeline to remind you of times you felt strongly attracted to women, to men, or to both.

- How early did you know that you felt differently from the girls around you, that you weren't attracted to the heterosexual images you saw?
- As an adolescent, did you date guys? Were you sexual with guys because you were trying to "prove" you had an attraction to males?
- How did you feel when you realized you did not feel an attraction?
- Have you fallen in love with men, women, or both?
- What is your history of sexual activity with others? Has it been with men, women, or both?
- Do you feel comfortable with your sexuality and like yourself sexually?
- Does your attraction to others vary depending on how you are feeling about yourself (your self-esteem)? Are there times when women just feel safer than men?
- What has your fantasy life been like? Is it predominately about heterosexual, lesbian, or bisexual relationships?
- Do you feel mostly attracted to other women but fear the rejection of your family, friends, or coworkers?
- Do you feel mostly attracted to other women but fear religious condemnation or censure?

Alfred Kinsey, the famous sex researcher, defined sexuality along a continuum from straight to gay, with "1" being entirely straight, and "6" being entirely gay. This continuum, commonly known as "the Kinsey scale," allows people to think of themselves as not simply gay *or* straight, but instead to understand their sexuality as a blending of gradations—perhaps being a straight 2 or a gay 4. Draw a line, numbering it from 1 to 6. Draw a circle around the number(s) that reflect your feelings about yourself.

Reflection

For many women, awareness of being attracted to other women emerges over time. Read through your responses and see how they match up with your Sexual History Timeline. Doing this exercise may make you think about words. It's important that you self-define—that you use words that are right for you. Some women identify as straight, others as lesbian or bisexual. Still others may say they are open, questioning, or "a woman who loves women."

Next Steps

- Consider talking with others who are nonjudgmental and supportive.
- Continue to learn about your sexual orientation.
- Read some of the books about lesbian/bisexual identity and relationships listed in the "Suggested Resources" section and visit some of the websites listed there.
- Many women find counseling very helpful as they explore and define their understanding of their orientation. Consider counseling as another form of support.

In completing this exercise, think about what you are committed to and how you lead your life. The commitments you make of your time, interests and energy ultimately define your life; no single act, no one fantasy or relationship, defines who you are. Embrace your totality.

Living in Your Skin: Ethnicity and Color

Just as every woman has a sexual history, every woman has attributes of skin color, geography, and ethnicity. Every woman comes from some group located on some part of the planet; African American, Asian, Indian, Scottish, Hispanic—everyone comes from somewhere. You may live in a country where your family goes back hundreds of years, or you may live in a country to which your family has recently immigrated. If you live in a country like the United States, where many races and ethnicities can be found, your family may have carefully preserved the customs of your ethnic identity, or you may come from a family who doesn't consider themselves ethnic at all. Even if you don't think of yourself ethnically, you may recognize that you think of yourself regionally—like "Southern," "Californian," "Midwesterner," or "New Yorker"—and adopt the region's values and customs.

We refer to the group you identify with, whether it's based on ethnicity, color, religion, or geographic location, as your "community." Your sexuality is influenced by your community, and by the perceptions of outsiders about your community, just as it is influenced by cultural/social influences.

In this exercise, you'll have a chance to reflect on how your community influenced your sexual development and how those influences continue as part of you today. You will not necessarily have had all these experiences or have had them in the order listed.

LIVING IN YOUR SKIN

Directions

This is a journaling exercise, so write down your thoughts as they come to you, before you have time to censor or edit. You may not think certain questions apply to you. If so, write down the question, leave a space after it, and go on to the next question. Later you may find that you have a memory that fits that unanswered question.

Now read through the questions listed below. Each question asks you to think about one aspect of how your family's ethnicity influenced your understanding and experience of sexuality. Think of an experience that reminds you of the question and write down that experience. If you're not sure of your exact age at the time, make your best guess. Because your ethnic community may have different views now than when you were growing up, we ask you to think about the influences on you as you grew up.

- What did your community teach you about sex education?
- If your religion is part of your ethnicity, what did your religion teach about women's sexuality?
- Did your religion teach this through your parents at home or through your church, temple, or mosque?

- Did your community view sexuality more conservatively than the larger culture?
- Did your community have a different standard about public modesty for women than for men?

- Did your community let you choose whom you dated?
- What were the rules about dating in your community?

- What were the rules about clothing or showing your body in your community?
- Did your community place value on a woman's physical beauty?
- How was beauty defined?
- Did your community place value on a woman's size, shape, or skin color?
- Did your community place value on a woman's role as a family member and caregiver?
- What did your community teach you about women's dress and make-up?

- How did your community feel about women shaving their body hair? About body piercing? About tattooing?

- What were the rules in your community about young women flirting?
- What were the rules in your community about older women flirting?
- What were the rules about flirting with others outside your community?

- How did your community feel about women enjoying sexual pleasure?
- Was masturbation ever discussed in your community?
- How did your community view sexual pleasuring, including oral sex?

- Did your community let you choose whom you married?
- How did your community feel about marriage with outsiders?

- What were your community's views about gays and lesbians?

- If you are bilingual, in which language do you make love?
- If bilingual, in which language do you think about sexual terminology?

- If your community is a minority within a larger culture, how did the larger culture's standard of beauty make you feel as you were growing up?
- How does the larger culture make you feel now?
- Growing up, did the larger culture hold negative views about the sexuality of women in your community?
- What were the views you thought the larger culture held about women of your ethnicity or color?

- To what extent have your values been influenced by your community?
- On a scale of 1 to 6, with 1 being the least and 6 being the most, rate your community's influence on you now.

Reflection

- Looking back through your answers, do you see areas of hurt or conflict?
- How have you handled the injuries or conflict?
- Did you find support within your community during hard times?
- Are there women with whom you could share stories and gain support for your ethnicity and sexuality?

Next Steps

- Your feelings about living in your skin may change over time, so periodically review these questions, perhaps thinking of other questions to ask yourself.
- Label two columns **My Community** and **Larger Culture**. List your answers under **My Community**. Now speculate how someone raised in the larger culture would answer the same questions about their upbringing and write those answers under **Larger Cul-**

ture. Compare your answers in each column. How do you feel about any differences? How do you feel about any similarities? Do you feel that your experience has been vastly different?
- Encourage a friend to do her own journaling about living in her skin. Share your notes and experiences. Even if you are of the same ethnic group, your experiences may have been very different.
- If you are in a partnership, what beliefs about color, ethnicity, and sexuality does your partner hold? Share your timeline and encourage your partner to make one too.
- If you are in a biracial marriage, discuss with your partner how the larger culture views sexuality for biracial couples.
- If you are a parent, what beliefs about color, ethnicity, and sexuality would you like to convey to your children?
- If you are a parent, ask your children how they experience their ethnicity and color.

This exercise may bring up painful memories of discrimination and misunderstanding. Perhaps this is the first time you've thought about your sexuality in this way. You may notice how different your experiences were from your parents' expectations. You may notice how much the larger culture has changed (or not changed) in relation to your ethnicity or color. By tracing the history of your body, your sexual development, and the messages from your community, you're ready to tackle the beliefs and attitudes you have about your sexuality.

Beliefs and Attitudes Exercise

Our beliefs about, and attitudes toward sex are shaped over our lifetime and exert a profound influence on our sexual behavior and satisfaction. Beliefs and attitudes shaped by negative experiences or faulty education can hold you back from having a better relationship with your partner and yourself.

In this next exercise you are asked to list your attitudes and beliefs about sexuality and to think about where those beliefs came from and whether they are still meaningful to you. Then, if you choose, you can update your sexual beliefs and attitudes.

BELIEFS AND ATTITUDES

Directions

- Make a list of the following developmental periods:

  Infancy
  Childhood
  Preadolescence
  Adolescence
  Late adolescence and early adulthood—18–29
  Adulthood—30s

Early middle years—40s
Middle years—50s
Later middle years adult years—60s
Older adult years—70s
Early old age—80s
Old age—90s

- Write down any sexual beliefs or attitudes you have for each developmental period. For instance, for "Infancy" you might write: "Infants are not sexual" or "A baby's sexuality should be protected."
- To help identify your beliefs and attitudes, read through your work from the other exercises ("Body Language," "Body History Timeline," "Sexual History Timeline," and "Living in Your Skin"). Think about the beliefs and attitudes you learned or developed as a result of these experiences.
- Next to each belief or attitude, write down where you think it came from—who or what influenced this belief or attitude?
- As you look at your list, do you see attitudes and beliefs that you'd like to revise, perhaps based on your life experience, reading this book, or talking with others?

Reflection

Reading through your list can be a periodic activity that recharges your awareness "batteries." You may want to ask a friend what she was taught and what she believes now about sex. If you're in a relationship, you can ask your partner about his or her attitudes and beliefs. If you're in contact with your siblings, ask them how their attitudes and beliefs were shaped by your family's environment. Try to be nonjudgmental in sharing and listening to yourself and others.

Next Steps

- Because attitudes and beliefs may change over time, periodically review your list and note any changes, even "small ones."
- If you're in a partnership, try to come up with a shared list of attitudes and beliefs.
- If you're a parent, ask yourself what beliefs you would like to convey to your children about female sexuality and sexual interaction. Think about initiating conversations with your children on this topic.
- If you're a parent, use your own sexual journey as an opportunity to provide sex education and values clarification for your children. Ask your children to articulate their views about sex. Discuss different sexual scenarios and how their beliefs about sex would apply. Share your own thoughts and beliefs in relation to the scenarios. Remember that this is a "discussion-in-process," not a "one time only" opportunity. When talking with anyone about his or her attitudes and beliefs, you are treading near the very core of that individual's personality and identity. You'll need to move gently, avoid preaching, and revisit the discussions regularly.

WAYS TO UNDERSTAND YOUR BODY

Following are two exercises to help you become more familiar and comfortable with your body.

Body Language Exercise

How you experience yourself as a person begins with the words you use to describe your body. Though everyone has a general language of body terms, we've discovered that some women have never developed an intimate, private language for their bodies, and many women never learned the proper terms for the sexual parts of their bodies. Some haven't taken time to think about what parts of their bodies are sexually responsive. When you think about and name the sexual parts of your body, you are acknowledging the importance of your sexuality. The following exercise is designed to help you develop your own body language.

BODY LANGUAGE

Directions

- Find a comfortable place to sit or stretch out. Have a pad of paper and a pen ready. Beginning with your toes, think of each part of your body, perhaps even touching that part, and then write down the name you use for that part of your body. Don't type this assignment—using your own handwriting is important.
- Look at your list, studying each word carefully. Did you leave any words out? What words did you use for your genitals? What do you call other sexual parts of your body?
- Circle any word that is a put-down or a negative word. Remember that words can be negative for some people, but not for others. For example, *boobs* or *pussy* may seem negative for one woman but very natural and positive for another woman.
- Cross out negative words and substitute more positive ones. Referring back to Chapter 3 may help you come up with alternative words.
- Take the words for the sexual parts of your body and rewrite them, putting the word *my* in front of each. Look at your list again. Do you like these words? If there are still words that you don't like, cross them out and write in the words that you want to start using for your body. There is no objective standard of right or wrong, only the words that are right or wrong *for you*.
- Trace your finger across each word in the completed list. These are the words that you use to describe your body. This is your personal "body language."

Reflection

- Are the words on your list ones you would want a lover to use?
- When you're mad at yourself, do you use negative or positive words for your body? For example, do you use "cunt" or "asshole" as a way to put yourself down?
- Make an effort to use your positive body language all the time.

Next Steps

- Review your list several times over the next few weeks. Make a conscious effort to use your body language when you talk to yourself about your body. Use these words with your lover as well.
- A further idea might be to ask a friend what words she uses in her body language.
- Continue to think about and use your body language to gain increased comfort with your sexual self.

Hands-On Exploration

The exercises you've completed thus far in this Appendix have asked you to look inward, remember, and reflect on the meaning of life experiences, beliefs and attitudes, and sexual language. The next exercise moves from the realm of thoughts, ideas, and words to the world of flesh and blood. We ask you to get close and personal as you examine your body.

Many women have been conditioned to have negative or even phobic reactions to their genitals—which, not surprisingly, often results in sexual avoidance and dissatisfaction. Knowledge of, and familiarity with, your genitalia can help desensitize these reactions.

EXPLORING YOUR BODY

Directions

Undress from the waist down and make yourself comfortable on your bed or sofa. Prop pillows behind your back. Spread your legs apart, and with a small mirror, study your vulva. Have this book alongside you, opened to the diagrams in Chapter 3.

- Identify your clitoris, labia majora, labia minora, perineum, and anus.
- After propping the mirror to free your hands, spread the labia apart and look for the urethra and examine the introitus (vaginal opening). Take your time, paying attention to the texture of the skin and whether the opening of your vagina is moist or dry.
- Slide back the prepuce (clitoral hood) and examine the exposed clitoris.
- Contract and relax your pelvic floor muscles. You may be able to see the perineum (the area between your vaginal opening and your anus) move in and out as you are contracting and relaxing. Your buttocks may squeeze together, but the goal is to notice the sensation of contracting the muscles around the vulva rather than the butt muscles, stomach, or thigh muscles. Depending upon your body size and your flexibility, you may not be able to see much, but you should be able to feel whether your muscles are appropriately contracting.

- Moisten a finger with saliva or a water-soluble lubricant and insert your finger in your vagina. Explore the interior of your vagina. Notice its ridges and wetness. If you have the physical flexibility to do so, press the upper wall of your vagina, about two inches inside, toward your pubic bone. Try rubbing back and forth. You may feel some pressure to urinate, and you may feel pleasant sensations. If you continue the stimulation, you may experience sexual arousal. The level of arousal will be different for different women and will be somewhat dependent upon how much experience you have had with stimulating your G spot. The goal is to be aware of the different areas of arousal of your body, not to achieve a specific level of stimulation.
- With your finger inserted in your vagina, contract your pelvic muscles. Note the pressure of the muscular contractions around your finger.
- Experiment with the sensation of contracting and relaxing the pelvic muscles.

Reflection

For many women, this exercise may be the first time that they have closely examined their genitals or perhaps the first time they have touched their genitals directly without using a towel, washcloth, or tissue. This can be a big step, and initially it may feel uncomfortable.

If you find yourself becoming anxious, stop for a few moments, close your eyes, do some deep breathing, and remind yourself that your exploration and touching is really no different than if you were examining your nose or ear. Remember, this is your body.

If you find this exercise overwhelming at first, break it down into steps that seem more manageable. For example, the first time, simply study your vulva in the mirror until you feel more comfortable. Perhaps the next time you repeat the exercise, add touch, but only touch your pubic hair and surface skin. Later, when you feel ready, you can explore the opening of your vagina. By slowly phasing in all the steps as you repeat the exercise over time, you will probably reduce your uncomfortable feelings.

Next Steps

Continue strengthening your sense of ease with your body. Each time you bathe or take a shower, rather than rushing through the process of washing your genitals, take a moment to pull back your clitoral hood and spread open your labia, study your exposed genitals, touch and stroke them lovingly as you rinse, and review your body language.

WAYS TO MAKE PEACE WITH YOUR BODY

The following exercises add to the ideas in Part III for making peace with your body, regardless of the cause of alienation, by presenting strategies for increasing body acceptance and the capacity to experience pleasure.

Sensory Journey

When sex becomes a source of conflict, fear, or discomfort, you may learn to distance yourself from all physical feelings, not just sexual sensations. But even if you're not alienated from your body, you may have similar difficulties with being out of touch with physical sensations. Do you take pride in being able to do two or three things at once, like entertaining your toddler with funny faces as you talk on the phone and empty the dishwasher? That's great in terms of efficiency, but it also means you've probably become an expert at ignoring your sensory cues in favor of outside demands and responsibilities. While making funny faces and managing the phone and dishwasher, you may have ignored the fact that your feet hurt, that you are bone-tired, and that you want to lie down. You tune *out* what your body is saying and tune *in* to what the outside world is demanding of you.

The goal of this exercise is to reverse the process of blindly responding to outside demands by ignoring physical sensations. Instead, you will be encouraged to respond to what your senses tell you.

SENSORY JOURNEY

Directions

This exercise is a sensory journey. You may want to read through it first so that you can plan this exercise out in advance. You will need to gather together different objects for the exercise, and you'll need a place where you can relax undisturbed. You should allow at least an hour for this exercise.

The exercise focuses on your five senses, beginning with sight, then sound, smell, taste, and touch.

- In advance, collect the following items: mirror, radio or CD/tape player with favorite music, and a clock that ticks. Put together some favorite scented items like incense, scented candles, perfume, a favorite bar of soap, a small pine or cedar branch, an orange, and cinnamon or some other spice. Gather a few favorite tastes like fruit or chocolate.
- To begin, undress slowly and take a leisurely bath or shower, noticing the feel of the water on your skin. Press your face against the cool side of the tub or shower, contrasting the soft warmth of the water with the hard coolness of the tile. Slide your hands gently all over your body, consciously focusing on the water wrapping around you.
- When you decide to end your shower or bath, move out of the tub slowly, noticing the feel of the air against your damp skin. Dry off carefully, focusing on the rough texture of the towel against your skin and the tingling feeling where rough and smooth meet.

SIGHT

- Now you're ready to begin the sensory exploration. While still naked, stand in front of a mirror and stretch both hands over your head and reach for the ceiling, first with one arm, then the other. Notice the comforting stretch of your muscles and watch in the mirror as your body moves with your arms.
- Let your arms come down to your sides and study your head and face. See your hair wet from the shower or bath. Look into your eyes and smile, really smile, at yourself. Think about how happy you were when there was a snow day and school was canceled, or when you found your favorite childhood doll in a box in the attic, and smile like you did then. Let your eyes look at all of you and, for once, just let your body be. This exercise is not about shape; it's about sense.
- Slowly turn around in front of the mirror, letting your eyes roam over all of you. Find the hollow where your shoulder blades meet. Look at other special places on your body. Find places you can affirm and, for once, don't criticize any part of you. This exercise is about your ability to see and to enjoy the sense of sight.

SOUND

- Move over to a soft place where you can sit or lie down. Concentrate on listening to the sounds around you. Are they familiar sounds? Listen to the sounds of a clock ticking, of noises coming from outside the room, of the stillness in the room. Listen to the sound of your body moving on the fabric where you are lying. Listen to the sound of your feet as you move them against each other. Listen to the sound of your fingers as you brush them against your skin. Listen to the sound of your own breathing. Try breathing in slow, even breaths.
- Put on a tape or CD of your favorite music or nature sounds. Listen to the blends of sounds and how the music is soft at times, then louder, sometimes gentle, and sometimes urgent and compelling.
- Check out the sound of your own voice. Start by saying your name out loud. Say a few other things like the names of your favorite foods, your best friends, or places you want to visit.
- Now focus on finding the range and variations of your voice. Hum a brief passage of the music you just heard. Next, softly hum a steady note with your lips closed. Now open your mouth and see how the sound changes.
- Make soft "la-la" sounds with your mouth open. Change the sound as your tongue taps the roof of your mouth. Change the pace of how fast you sing "la-la-la" and let a little more sound out.
- Sing "Doe, a deer . . . " Each musical note in the song has a different vowel sound. Skip the words and concentrate on the sounds. For example "doe" becomes "ooohh," "ray" becomes "aaaehh," "me" becomes "eeeee," and "fa," "aaaaah." Think of how the sounds are similar to lovemaking sounds. Practice whispering the sounds as well as saying them out loud.
- Now try saying sexual words out loud. Maybe these are words from your body language list, or things you'd like to try with your lover. Saying the words out loud when

you're alone is good rehearsal for asking for what you want when you're having sex with your partner. If you feel self-conscious about saying the sex words out loud, practice whispering them.

SMELL

- Remember those items you collected in the smell category before beginning this exercise? Now's the time to focus on them. Notice the different scents and concentrate on your responses to each one. Let your mind wander freely. What do the scents remind you of? Where were you when you last smelled that scent?
- Now take your fingers and slowly slide them over your vulva and into your vagina. Let your fingers come into contact with your vaginal secretions.
- Now bring your fingers to your nose and inhale. This is your body's natural human scent. What does this smell like to you?

TASTE

- Repeat the last exercise using the foods you've selected. Roll these foods around in your mouth. Concentrate on their unique flavor and the way you respond to them. Let your mind wander to other times you've enjoyed tasting these particular flavors.
- If you're comfortable with this, insert your finger into your vagina and then slide your finger into your mouth. What do you taste like? Some women say this is a chalky taste. Others think it's slightly salty. You get to be the expert on youself.

TOUCH

- Take time to touch yourself slowly and carefully, starting with your toes and ending by sliding your fingers through your scalp. Concentrate on your response to this touch. Where do you like to touch yourself? Are there places that are ticklish or uncomfortable? Are there places that you're comfortable touching but don't want a partner to touch?
- End the touch exercise by gently touching and massaging your face. Stroke your eyes, your forehead, your cheeks, and finally your mouth.

REFLECTION

- As you moved through each section of the exercise, what were your reactions? Was it hard to move from the more "passive" part of the exercise involving sight to the more active parts, like making sounds and singing? What thoughts crossed your mind as you did this exercise? Was any part of the exercise distasteful?
- Were your thoughts strongly negative (e.g., *I hate doing this*, or *This is disgusting*, or *I just can't do this*)? If so, where do you think the response came from?
- If you want to work on the negative thoughts or feelings, you can try substituting more positive thoughts, like, *Even though this feels a little funny at first, I can do this*, or

I can try it a few times and if I don't like it, I'll try making up some sensory experiences that are more comfortable for me.

NEXT STEPS

- If you liked increasing your sensory awareness, make up some of your own exercises using your five senses.
- If you would like to become more familiar and comfortable with your genitals or would like suggestions on how to experiment with self-pleasuring, look at the exercises in Chapter 15, "Body Work—Up Close and Personal" and "Masturbation."

Investing Time in Your Sexual Self

An important step in making peace with your body is actively seeking out, rather than shying away from, opportunities to be sensual. The more intentional, or thoughtful, you are about your sexual expression, the more satisfaction you will experience from it. Many women fear that if they plan their sexuality, they'll lose spontaneity. Just the opposite is true: with planning, more opportunities become available for spontaneous things to happen. Planning time for your sexuality doesn't mean you are overvaluing sex, and being intentional about sexuality is not just for women with partners. Learning to take time for your sexuality is important to all women.

INVESTING TIME IN YOUR SEXUAL SELF

Directions

- Think realistically about how often you'd like to feel sexual pleasure in a day, in a week, in a month. Decide how often you'd like that sexual pleasure to come through fantasy, how often through sensual touch or masturbation, and, if you have a partner, how often you'd like to include your partner. Can you find sexual pleasure in sensual thoughts and feelings, or must orgasm be present in order to qualify as sexual pleasure? Each woman is different.
- Once you've decided how often to have a sexual experience, you can figure out where you can schedule time for it during the course of a day or week. Most women's lives are busy, and it will take prioritizing and determination to increase your time to be sexual. Keep in mind that you can vary the time you spend on a sexual activity. Not every sexual interlude needs to be two hours! If necessary, make a list of these times as a reminder of your priorities.

Reflection

- After a week of planning and prioritizing sex, evaluate your response. Did you like knowing when you were going to have time to concentrate on sex? Did you feel disappointed that the element of unplanned spontaneity was missing? Or did you enjoy the pleasure of anticipation as well as the pleasure of the event? Did you find yourself feeling that it was okay to plan some things, like sex with your partner, but not okay to plan other things, like sexual fantasies or masturbating?
- Pay attention to your thoughts and reactions. Were you critical or judgmental about yourself? If you were, it may be helpful to read Chapter 13 on analyzing, challenging, and modifying self-defeating thinking.

Next Steps

- Continue to find time each week to explore and enjoy your sexuality.
- If you're enjoying this sexual growth, here are some additional ideas to try over time:
  —Read other books about sex.
  —Try using a vibrator while masturbating.
  —Develop favorite sexual fantasies. If you're passive in the fantasy, try being active. If you're always the active one, try reversing the roles.
  —Rent an erotic movie.
  —Read a romance novel.
  —Write yourself a letter expressing appreciation of your sexuality.

WAYS TO CREATE A BETTER SEXUAL RELATIONSHIP

Most couples want a satisfying, perhaps even a vibrant and exciting, sex life. They may be willing to settle for periods of abstinence, delays in frequency, and even a few boring interludes, but overall, they want sex to be an enjoyable, fulfilling part of their relationship.

What does it take to create a more satisfying sexual relationship? What creates passion is *involvement*. To experience loving sex, it's important for both partners to commit themselves fully to talking honestly and openly about sexuality, being respectful of each other's sexual needs and vulnerabilities, and making sexual intimacy a priority in their relationship.

Following is a series of exercises to help you and your partner enrich your sexual relationship. We suggest that you approach these exercises like you would a trip or vacation. Enjoy not only the actual trip but also the anticipation as you plan it as well as the memories that remain long after the trip is over. Take time to plan the exercises. Be curious about them, talk about them, even laugh about them. When doing the exercises, involve yourselves fully. Tune in to each other and tune out extraneous distractions. Enjoy the fact that you are doing something sensual together. Afterward, share your reactions to the exercises and take pleasure in the memories.

If there's tension in your relationship, we would advise moving slowly, being clear with each other about what each wants out of each exercise, and keeping expectations reasonable. Finally, remember to keep trying. Patience, respect, and mutual commitment can create important change in a relationship.

What's in a Name?

All too often, talking about sex, even with a long-term partner, can be intimidating. Many of us have been raised to believe that nice people don't talk about sex, certainly not in a way that might sound "vulgar." This exercise is designed to help desensitize sexual language. You and your partner will be encouraged to say aloud every sexual slang word or phrase you can think of. The purpose is to "break the ice" so that you and your partner can begin to build a framework for healthy sexual communication.

WHAT'S IN A NAME?

Directions

- Schedule time alone together when both of you are feeling relaxed and unrushed. Start with the word *penis* and brainstorm for slang terms. Go back and forth, taking turns voicing slang expressions. When you run out of ideas, repeat the exercise with each of the following words: *vulva, vagina, breasts, masturbation, intercourse,* and *oral sex.*
- When you finish going through all of the above terms, take turns answering the following questions:
  —How did I feel about doing these exercises?
  —Were there any slang expressions I didn't like or found offensive? Which ones?
  —Which words do I feel most comfortable using when talking about sex and body parts?

Reflection

- When doing this exercise, did you feel embarrassed or ashamed? If so, can you trace these reactions back to earlier experiences in your life? Share your reflections with your partner.
- Some people may find this exercise exciting. The excitement can come from the novelty of using language that may have been forbidden in our childhood. There is often a natural attraction to outrageous and risqué behavior. Also, feeling liberated from a longstanding sexual prohibition can be exciting.

Next Steps

Be sure to respect each other's sensitivities about language. If you or your partner finds certain terms to be demeaning or offensive, it's important that these responses be respected in future discussions.

Let's Talk

So the ice is broken: you can use the anatomical words, including the slang versions. But can you express the feelings—the wants, the fears, and the excitement—that sex brings out in you? For many couples, that's a big challenge. Just starting this type of conversation can seem daunting. *How do I bring the subject up*? *What if I shock him*? *Will she think I'm obsessed with sex*? This exercise has been designed to help the two of you start talking about sex. By answering the questions listed in the exercise and sharing your answers with one another, you will begin to explore issues important in all sexual relationships. Our hope is that you'll continue throughout your lives to talk openly and honestly about your sexual relationship.

LET'S TALK

Directions

Make two copies of the following open-ended statements:

- My most exciting sexual moment with you was ____________.
- The part of my body I feel most self-conscious about is ____________.
- The sexiest part of your body is ____________.
- The thing about sex that I am most uncomfortable with is ____________.
- The most exciting place for us to make love would be ____________.
- My favorite part of lovemaking with you is ____________.
- Things that make lovemaking exciting for me are ____________.
- The sexiest thing about you is ____________.
- The thing you do sexually that turns me on the most is ____________.

Reflection

Reflect on the following questions and share your responses with one another:

- How difficult was this exercise?
- As the two of you went back and forth sharing your answers, did the exercise become easier?

- Were you surprised by anything your partner said?
- What can both of you do to ensure that more talks like this happen in the future?
- Based on what you heard from your partner, are there any action steps you want to take to help make sex more exciting and satisfying for both of you?

Next Steps

- If any action steps came up as a result of this discussion, try to follow through on them.
- Keep talking.

Sensual Massage

Far too many couples have lost their ability to fully enjoy lovemaking. Rather than making sex an exciting experience that awakens and stimulates all of their senses, couples often fall into a predictable routine. To make matters worse, the routine often deprives women of the emotional and physical stimulation that is most effective in leading to their sexual excitement and satisfaction. The following exercise is designed to help you and your partner return to the basics. Rather than focusing on genital arousal, the two of you are encouraged to rediscover the joy that can come from flesh touching flesh, using all of your senses as you enjoy quiet, intimate time together.

SENSUAL MASSAGE

Directions

Find quiet, private time together and go through the following steps:

- Set a comfortable mood with music, soft lighting, scented candles, and perhaps wine, or special mineral water, or sensuous fruit.
- Undress each other, taking your time and focusing on your senses.
- Have your partner lie face down. Begin a slow, sensuous body massage. If you want to, experiment with body oil. Pay attention to all of your senses. Take in the scent of the burning candles (if you're using them to create a mood) or the essence of your partner's cologne. Feel the texture of your partner's skin. Hear the music; listen to your partner's sighs and moans. Look at your partner's face, hair, and body, and appreciate the curves, lines, angles, and shapes that make him or her unique.
- After slowly moving from head to toe, have your partner roll over. Repeat the massage,

starting with the facial muscles and working your way down to the feet. For now, skip the genital area.

- When finished providing a massage, switch roles and allow your partner to massage you, back and front. Give yourself permission to relax and to indulge in pleasure. This is not the time to worry about whether your partner is enjoying him- or herself—these are a few moments for you to be selfish.
- When your partner's finished, take a few more moments and hold each other. Enjoy the silence together or talk about your reactions to the experience you just shared.

Reflection

Did you feel self-conscious while doing this exercise? If so, what may have caused your feelings of awkwardness or discomfort? Were you concerned about your appearance? Were you afraid that your partner was not enjoying the exercise? Did you feel like you were doing something wrong? If you're willing, share your reflections on these questions with your partner.

Next Steps

Repeat the above steps, adding genital stimulation. Experiment with ways of stimulating each other without relying on intercourse. Try using your hand, tongue, thigh, breasts, a feather, or a vibrator.

Let's Experiment

One valuable way to avoid letting your sexual relationship drift into autopilot is to add variety and excitement to your lovemaking. By making use of your imagination, creativity, and sense of adventure, you and your partner can introduce playful, sensual, mutually enjoyable variations into your sex life. This exercise provides a safe format for you and your partner to look at a range of novel sexual experiences without having to feel particularly threatened. If you identify only one new mutually acceptable behavior as a result of the exercise, wonderful. Try it, enjoy it, and learn from it. Over time, keep revisiting this exercise. Things you would never consider doing right now may become more acceptable in the future as both your sexual comfort and your sexual relationship continue to grow.

A final note about experimentation. It's important that both people want to try the new behavior. If one person is turned off by the idea but agrees to try it to accommodate the partner, trouble is inevitable. Remember, the goal of experimentation is to keep excitement and passion alive, not to create resentment and discomfort.

LET'S EXPERIMENT

Directions

- Take two sheets of paper and make three columns on each sheet. On top of the first column, write "**New Activity**," on top of the middle column, write "**Let's Try It**," and on the third column, "**Pass**."
- Underneath column one list the following:
  Shower together
  Fellatio
  Cunnilingus
  Masturbation in front of each other
  Anal sex
  New positions for intercourse
  Strip poker
  Phone-sex with each other (explicit talk about sex over the telephone)
  Role-play a fantasy
  Watch an erotic movie
  Watch an erotic dance performance
  Use sex toys
- Both of you take a copy of the above list and check off which of the activities you're willing to try (column two) and which you want to skip (column three).
- Compare your lists and see which activities both of you want to try. Neither of you has to explain or defend his or her choices.
- Pick an activity you're both willing to try and start planning when and how to do it.

Reflection

Did you feel that you had to defend any of your choices? It is important that each partner's personal tastes and comfort level are respected. If you're feeling pressured or criticized by your partner, try discussing these feelings with him or her—and be sure to monitor your own responses to your partner for any stray criticalness or pressure.

Next Steps

- Periodically revisit this exercise. Options you decline now may become more acceptable in the future. Perhaps the two of you will think of additional possibilities to put on the list.
- Continue to be open to experimentation and novelty, but never allow yourself to be pressured into trying something that exceeds your comfort level or violates your values—and never allow yourself to pressure your partner.

Suggested Resources

BODY IMAGE

Blank, H. (2000). *Big big love: A sourcebook on sex for people of size and those who love them.* Emoryville, CA: Greenery Press.

Brumberg, J. J. (1997). *The body project: An intimate history of American girls.* New York: Random House.

Erdman, C. K. (1995). *Nothing to lose: A guide to sane living in a large body.* San Francisco: Harper San Francisco.

Greene, B., & Winfrey, O. (1996). *Make the connection: Ten steps to a better body and a better life.* New York: Hyperion.

Hirschmann, J. R., & Munter, C. H. (1995). *When women stop hating their bodies: Freeing yourself from food and weight obsession.* New York: Fawcett Columbine.

Northrup, C. (1998). *Women's bodies, women's wisdom: Creating physical and emotional health and healing.* New York: Bantam Doubleday Dell.

Pipher, M. (1995). *Reviving Ophelia: Saving the selves of adolescent girls.* New York: Ballantine Books.

Wolf, N. (1992). *The beauty myth.* New York: Anchor.

BODY MASSAGE/BODY WORK

Books

Berry, C. R. (1993). *Your body never lies.* Berkeley, CA: Pagemill Press.

Braddock, C. (1995). *Body voice: Using the power of breath, sound and movement to heal and create new boundaries.* Berkeley, CA: Pagemill Press.

Caldwell, C. (1997). *Getting in touch: The guide to new body-centered therapies.* Teterboro, NJ: Quest.

Leonard, G., & Murphy, M. (1995). *The life we are given: A long-term program for realizing the potential of body, mind, heart and soul.* New York: Tarcher.

Institutes and Workshops

Alive and Well! Institute of Conscious Body
100 Shaw Drive
San Anselmo, CA 94960
(888) 259-5961
www.alivewell.com

Foundation of Human Enrichment
PO Box 1872
Lyons, CO 80540
(303) 823-9524
www.traumahealing.com

COUPLES COMMUNICATION AND INTIMACY

Barbach, L. (1984). *For each other: Sharing sexual intimacy.* New York: New American Library.

Christensen, A. & Jacobson, N. (1999). *Reconcilable differences.* New York: Guilford Press.

Gottman, J. (1999). *The seven principles for making marriage work.* New York: Crown.

Hendricks, G., & Hendricks, K. (1990). *Conscious loving: The journey to co-commitment.* New York: Bantam Books.

Hendrix, H. (1990). *Getting the love you want: A guide for couples.* New York: HarperPerennial.

Klein, M. (1988). *Your sexual secrets: When to keep them, when and how to tell.* New York: Pacifica Press.

Lerner, H. G. (1989). *The dance of intimacy: A woman's guide to courageous acts of change in key relationships.* New York: HarperCollins.

Schnarch, D. (1997). *Passionate marriage: Sex, love and intimacy in emotionally committed relationships.* New York: Norton.

Stanley, S., Blumberg, S., Markman, H., & Edell, D. (1996). *Fighting for your marriage.* San Francisco: Jossey-Bass.

Vaughn, P. (1998). *The monogamy myth: A personal handbook for recovering from affairs.* New York: Newmarket Press.

DESIRE AND AROUSAL

Birch, R. W. (1996). *Oral caress: The loving guide to exciting a woman: A comprehensive illustrated manual on the joyful art of cunnilingus.* Blacksburg, VA: PE Central.

Hastings, A. S. (1998). *Treating sexual shame: A new map for overcoming dysfunction, abuse, and addiction.* Northvale, NJ: Jason Aronson.

DISABILITY AND ILLNESS

Books

Kaufman, M. (1995). *Easy for you to say: Q & A's for teens living with chronic illness or disability.* Toronto: Key Porter Books.

Papadopoulos, C. (1989). *Sexual aspects of cardiovascular diseases.* New York: Praeger.

Schover, L. (1997). *Sexuality and fertility after cancer.* New York: Wiley.
Schover, L. (1988). *Sexuality and cancer: For the woman who has cancer and her partner.* New York: American Cancer Society.
Sipski, M., & Alexander, C. (1997). *Sexual function in people with disability and chronic illness: A health professional's guide.* Frederick, MD: Aspen.
Woodward, J. (1979). *Signs of sexual behavior: An introduction to some sex-related vocabulary in American Sign Language.* Silver Springs, MD: TJ Publishers.

Organizations and Websites

American Cancer Society
(800) 227-2345
www.cancer.org

Association of Cancer Online Resources (ACOR)
www.acor.org

The Disability Resources (DRM WebWatcher)
www.DisabilityResources.org

National Alliance for the Mentally Ill (NAMI)
Colonial Place Three
2107 Wilson Boulevard, Suite 300
Arlington, VA 22201
(703) 524-7600; (800) 950-6264
www.nami.org

National Clearinghouse on Women and Girls with Disabilities
Educational Equity Concepts, Inc.
114 East 32nd Street, Suite 701
New York, NY 10016
(212) 725-1803
www.edequity.org

The Sexual Health Network, Inc.
www.sexualhealth.com

Sexuality Information and Education Council of the United States (SIECUS)
130 West 42nd Street, Suite 350
New York, NY 10036
(212) 819-9770
www.siecus.org

EROTICA AND FANTASY

Barbach, L. (Ed). (1985). *Pleasures: Women write erotica.* New York: HarperCollins.
Barbach, L. (Ed). (1995). *Erotic interludes: Tales told by women.* New York: Plume/Penguin.
Barbach, L. (Ed). (1996). *The erotic edge.* New York: Plume/Penguin.

Bright, S. (Ed). (2000). *Best American erotica 2000*. New York: Touchstone Books.

Decosta-Willis, M., Martin, R., & Bell, R. (Eds). (1992). *Erotique noire: Black erotica*. New York: Doubleday.

Friday, N. (1998). *My secret garden: Women's sexual fantasies*. New York: Pocket Books. (Friday has many good books on sexual fantasy, including *Women on Top* and *Forbidden Flowers*.)

Kudaka, G. (Ed). (1995). *On a bed of rice: An Asian American erotic feast*. New York: Anchor.

Martin, R. (Ed). (1997). *Dark Eros: Black erotic writings*. New York: St. Martin's Press.

Queen, C., & Davis, J. (Eds). (1998). *Sex spoken here: Good vibrations erotic reading circle selections*. San Francisco: Down There Press.

EROTIC POWER PLAY (SAFE, SANE, AND CONSENSUAL)

Books

Bannon, R. (1993). *Learning the ropes: A basic guide to safe and fun S/M lovemaking*. San Francisco: Daedalus.

Brame, G. G., Jacobs, J., & Brame, W. (1996). *Different loving: The world of sexual dominance and submission*. New York: Villard/Random Books.

Easton, D., & Liszt, C. A. (1994). *The bottoming book: How to get terrible things done to you by wonderful people*. Emeryville, CA: Greenery Press.

Easton, D., & Liszt, C. A. (1996). *The topping book: Or getting good at being bad*. Emeryville, CA: Greenery Press.

Green, L. (1998). *The sexually dominant woman: A workbook for nervous beginners*. Emeryville, CA: Greenery Press.

Moser, C., & Madeson, J. J. (1998). *Bound to be free: The SM experience*. New York: Continuum.

Scott, G. G. (1997). *Erotic power: An exploration of dominance and submission*. Secaucus, NJ: Citadel/Carol.

Taormino, T. (1997). *The ultimate guide to anal sex for women*. San Francisco: Cleis Press.

Wiseman, J. (1998). *SM 101: A realistic introduction*. San Francisco: Greenery Press.

Websites

Deviant Desires
www.deviantdesires.com

GENERAL SEXUALITY INFORMATION

Books

Anderson, D., & Berman, M. (1997). *Sex tips for straight women from a gay man*. New York: HarperCollins.

Angier, N. (1999). *Woman: An intimate biography*. New York: Random House.

Barbach, L. (1984). *For each other: Sharing sexual intimacy*. New York: New American Library.

Barbach, L. (1998). *Turn ons: Pleasing yourself while you please your lover*. New York: Plume/Penguin.

Bauer, J. (1993). *Impossible love: Or why the heart must go wrong*. Woodstock, CT: Spring.

Boston Women's Health Book Collective. (1998). *Our bodies, ourselves: For the new century.* New York: Touchstone.

Daniluk, J. C. (1998). *Women's sexuality across the lifespan: Challenging myths, creating meanings.* New York: Guilford Press.

Joannides, P., & Gross, D. (1998). *The guide to getting it on: The universe's coolest and most informative book about sex.* West Hollywood, CA: Goofy Foot Press.

Kitzinger, S. (1985). *Woman's experience of sex.* New York: Viking Press.

Love, P., & Robinson, J. (1999). *Hot monogamy: Essential steps to more passionate, intimate lovemaking.* New York: Plume/Penguin.

McCarthy, B., & McCarthy, E. (1989). *Female sexual awareness: Achieving sexual fulfillment.* New York: Carroll & Graf.

McCarthy, B., & McCarthy, E. (1998). *Couple sexual awareness: Building sexual happiness.* New York: Carroll & Graf.

Michael, R. T., Ganon, J. H., Laumann, E. O., & Kolata, G. (1995). *Sex in America: A definitive survey.* New York: Warner Books.

Morin, J. (1998). *Anal pleasure and health: A guide for men and women.* San Francisco: Down There Press.

Ogden, G. (1999). *Women who love sex: An inquiry into the expanding spirit of women's erotic experience.* Cambridge, MA: Womanspirit Press.

Paget, L. (2000). *How to give her absolute pleasure: Totally explicit techniques every woman wants her man to know.* New York: Bantam Doubleday Dell.

Penner, C. (1982). *The gift of sex: A guide to sexual fulfillment.* Nashville, TN: Word Books.

Penner, C., & Penner, J. (1995). *Getting your sex life off to a great start: A guide for engaged and newlywed couples.* Nashville, TN: Word Books.

Reinsch, J. M. (1991). *The Kinsey Institute new report on sex: What you must know to be sexually literate.* New York: St. Martins Press.

Schwartz, P., & Lever, J. (2000). *The great sex weekend: A 48-hour guide to rekindling sparks for bold, busy, or bored lovers.* New York: Perigee/Penguin.

Steward, F., Stewart, F. H., Stewart, G., & Hatcher, R. (1990). *Understanding your body: Every woman's guide to gynecology and health.* New York: Bantam Doubleday Dell.

Tiefer, L. (1995). *Sex is not a natural function.* New York: Westview Press.

Westheimer, R. K. (1995). *Sex for dummies.* Foster City, CA: IDG Books.

Westheimer, R. K. (1999). *Dr. Ruth's pregnancy guide for couples.* New York: Routledge.

Winks, C., & Semans, A. (1997). *The new good vibrations guide to sex: How to have safe, fun sex.* San Francisco: Cleis Press.

Wiseman, J. (1998). *More than 125 tricks to make good sex better (Vols. 1 & 2).* (Order from author: PO Box 1261, Berkeley, CA 94701)

Zoldbrod, A. (1998). *Sex smart: How your childhood shaped your sexual life and what to do about it.* Oakland, CA: New Harbinger.

Organizations and Websites

AASECT (American Association of Sex Educators, Counselors, and Therapists)
PO Box 5488
Richmond, VA 23220-0488
(804) 644-3288
www.aasect.org

Columbia University's Health Education Program
www.goaskalice.columbia.edu

The Kinsey Institute for Research in Sex, Gender, and Reproduction
313 Morrison Hall, Indiana University
Bloomington, IN 47405
(812) 855-7686
www.kinseyinstitute.org

Libida
www.libida.com

Masters and Johnson Institute
16216 Baxter Road, Suite 399
Chesterfield, MO 63017
(314) 781-1112
www.mastersandjohnson.com

Planned Parenthood
(800) 230-7526
www.plannedparenthood.org

Sexuality Information and Education Council of the United States (SIECUS)
130 West 42nd Street, Suite 350
New York, NY 10036
(212) 819-9770
www.siecus.org

Society for Human Sexuality
www.sexuality.org

Women's Sexual Health
www.womenshealth.com

G SPOT

Ladas, A., Whipple, B., & Perry, J. (1983). *The G spot: And other discoveries about human sexuality.* New York: Bantam Doubleday Dell.

Winks, C. (1998). *The good vibrations guide to the G-spot.* San Francisco: Down There Press.

INFERTILITY

Domar, A. D., & Dreher, H. (1997). *Healing mind, healthy woman: Using the mind-body connection to manage stress and take control of your life.* New York: Holt.

Zoldbrod, A. (1990). *Getting around the boulder in the road: Using imagery to cope with fertility problems.* Lexington, MA: The Center for Reproductive Problems. (Available from author: 12 Rumford Road, Lexington, MA 02420)

Zoldbrod, A. (1992). *Men, women, and infertility: Intervention and treatment strategies*. New York: Lexington Books.

LESBIAN, BISEXUAL, TRANSGENDER, AND INTERSEX

Books

Bright, S. (1999). *Susie sexpert's lesbian sex world*. San Francisco: Cleis Press.

Caster, W. (1993). *The lesbian sex book*. Boston: Alyson.

Clunis, D. M. (2000). *Lesbian couples: A guide to creating healthy relationships*. Seattle, WA: Seal Press.

Devor, H. (1997). *FTM: Female-to-male transsexuals in society*. Bloomington, IN: Indiana University Press.

Dreger, A. (1999). *Intersex in the age of ethics*. Hagerstown, MD: University Publishing Group.

Haeberle, E. J., & Gindorf, R. (Eds.). (1998). *Bisexualities: The ideology and practice of sexual contact with both men and women*. New York: Continuum.

Hutchins, L., & Ka'ahumanu, L. (1991). *Bi any other name: Bisexual people speak out*. Boston: Alyson.

Loulon, J. (1987). *Lesbian passion: Loving ourselves and each other*. Duluth, MN: Spinster's Ink.

Morris, K. E. (1996). *Speaking in whispers*. Chicago: Third Side Press. (African American lesbian erotica)

Newman, F. (1999). *The whole lesbian sex book: A passionate guide for all of us*. San Francisco: Cleis Press.

Newman, L. (Ed). (1998). Pillow talk: Lesbian stories between the covers. Boston: Alyson.

Queen, C., & Schimel, L. (Eds). (1996). *Switch hitters: Lesbians write gay male erotica and gay men write lesbian erotica*. San Francisco: Cleis Press.

Sang, B., Warshow, J. K., & Smith, A. J. (1991). *Lesbians at midlife: The creative transition*. Duluth, MN: Spinsters Ink.

Taormino, T. (1996–2000). *Best lesbian erotica*. San Francisco: Cleis Press. (Annual series)

Organizations and Websites

Bisexual Resource Center
www.biresource.org

Dykesworld
www.dykesworld.de

Gay.com
www.gay.com

Gender Education and Advocacy
www.gender.org

Harry Benjamin International Gender Dysphoria Association
www.hbigda.org

Human Rights Campaign
919 18th Street, Suite 800
Washington, DC 20005
(202) 628-4160
www.hrc.org

International Foundation for Gender Education (IFGE)
www.ifge.org

Intersex Society of North America (ISNA)
www.isna.org

Lesbian.org: Promoting Lesbian Visibility on the Internet
www.lesbian.org

Lesbian's Safer Sex Guide
www.safersex.org/women/lesbians.html

National Gay and Lesbian Task Force
1700 Kalorama Road
Washington, DC 20009
(202) 332-6483
www.ngltf.org

Parents, Families and Friends of Lesbians and Gays (PFLAG)
1726 M Street, NW
Washington, DC 20036
(202) 467-8180
www.pflag.org

Queer Net
www.queernet.org

MALE SEXUALITY

Milstein, R., & Slowinski, J. (1999). *The sexual male: Problems and solutions.* New York: Norton.
Zilbergeld, B. (1999). *The new male sexuality: A guide to sexual fulfillment.* New York: Bantam Doubleday Dell.

MASTURBATION

Blank, J. (Ed). (199s6). *First person sexual.* San Francisco: Down There Press.
Blank, J. (1998). *I am my lover: Women pleasure themselves.* San Francisco: Down There Press.
Dodson, B. (1996). *Sex for one: The joy of self-loving.* New York: Three Rivers Press.

MENOPAUSE AND AGING

Books

Anderson, C. M., & Stewart, S. (1995). *Flying solo: Single women in midlife.* New York: Norton.

Barbach, L. (1995). *The pause: Positive approaches to menopause.* New York: Plume/Penguin.

Blank, J. (2000). *Still doing it: Women and men over 60 write about their sexuality.* San Francisco: Down There Press.

Block, J. D., & Crain Bakos, S. (1999). *Sex over 50.* New York: Prentice Hall.

Friedan, B. (1993). *The fountain of age.* New York: Simon & Schuster.

Levine, S. (1998). *Sexuality in mid-life.* New York: Plenum.

Rako, S. (1996). *The hormone of desire: The truth about sexuality, menopause, and testosterone.* New York: Three Rivers Press.

Rosenthal, S. (1999). *The new sex over 40.* New York: Tarcher.

Siegal, D. L., Doress-Worters, P. B., & Sanford, W. (1994). *The new ourselves, growing older: Women aging with knowledge and power.* New York: Touchstone/Simon & Schuster.

Taetzsch, L. (Ed). (1995). *Hot flashes: Women writers on the change of life.* Boston: Faber & Faber.

Tallmer, M. (1995). *Questions and answers about sex in later life.* Philadelphia: Charles Press.

Organizations and Websites

As We Change catalogs
(800) 203-5585
www.aswechange.com

Senior Care Web
www.seniorcareweb.com

ORGASM

Books

Barbach, L. (1994). *For yourself: The fulfillment of female sexuality.* New York: New American Library.

Heiman, J., & LoPiccolo, J. (1988). *Becoming orgasmic: A sexual growth program for women.* New York: Simon & Schuster.

Swift, R. (1993). How to have an orgasm—as often as you want. New York: Carroll & Graf.

Video

Becoming Orgasmic
Sinclair Intimacy Institute
PO Box 8865
Chapel Hill, NC 27515
(800) 843-0305
www.bettersex.com

PAIN

Books

Catalano, E., Hardin, K., & Tupper, S. (1996). *The chronic pain workbook: A step by step guide for coping with and overcoming pain.* Oakland, CA: New Harbinger.

Goodwin, A. J., & Agronin, M. (1997). *A woman's guide to overcoming sexual fear and pain.* Oakland, CA: New Harbinger.

Sternbach, R. (1995). *Mastering pain: A twelve-step program for coping with chronic pain.* New York: Ballantine Books.

Websites

International Pelvic Pain Association
www.pelvicpain.org

National Vulvodynia Association (NVA)
www.nva.org

University of Michigan Center for Vulvar Disease
www.med.umich.edu/obgyn/vulva/

Vulvar Pain Foundation
PO Drawer 177
Graham, NC 27253
(336) 226-0704
www.vulvarpainfoundation.org

POLYAMORY

Easton, D., & Liszt, C. (1998). *The ethical slut: A guide to infinite sexual possibilities.* San Francisco: Greenery Press.

RACE, ETHNICITY, AND SEXUALITY

Books

Alarcon, A. C., & Moraga, C. (1992). *The sexuality of Latinas.* Berkeley, CA: Third Woman Press.

Villarosa, L. (Ed). (1994). *Body and soul: The black woman's guide to physical health and emotional well-being.* New York: HarperPerennial.

White, E. C. (Ed). (1994). *The black woman's health book: Speaking for ourselves.* Seattle, WA: Seal Press.

Organizations and Websites

Cultural Diversity in Sexuality—Website Links
http://pages.prodigy.net/sixx/links.htm

Native American Women's Health Education Resource Center
PO Box 572
Lake Andes, SD 57356
(605) 487-7072

SEX EDUCATION FOR CHILDREN AND TEENS

Books

Andry, A., Schepp, S., & Hampton, B. (1984). *How babies are made.* New York: Little, Brown.

Bass, E., & Kaufman, K. (1996). *Free your mind: The book for gay, lesbian, and bisexual youth and their allies.* New York: HarperCollins.

Bell, R. (1988). *Changing bodies, changing lives: A book for teens on sex and relationships.* New York: Times Books.

Cole, J. (1988). *Asking about sex and growing up: A question and answer book for boys and girls.* New York: William Morrow.

Eyre, L., & Eyre, R. M. (1998). *How to talk to your child about sex: It's best to start early, but it's never too late—a step by step guide for every age.* New York: St. Martin's Press.

Fenwick, E., & Walker, R. (1996). *How sex works.* New York: Dorling Kindersley.

Gardner-Loulan, J., Lopez, B., & Quackenbush, M. (1991). *Period.* Volcano, CA: Volcano Press.

Gordon, S., & Gordon, J. (1989). *Raising a child conservatively in a sexually permissive world.* New York: Simon & Schuster.

Gravelle, K., & Gravelle, J. (1996). *The period book: Everything you don't want to ask but need to know.* New York: Walker & Co.

Harris, R. H., (1996). *It's perfectly normal: Changing bodies, growing up, sex and sexual health.* Cambridge, MA: Candlewick Press.

Harris, R. H. (1999). *It's so amazing! A book about eggs, sperm, birth, babies, and families.* Cambridge, MA: Candlewick Press.

Jukes, M. (1996). *It's a girl thing: How to stay healthy, safe, and in charge.* New York: Knopf.

Jukes, M. (1998). *Growing up: It's a girl thing—straight talk about first bras, first periods, and your changing body.* New York: Knopf.

Madaras, L. (2000). *What's happening to my body? A book for girls.* New York: Newmarket Press.

Mayle, P. (1999). *Where did I come from?* Secaucus, NJ: Carol Publishing Group.

Moglia, R. (1997). *All about sex: A family resource on sex and sexuality.* New York: Crown.

Schoen, M. (1990). *Belly buttons are navels.* Buffalo, NY: Prometheus.

Websites

American Social Health Association
www.iwannaknow.org

Planned Parenthood—Teens
www.teenwire.com

Sex, Etc.—A Website for Teens by Teens
The Network for Family Life Education
School of Social Work, Rutgers University
www.sxetc.org

SEX TOYS, VIDEOS, AND THE INTERNET

Books

Blank, J. (2000). *Good vibrations: The complete guide to vibrators*. San Francisco: Down There Press.

Semans, A., & Winks, C. (1999). *The woman's guide to sex on the web*. San Fransico: HarperEdge.

Winks, C. (1998). *The good vibrations guide to adult videos*. San Francisco: Down There Press.

Mail Order

Adam and Eve
PO Box 800
Carrboro, NC 27510
(800) 293-4654
www.aeonline.com
www.adameve.com

Blowfish
2261 Market Street, #284
San Francisco, CA 94114-1600
(415) 285-6064; (800) 325-2569
www.blowfish.com

Condomania
Attention: Mail Order
647 Poinsetta Place
Los Angeles, CA 90036
(800) 926-6366
www.condomania.com

Eve's Garden
119 West 57th Street, Suite 1201
New York, NY 10019
(212) 757-8651; (800) 848-3837
www.evesgarden.com

Good Vibrations/Sexuality Library/Down There Press (Open Enterprises)
938 Howard Street, Suite 101
San Francisco, CA 94103
(415) 974-8990
(800) 289-8423
www.goodvibes.com

Grand Opening!
318 Harvard St. #32, Arcade Building
Coolidge Corner
Brookline, MA 02446
(617) 731-2626
www.grandopening.com

Sinclair Intimacy Institute
PO Box 8865
Chapel Hill, NC 27515
(800) 843-0305
www.bettersex.com

Stormy Leather
1158 Howard Street
San Francisco, CA 94103
(415) 626-1672
www.stormyleather.com

Toys in Babeland
711 East Pike Street
Seattle, WA 98122
(206) 328-2914; (800) 658-9119
www.babeland.com

SPIRITUALITY AND SEX

Books

Gach, M. R. (1997). *Acupressure for lovers: Secrets of touch for increasing intimacy.* New York: Bantam Doubleday Dell.

Lacroix, N. (1997). *Art of tantric sex.* New York: Dorling Kindersley.

Muir, C., & Muir, C. (1990). *Tantra: The art of conscious loving.* St. Paul, MN: Mercury House.

Stubbs, K. R. (1999). *Erotic massage: The tantric touch of love.* New York: Tarcher.

Websites

Tantra.com
www.tantra.com

STDs AND SAFER SEX

Books

Whipple, B., & Ogden, G. (1989). *Safe encounters: How women can say yes to pleasure and no to unsafe sex.* New York: McGraw-Hill.

Organizations and Websites

American Social Health Association—Herpes/HPV Resource Center
PO Box 13827
Research Triangle Park, NC 27709
National Herpes Hot Line (919) 361-8488
(800) 230-6039
www.ashastd.org

Café Herpe
www.cafeherpe.com

Centers for Disease Control and Prevention
National STD Hotline: (800) 227-8922
www.CDC.gov

Hepatitis Information Network (HepNet)
(800) 223-0179
www.hepnet.com

HIV/AIDS Information and Resources
www.thebody.com

Journal of the American Medical Association (JAMA) HIV/AIDS Information
www.ama-assn.org

National HIV/AIDS Hotline
English: (800) 342-2437, 24 hours a day
Spanish: (800) 344-7432, from 8 A.M. until 2 A.M. (EST)

Safer Sex Institute: Women's Safer Sex Guide
www.safersex.org/women.safersex

Unspeakable: The Naked Truth about STDs
www.unspeakable.com

TRAUMA

Books

Carter, C. (1997). *The other side of silence: Women tell about their experience with date rape*. Gilsum, NH: Avocus.

Haines, S. (1999). *The survivor's guide to sex: How to have an empowered sex life after child sexual abuse*. San Francisco: Cleis Press.

Herman, J. (1992). *Trauma and recovery: The aftermath of violence—from domestic abuse to political terror.* New York: Basic Books.

Levine, P. A. (1997). *Waking the tiger: Healing trauma—the inner capacity to transform overwhelming experiences*. Berkeley, CA: North Atlantic Books.

Levy, B. (1998). *In love and in danger: A teen's guide to breaking free of abusive relationships*. Seattle, WA: Seal Press.

Lindquist, S. (2000). *The date rape prevention book: The essential guide for girls and women*. Trabuco Canyon, CA: Sourcebooks.

Maltz, W. (2001). *The sexual healing journey: A guide for survivors of sexual abuse*. New York: HarperPerennial.

Maltz, W., & Holman, B. (1987). *Incest and sexuality: A guide to understanding and healing*. Lexington, MA: Lexington Books.

Nicarthey, G., & Davidson, S. (1997). *Getting free: You can end abuse and take back your life*. Seattle, WA: Seal Press.

Pierce-Baker, C. (1998). *Surviving the silence: Black women's stories of rape*. New York: Norton.

Warshaw, R. (1994). *I never called it rape: The Ms. report on recognizing, fighting and surviving date and acquaintance rape*. New York: HarperPerennial.

Westerlund, E. (1992). *Women's sexuality after childhood incest*. New York: Norton.

Wiehe, V. R., & Richards, A. L. (1995). *Intimate betrayal: Understanding and responding to the trauma of acquaintance rape*. Thousand Oaks, CA: Sage.

Organizations and Websites

Jim Hopper Child Sexual Abuse Resource Page
www.jimhopper.com

The Trauma Center
www.traumacenter.org

VOICES (Victims of Incest Can Emerge Survivors) in Action, Inc.
PO Box 148309
Chicago, IL 60614
www.voices-action.org

References

Administration on Aging, U.S. Department of Health and Human Services. (2000). *A profile of older Americans: 2000.* Washington, DC: Author.

American Psychiatric Association. (1994). *Diagnostic and statistical manual of mental disorders (4th ed.).* Washington, DC: Author.

American Social Health Association. (1995). *Gallup study: Teenagers know more than adults about STDs, but STD knowledge among both groups is low.* Research Triangle Park, NC: Author.

Angier, N. (1999). *Woman: An intimate geography.* New York: Houghton Mifflin Co.

Boston Women's Health Collective. (1992). *The new our bodies, ourselves: A book for and about women.* New York: Touchstone Books.

Brumberg, J. (1997). *The body project: An intimate history of American girls.* New York: Random House.

Burns, D. (1999). *The feeling good handbook (rev. ed.).* New York: Plume.

Cates, W. (1999). Estimates of the incidence and prevalence of sexually transmitted diseases in the United States. *Sex Trans Disease, 26*(Suppl.), S2–S7.

Davis, K. (1995). *Reshaping the female body: The dilemma of cosmetic surgery.* New York: Routledge.

de Bruijn, G. (1982). From masturbation to orgasm with a partner: How some women bridge the gap—and why others don't. *Journal of Sex and Marital Therapy, 8*, 151–167.

DuPont, R., Dupont-Spencer, E., & DuPont, C. (1998). *The anxiety cure: An eight-step program for getting well.* New York: Wiley.

Eng, T., & Butler, W. (Eds.). (1997). *The hidden epidemic: Confronting sexually transmitted diseases.* Washington, DC: National Academy Press.

Feldman, H. A., Goldstein, I., Hatzichristou, G., Krane, R. J., & McKinlay, J. B. (1994). Impotence and its medical and psychosocial correlates: Results of the Massachusetts male aging study. *Journal of Urology, 151*, 54–61.

Friedan, B. (1994). *The fountain of age.* New York: Simon & Schuster.

Gottman, J. (1999). *The seven principles for making marriage work.* New York: Crown.

Greene, B., & Winfrey, O. (1996). *Make the connection: Ten steps to a better body, and a better life.* New York: Hyperion.

Greenspan, J. R., & Nakashima, A. K. (1994). *Sexually transmitted disease surveillance, 1993.* Atlanta, GA: U.S. Department of Health and Human Services, Centers for Disease Control and Prevention.

Haines, S. (1999). *The survivor's guide to sex: How to have an empowered sex life after child sexual abuse.* San Francisco: Cleis Press.

Heiman, J., & LoPiccolo, J. (1988). *Becoming orgasmic: A sexual and personal growth program for women.* New York: Simon & Schuster.

Hemingway, E. (1929). *A farewell to arms.* New York: Simon & Schuster

Hyde, J. S. (2000). *Understanding human sexuality.* New York: McGraw-Hill.

Kenney, J. W., Reinholtz, C., & Angelini, P. J. (1998). Sexual abuse, sex before age 16, and high-risk behaviors of young females with sexually transmitted diseases. *Journal of Obstetric, Gynecologic, and Neonatal Nursing, 27*(1), 54–63.

Kinsey, A., Pomeroy, W., Martin, C., & Gebhard, P. (1953). *Sexual behavior in the human female.* Philadelphia: Saunders.

Kitzinger, S. (1985). *The complete book of pregnancy and childbirth.* New York: Knopf.

Laan, E., Everaerd, W., Bellen, G., & Hanewald, G. (1994). Women's sexual and emotional responses to male- and female-produced erotica. *Archives of Sexual Behavior, 23,* 153–170.

Ladas, A. K., Whipple, B., & Perry, J. D. (1983). *The G spot and other discoveries about human sexuality.* New York: Dell.

Laumann, E., Gagnon, J., Michael, R., & Michaels, S. (1994). *The social organization of sexuality.* Chicago: University of Chicago Press.

Maltz, W. (1991). *The sexual healing journey: A guide for survivors of sexual abuse.* New York: HarperCollins.

Masters, W., & Johnson, V. (1966). *Human sexual response.* Boston: Little, Brown.

Masters, W., & Johnson, V. (1979). *Homosexuality in perspective.* Boston: Little, Brown.

Meadow, R., & Weiss, L. (1992). *Good girls don't eat dessert: Women's conflict about eating and sexuality.* New York: Harrington Park Press.

National Campaign to Prevent Teen Pregnancy. (2000). *Not just another thing to do.* Retrieved June 30, 2000 from the World Wide Web: www.teenpregnancy.org.

Northrup, C. (1994). *Women's bodies, women's wisdom: Creating physical and emotional health and healing.* New York: Bantam Books.

Perry, J. D., & Whipple, B. (1981). Pelvic muscle strength of female ejaculators: Evidence in support of a new theory of orgasm. *Journal of Sex Research, 17,* 22–39.

Reinisch, J. M. (1991). *The Kinsey Institute new report on sex: What you must know to be sexually literate.* New York: St. Martin's Press.

Schnarch, D. (1997). *Passionate marriage: Sex, love, and intimacy in emotionally committed relationships.* New York: Norton.

Sipski, M. L., & Alexander, C. J. (1997). *Sexual function in people with disability and chronic illness.* Gaithersburg, MD: Aspen.

Strong, B., & DeVault, C. (1988). *Understanding our sexuality.* New York: West.

Walsh, F. (1991). Promoting healthy functioning in divorced and remarried families. In A. Gurman & D. Kniskern (Eds.), *Handbook of family therapy, Volume II* (pp. 525–545). New York: Brunner/Mazel.

Whipple, B., & Komisaruk, B. R. (1998). Beyond the G spot: Recent research on female sexuality. *Medical Aspects of Human Sexuality, 1*(3), 19–23.

Wilson, R. (1996). *Don't panic: Taking control of anxiety attacks.* New York: HarperPerennial.

Wolf, N. (1991). *The beauty myth: How images of beauty are used against women.* New York: Doubleday.

Wolf, N. (1997). *Promiscuities: The secret struggle for womanhood.* New York: Ballantine Books.

Worden, J. W. (1991). *Grief counseling and grief therapy* (2nd ed.). New York: Springer.

Zoldbrod, A. (1993). *Men, women and infertility: Intervention and treatment strategies.* New York: Lexington Books.

Index

About the Authors

Sallie Foley, MSW, a certified sex therapist, educator, and supervisor, is a Senior Clinical Social Worker at the University of Michigan's Sexual Health Counseling Services and is on the faculty at the University of Michigan Graduate School of Social Work. Respected for her expertise in couple and sex therapy, she writes and lectures nationally and is frequently interviewed by the media on the subject of human sexuality. Ms. Foley has a private practice in Ann Arbor, Michigan, where she lives with her husband, Steve, and their two daughters and son.

Sally A. Kope, MSW, is in private practice in Ann Arbor, Michigan, as a couple counselor and certified sex therapist, and is a recognized expert in sexual health, providing training at a national level. She has written chapters and articles on various aspects of sexuality, is a lecturer at the University of Michigan Medical School's Department of Human Genetics, and is the past program director of the University of Michigan's Sexual Health Counseling Services. Ms. Kope and her husband, Marty, are parents of four, parents-in-law of three, and grandparents of four children. She provided the illustrations for *Sex Matters for Women.*

Dennis P. Sugrue, PhD, is a Clinical Associate Professor of Psychiatry at the University of Michigan Medical School. He is the founder and former codirector of the Henry Ford Center for Human Sexuality in Farmington Hills, Michigan. Recognized as a leader in the field of human sexuality, he was elected president for 2001–2002 of the American Association of Sex Educators, Counselors, and Therapists (AASECT), the nation's largest credentialing organization for professionals specializing in sex education and therapy. Dr. Sugrue has a private practice in Bloomfield Hills, Michigan.